CANCER ETIOLOGY, DIAGNOSIS AND TREATMENTS

DIFFUSE LARGE B-CELL LYMPHOMA (DLBCL)

SYMPTOMS, TREATMENT AND PROGNOSIS

CANCER ETIOLOGY, DIAGNOSIS AND TREATMENTS

Additional books in this series can be found on Nova's website under the Series tab.

Additional e-books in this series can be found on Nova's website under the e-book tab.

CANCER ETIOLOGY, DIAGNOSIS AND TREATMENTS

DIFFUSE LARGE B-CELL LYMPHOMA (DLBCL)

SYMPTOMS, TREATMENT AND PROGNOSIS

HAIPENG SHAO
EDITOR

NOVA BIOMEDICAL

New York

Library of Congress Cataloging-in-Publication Data

ISBN: 978-1-63484-402-4

Library of Congress Control Number: 2015959363

Published by Nova Science Publishers, Inc. † New York

Contents

PREFACE

Diffuse large B-cell lymphoma (DLBCL) is the most frequently treated non-Hodgkin lymphoma by oncologists during daily practice. While the diagnosis and chemotherapy regimens for DLBCL are well-established, advances in the past decade have identified increasingly diverse specific entities and prognostic markers in DLBCL. The subtypes or specific entities of DLBCL have distinctive clinical, pathologic or genetic features that often require tailored treatment strategy. New immunochemotherapy agents are continuously been developed and some have shown promise in the treatment of relapsed or refractory DLBCL. In the era of personalized medicine, it is important for the pathologists and clinicians to keep up with the most recent development in the field, and to provide optimal care for the patients with DLBCL.

This book is compiled from a series of chapters covering the pathologic features, diagnosis, prognosis and treatment strategies of DLBCL. The goal of the book is to offer people involved in the management of patients with DLBCL a quick and updated review of the current state of the art in the diagnosis, prognostic stratification and treatment of DLBCL. The pathologic features including morphology, immunophenotype, molecular cytogenetics of DLBCL, NOS and specific subtypes are covered in Chapter 1. The chemotherapeutic regimens and future directions in the treatment of DLBCL are discussed in Chapter 2. The roles of radiation therapy and hematopoietic stem cell transplant in the treatment of DLBCL are addressed in Chapters 3 and 4. The last five chapters cover the ins and outs of treatment of the most common subtypes of DLBCL. The field of lymphoma diagnosis and treatment is continuously evolving, and it is the authors' hope that this book not only provides current knowledge in DLBCL but also serves as a foundation for readers to keep up with new findings in the literature.

I would like to express my deep appreciation for the contributing authors for taking the time out of their busy clinical service to write for this book. The collaboration reflected in the publication of this book between pathologists and clinicians is essential for the successful treatment of patients with lymphoma. As a pathologist, I have learned a great deal from my colleagues on the clinical side. I hope residents, fellows and physicians find the information provided in this book useful for their education as well.

The terminology of the subtypes or specific entities of DLBCL is based on the 2008 WHO classification. The terminology of a couple of the subtypes/entities will be changed in the upcoming 2016 WHO classification, and the readers are advised to refer to the new terminology once the 2016 WHO classification becomes available.

Lastly, I would like to thank my family (Ying, Richard and Sophia) for their support on my effort devoted to this book.

In: Diffuse Large B-Cell Lymphoma (DLBCL)
Editor: Haipeng Shao
ISBN: 978-1-63484-402-4

Chapter 1

PATHOLOGIC DIAGNOSIS AND PROGNOSTIC MARKERS OF DIFFUSE LARGE B-CELL LYMPHOMA

Jinming Song, Ling Zhang and Haipeng Shao*

Department of Hematopathology and Laboratory Medicine, H. Lee Moffitt Cancer Center and Research Institute, Tampa, FL, US

ABSTRACT

Diffuse large B-cell lymphoma (DLBCL) is the most common type of non-Hodgkin lymphoma worldwide. DLBCL is clinically aggressive but often treatable with current regimens of chemotherapy. DLBCL is defined pathologically by diffuse infiltrate of medium to large lymphoma cells, and comprises a heterogeneous group of lymphomas with variable clinicopathologic and genetic features, ranging from ones with good response to chemotherapy to the so called "double hit" lymphoma with extremely aggressive clinical course and poor prognosis. The advancement in the understanding of the pathogenesis of DLBCL through the application of phenotypic and molecular genetic studies has led to the recognition of an expanded list of subtypes of DLBCL with distinct clinicopathologic features and prognosis. Accurate diagnosis and classification are essential for appropriate treatment and prognostic stratification. This chapter focuses on the pathologic diagnosis of DLBCL, including morphologic, phenotypic and genetic features of various subtypes of DLBCL. The clinical presentation, diagnostic criteria and differential diagnosis of each subtype of DLBCL are discussed. Application of commonly available techniques is addressed for the diagnosis of each entity. The clinically proven prognostic markers will be emphasized in the category of DLBCL, NOS.

* Corresponding author: Haipeng Shao. E-mail: Haipeng.shao@moffitt.org, phone: 813-745-2672, fax: 813-745-1708.

INTRODUCTION

Diffuse large B-cell lymphoma (DLBCL) is defined morphologically as a mature B-cell neoplasm with diffuse infiltrate by medium sized or large lymphoid cells with nuclear size equal or larger than that of benign histiocytes or over twice the size of small mature lymphocytes [1]. In early Kiel classification and the working formulation, DLBCL was subclassified into intermediate grade centroblastic (large noncleaved cells) and high grade immunoblastic lymphomas [2, 3]. The low reproducibility of distinguishing between centroblastic and immunoblastic lymphomas by practicing pathologists prompted a single entity of DLBCL proposed by the Revised European American Lymphoma (REAL) classification and the 2001 World Health Organization (WHO) classification [4, 5]. The 2001 WHO classification also recognized the existence of a number of clinicopathologically distinct subtypes of DLBCL [5]. Along the line of classification of lymphomas into biologically and clinically relevant entities, the 2008 WHO classification proposed several distinct variants and subgroups of DLBCL based on location, clinicopathologic, immunophenotypic and molecular genetic features. Recent advances furthered the list of distinct variants of DLBCL (Table 1). The vast majority of DLBCL still cannot be classified into these distinct variants, and is categorized as DLBCL, not otherwise specified (NOS) according to the 2008 WHO classification [1].

EPIDEMIOLOGY AND CLINICAL FEATURES

DLBCL is the most common non-Hodgkin lymphoma (NHL), accounting for 25-30% of cases of NHL in Western countries [6, 7]. The median age at diagnosis is 64 years with a slight male predominance [6], but DLBCL can also be seen in pediatric population [8, 9]. Patients usually present with rapidly enlarging mass lesion(s) in nodal or extranodal sites.

Approximately half of the patients present with stage I-II disease, B symptoms are present in about a third of the patients [7]. The majority of DLBCL are nodal disease, while approximately 40% of DLBCL presents in extranodal sites initially [4]. The most common extranodal sites include gastrointestinal tract (especially stomach and ileocecal region), central nervous system (CNS), bone and skin. DLBCLs in specific extranodal sites, particularly CNS and skin show distinctive clinicopathologic features and are recognized as specific subtypes in 2008 WHO classification (discussed later in this chapter). Bone marrow involvement is uncommon (11-27%) [10], and can be concordant with involvement by large lymphoma cells or discordant with involvement by low grade B-cell lymphoma, such as follicular lymphoma [11]. DLBCL lymphoma cells can be found in the peripheral blood of approximately a third of the patients when BM is involved by DLBCL [12]. DLBCL typically occurs *de novo*, but can result from transformation of low grade B-cell lymphomas, including chronic lymphocytic leukemia/small lymphocytic lymphoma, follicular lymphoma, marginal zone lymphoma, lymphoplasmacytic lymphoma or nodular lymphocyte-predominant Hodgkin lymphoma. An association with classical Hodgkin lymphoma in rare cases has also been reported [13]. The risk factors for the development of DLBCL are largely unknown. A small subset of DLBCLs, usually associated with Epstein-Barr virus, occurs in patients with underlying immune dysfunction, such as human immunodeficiency virus (HIV) infection, primary immune disorders, transplantation, iatrogenic agents (i.e., methotrexate, infliximab, fludarabine), immunosenescence in elderly patients, and T-cell dysfunction in angioimmunoblastic T-cell lymphoma [14-19]. Long-standing chronic inflammation in body cavities and narrow spaces can result in rare cases of DLBCL [20], and such cases are recognized as a distinct entity by 2008 WHO classification.

MORPHOLOGIC AND IMMUNOPHENOTYPIC FEATURES

The tissue sections show effacement of underlying architecture by diffuse infiltrate of lymphoma cells, with frequent invasion into adjacent tissues. Areas of coagulation necrosis can be seen, and in some cases can be extensive with complete nodal infarction and no viable lymphoma cells [21-23].

Table 1. Classification of Diffuse Large B-cell Lymphoma

<table>
<tr><td colspan="2">DLBCL, Not Otherwise Specified</td></tr>
<tr><td>• Common morphologic variants
Centroblastic
Immunoblastic
Anaplastic
• Rare morphologic variants
• Molecular subgroups
Germinal center B-cell-like
Activated B-cell-like</td><td>• Cytogenetic subgroups
Double/triple hit lymphoma*
DLBCL with IG/IRF4 translocation
• Immunohistochemical subgroups
CD5-positive de novo DLBCL
Germinal center B-cell-like
Non-Germinal center B-cell-like
DLBCL with MYC/BCL2 co-expression</td></tr>
<tr><td colspan="2">DLBCL Subtypes</td></tr>
<tr><td>• T-cell/histiocyte-rich large B-cell lymphoma
• Primary DLBCL of the central nervous system</td><td>• Primary cutaneous DLBCL, leg type
• EBV-positive DLBCL of the elderly</td></tr>
<tr><td colspan="2">DLBCL, Other Entities</td></tr>
<tr><td>• Primary mediastinal (thymic) large B-cell lymphoma
• Intravascular large B-cell lymphoma
• DLBCL associated with chronic inflammation
• Lymphomatoid granulomatosis</td><td>• ALK + large B-cell lymphoma
• Plasmablastic lymphoma
• Large B-cell lymphoma arising in HHV8-associated multicentric Castleman's disease
• Primary effusion lymphoma</td></tr>
<tr><td colspan="2">Borderline Cases</td></tr>
<tr><td colspan="2">B-cell lymphoma, unclassifiable, with features intermediate between DLBCL and Burkitt lymphoma
B-cell lymphoma, unclassifiable, with features intermediate between DLBCL and classical Hodgkin lymphoma</td></tr>
</table>

DLBCL, diffuse large B-cell lymphoma; IG, immunoglobulin loci; EBV, Epstein-Barr virus; ALK, anaplastic lymphoma kinase; HHV8, human herpesvirus 8; *Double/triple hit lymphoma is currently classified under "B-cell lymphoma, unclassifiable, with features intermediate between DLBCL and Burkitt lymphoma."

Partial involvement is occasionally seen in lymph nodes with sinusoidal or interfollicular pattern (Figure 1 and 2) [24]. Intravascular large B-cell lymphoma shows exclusive localization of lymphoma cells in the vascular spaces. Some DLBCLs, especially in the mediastinal and retroperitoneal regions, are usually associated with prominent sclerosis (Figure 3) [25, 26]. "Starry sky" pattern with interspersed tingible body macrophages can be seen in DLBCL with very high proliferation index [27].

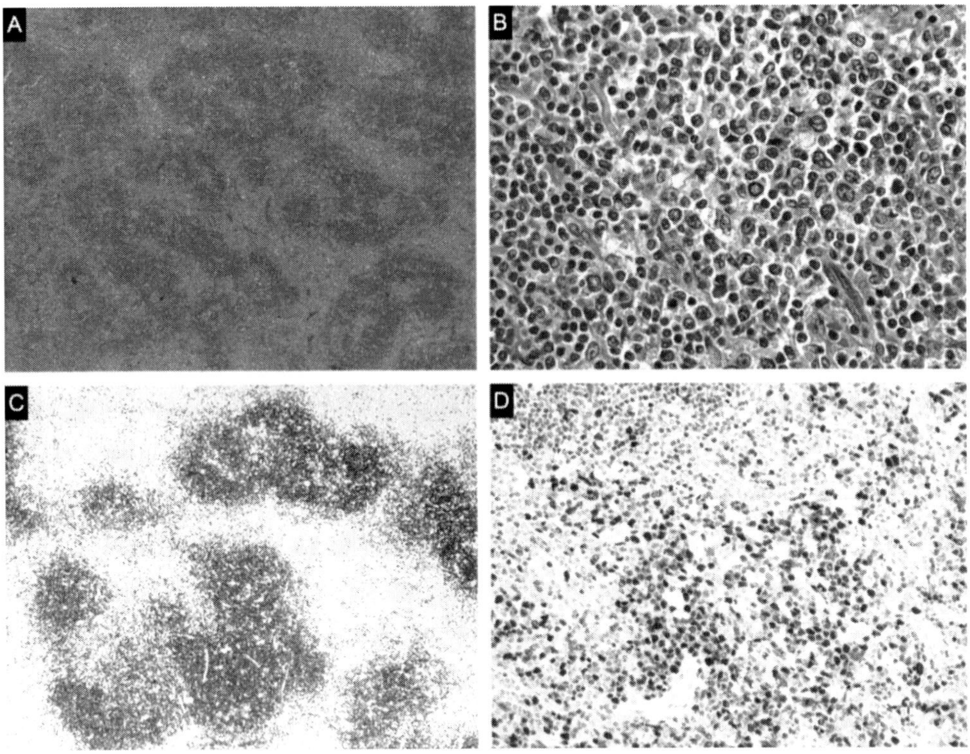

Figure 1. DLBCL with interfollicular growth pattern. (A), The lymph node shows many large irregular lymphoid follicles (H&E). (B), The interfollicular areas show large clusters and sheets of large atypical lymphoid cells (H&E). (C), IgD highlights the expanded benign mantle zones in follicles. (D), OCT2 shows the large B-cells in the interfollicular areas.

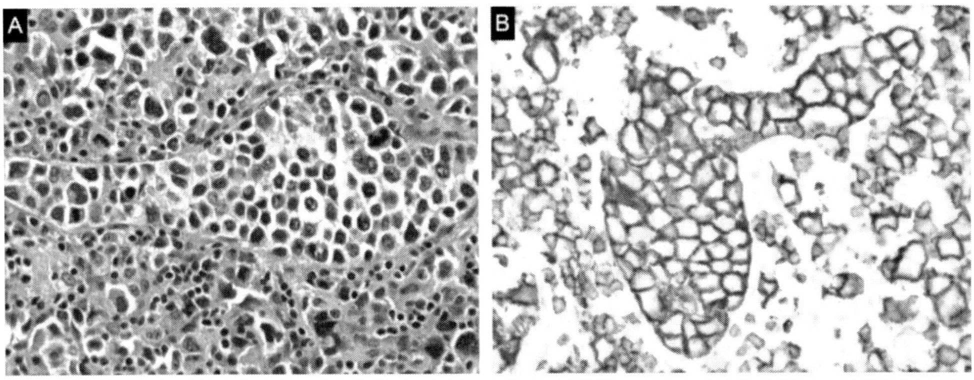

Figure 2. DLBCL with intrasinusoidal growth pattern. (A). Clusters of large lymphoma cells within a sinus (H&E). (B). CD20 highlights the clusters of large B-cells within a sinus.

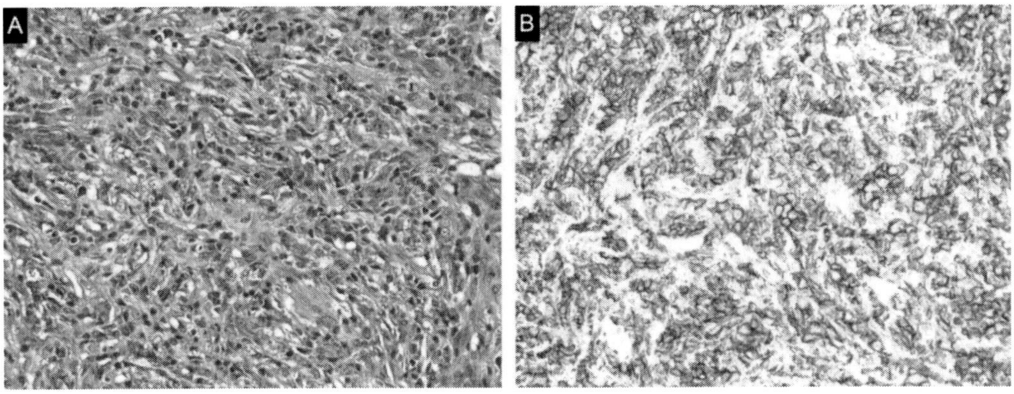

Figure 3. Retroperitoneal DLBCL associated with sclerosis. (A). DLBCL cells associated with fibrosis (H&E). (B). CD20 highlights the large B-cells.

In DLBCL transformed from low grade B-cell lymphomas, the low grade lymphoma can be found coexistent with DLBCL in the same tissue (Figure 4).

Cytologically, the lymphoma cells are medium to large with nuclear size equal or larger than that of benign histiocytes. If benign histiocytes are difficult to identify, the size of the lymphoma cells can be inferred by comparing with background small mature lymphocytes. The nuclei of the DLBCL cells are over twice the size of small mature lymphocytes. Three common morphologic variants have been identified: centroblastic, immunoblastic, and anaplastic variants (Figure 5). The centroblastic variant is most common in DLBCL. The centroblasts are large with round to oval nuclei, open chromatin, 2 to 4 small nucleoli attached to the nuclear membrane and scant amphophilic to basophilic cytoplasm. The centroblasts can have multilobated or angulated nuclei. Most cases of centroblastic variant of DLBCL show heterogeneous population of centroblasts and immunoblasts, with immunoblasts comprising <90% of the cells. The immunoblastic variant of DLBCL is defined by >90% immunoblasts. The immunoblasts are large with round nuclei, open chromatin, a single prominent centrally located nucleolus and moderate to abundant basophilic cytoplasm, some with plasmacytoid differentiation. The distinction between centroblasts and immunoblasts is not always clear-cut, and lymphoma cells with hybrid features are frequently seen. The anaplastic variant of DLBCL is characterized by large bizarre pleomorphic nuclei and abundant cytoplasm. These anaplastic cells may resemble Reed-Sternberg/Hodgkin cells or anaplastic large cell lymphoma cells. They may show sinusoidal or cohesive growth pattern. DLBCL with predominantly medium-sized blastoid cells is usually high grade with high proliferation index and is often the so-called "double hit" lymphoma [28]. Rare cases DLBCL show unusual morphologic features including variants with myxoid stroma, spindle cells, signet ring cells, fibrillary matrix, alveolar pattern, increased eosinophils, microvillous DLBCL, admixed crystal-storing histiocytosis and intrasinusoidal pattern. Variable numbers of background reactive cells are commonly seen in DLBCL, including small mature T-lymphocytes, plasma cells, histiocytes, and rarely granulocytes. On cytological smears, the DLBCL cells are typically large with round to irregular nuclei, variably prominent nucleoli, and moderate to abundant basophilic cytoplasm, sometimes with cytoplasmic vacuoles. The chromatin of the nuclei can be finely dispersed to coarsely clumped. Occasionally the DLBCL cells are cytologically indistinguishable from myeloblasts in acute myeloid leukemia with blastoid chromatin and pale basophilic cytoplasm.

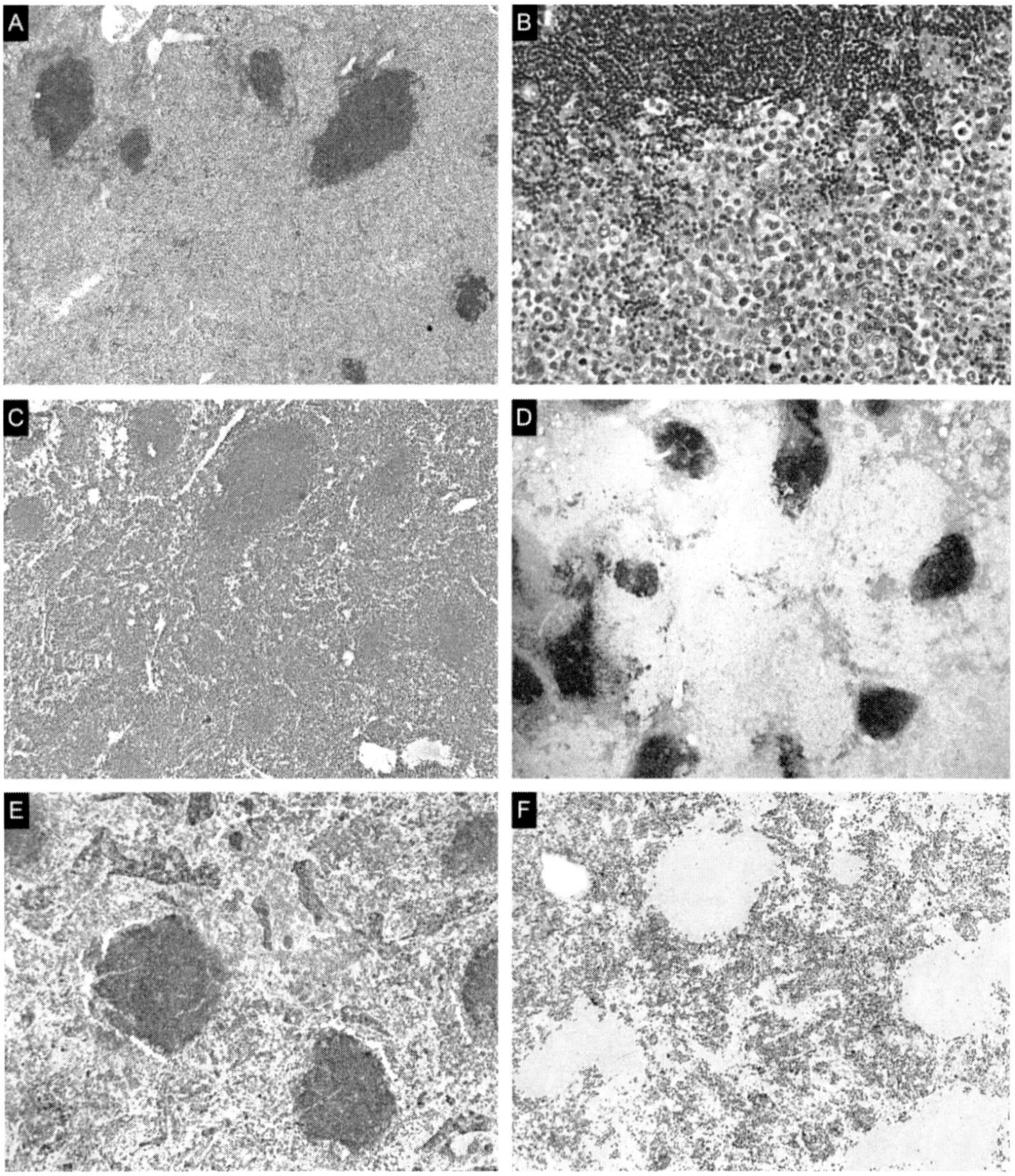

Figure 4. DLBCL with concurrent low grade follicular lymphoma. (A). The lymph node shows multiple lymphoid nodules and sheets of large lymphoid cells (H&E). (B). The lymphoid nodules (upper portion) are composed of small mature lymphoid cells, while the cells between the lymphoid nodules are large atypical lymphoid cells (H&E). The small lymphoid cells in lymphoid nodules are positive for CD20 (C), BCL6 (D), BCL2 (E), and negative for MUM1 (F). The large lymphoma cells are positive for CD20 (C), BCL2 (E), and MUM1 (F), and negative for BCL6 (D).

Flow cytometry and/or immunohistochemistry studies are essential to determine the immunophenotype of lymphoma cells for the diagnosis of DLBCL. DLBCL cells always express CD45 and pan B-cell markers CD19, CD20, CD22, CD79a, PAX5, OCT-2 and BOB.1. In relapsed DLBCL previously treated with rituximab (anti-CD20 antibody), CD20 expression is lost in approximately 60% cases [29].

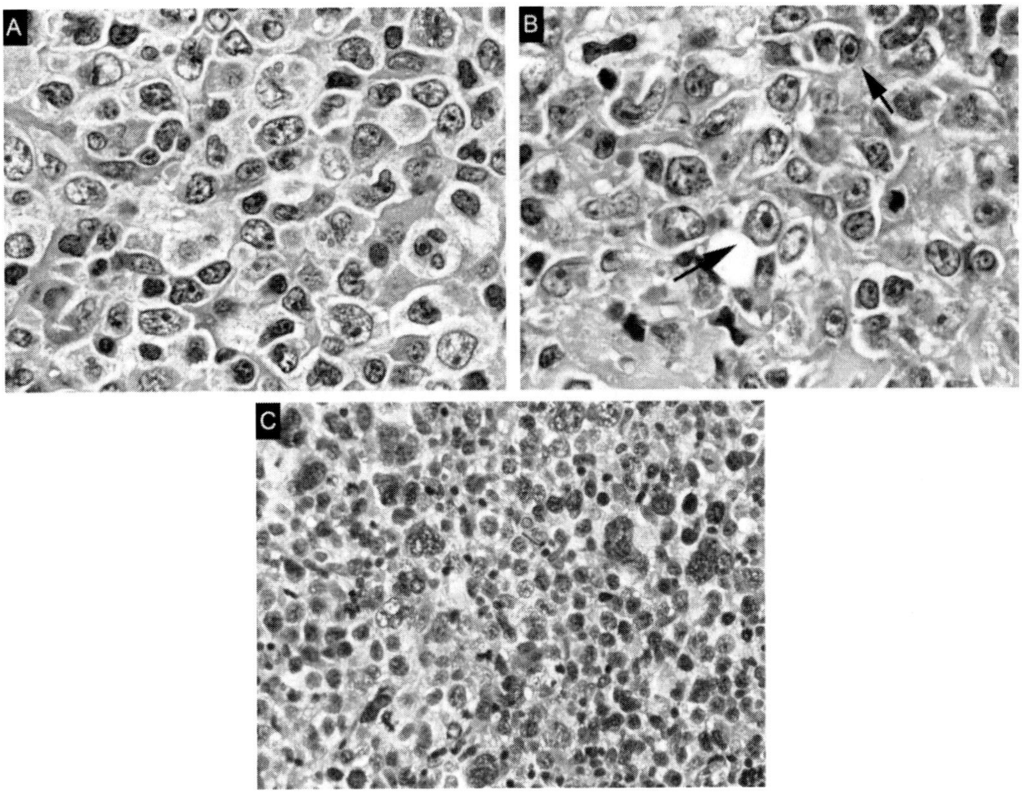

Figure 5. Cytological variants of DLBCL. (A). Centroblasts (H&E). (B). Immunoblasts (arrowheads) admixed with centroblasts (H&E). (C). Anaplastic cells with large bizarre nuclei (H&E).

Clonal surface and cytoplasmic immunoglobulin heavy and light chains are commonly expressed. Occasional cases of DLBCL may show lack of surface immunoglobulin light chain expression [30]. With the exception of CD5, pan-T cell markers are negative, although occasional cases with coexpression of CD3, CD2, CD4, CD7 or CD8 on the neoplastic B-cells have been reported [31, 32]. CD5 is expressed in approximately 10% *de novo* DLBCL [33]. CD10 is expressed in approximately 30-40% of cases and associated with germinal-center B-cell type and often t(14;18)(q32;q21) [34-38]. Approximately 60-70% cases are BCL6 positive [39-41]. BCL2 expression is present in approximately 50% cases, and often associated with t(14;18)(q32;q21) [36, 39, 42-44]. Post germinal center or plasma cell associated antigens such as MUM1 and CD38 are present in a subset of cases [45], while CD138 is only expressed in cases with plasmacytic differentiation. The activation marker CD30 is expressed in a small subset of DLBCL, but usually heterogeneous in terms of the level of expression [46]. The proliferation index as determined by Ki-67 expression is usually high (30-80%), and approaching 100% in some highly aggressive cases [47-50]. MYC is expressed in approximately 30% cases and in both GCB and ABC subtypes with similar frequency [51]. The MYC protein expression does not always correlate with *c-Myc* gene rearrangement. In immunocompetent patients, EBER (Epstein-Barr virus-encoded RNA) is positive in <5% DLBCL in Western countries and approximately 10% cases in East Asians, usually in the elderly patients [52]. EBV positive DLBCL is usually extranodal, with some degree of plasmacytoid morphology and associated with necrosis and CD30 expression.

Differential Diagnosis

The diagnosis of DLBCL is usually straightforward based on morphologic and phenotypic features. The unusual morphologic variants such as spindle cells and signet ring cells and sometimes cohesive or alveolar growth patterns of DLBCL would raise the differential diagnosis of a nonhematopoietic malignancy such as carcinoma or sarcoma. The diffuse infiltrate by large neoplastic cells is also seen in melanoma or seminoma. Immunophenotyping with a panel of antibodies including CD45 and pan-B cell markers will easily lead to the correct diagnosis. When fine needle aspirate and/or touch prep are available, the DLBCL cells are discohesive and show basophilic or amphophilic cytoplasm, often with lymphoglandular bodies (cytoplasmic break-down from smudged lymphocytes) in the background. These cytological features can guide subsequent flow cytometric analysis with appropriate antibody panels, especially when tissue biopsies are not taken.

The florid reactive immunoblastic proliferation in infectious mononucleosis, cytomegalovirus infections, drug induced lymphadenopathy, postvaccination reaction, early stage of Kikuchi disease and rare cases of acute inflammation can mimic DLBCL on Haematoxylin and Eosin (H&E) sections [53-56]. In these reactive conditions, the underlying architecture is distorted but not effaced. Necrosis can be seen focally with or without some Reed-Sternberg/Hodgkin-like cells. In infectious mononucleosis, the large cells are usually polymorphic with various differentiations into plasma cells/plasmacytoid cells. By immunohistochemical staining, the large lymphocytes consist of mixture of CD3 and CD20 positive immunoblasts. The B immunoblasts usually show heterogeneous expression of CD20 and some CD30 positive cells. Flow cytometry and polymerase chain reaction (PCR) studies for B-cell gene rearrangements show no clonal B-cells [57]. The immunoblasts are positive for EBV by the Epstein–Barr virus-encoded small RNAs (EBER) assay in infectious mononucleosis. The retained underlying architecture, clinical presentation and serologic studies (Heterophile antibody) will confirm the diagnosis of infectious mononucleosis. In drug induced lymphadenopathy, postvaccination reaction, and early stage of Kikuchi disease, the large lymphoid cells are predominantly CD3 positive T-immunoblasts with predominance of cytotoxic CD8 + T-cells. In rare cases associated with acute inflammation, the immunoblastic proliferation may be exuberant, but they do not form mass lesions and the underlying architecture is intact.

The anaplastic variant of DLBCL can be confused with anaplastic large cell lymphoma (ALCL) due to predominance of pleomorphic lymphoma cells and sometime sinusoidal or cohesive pattern. The ALCL cells are positive for CD30, T-cell markers and cytotoxic proteins (TIA1 and granzyme B). The anaplastic DLBCL is positive for pan B-cell markers and negative for T-cells and cytotoxic markers. ALK is not a useful marker herein, as it could be seen in either ALCL or ALK positive DLBCL (see the section on ALK positive DLBCL).

The pleomorphic variant of mantle cell lymphoma is morphologically indistinguishable from DLBCL, especially the anaplastic variant. Immunohistochemical stains for CD5, cyclin D1 and SOX11 are essential for the differential diagnosis. Approximately 10% DLBCLs are positive for CD5, but they are negative for cyclin D1 and SOX11. Rare cases of DLBCL are positive for cyclin D1 but show no *IGH/CCND1* translocation [58]. The cyclin D1 positive DLBCLs are always negative for SOX11 and usually negative for CD5. FISH study for *IGH/CCND1* translocation should be performed in equivocal cases to confirm the diagnosis.

In DLBCL composed predominantly of medium-sized lymphoid cells, including the B-cell lymphoma, unclassifiable, with features intermediate between DLBCL and Burkitt lymphoma, the differential diagnosis includes Burkitt lymphoma, B-lymphoblastic lymphoma and blastoid mantle cell lymphoma. These DLBCLs may have abundant apoptotic bodies, extremely high proliferation index and scattered tingible body macrophages in a "starry sky" pattern, closely mimicking Burkitt lymphoma. The Burkitt lymphoma cells are monomorphic with more coarse chromatin and squared cell borders. The Burkitt lymphoma cells are characteristically BCL2 negative and show germinal center phenotype with expression of CD10 and BCL6, and extremely high proliferation index by Ki-67 (almost 100%) [59]. The DLBCLs are often strongly positive for BCL2. When cytogenetic studies are performed, the Burkitt lymphoma is characterized by *MYC* rearrangement to an immunoglobulin heavy or light chain loci and a simple karyotype, while in DLBCL the *MYC* gene may be rearranged but the partner gene is usually not immunoglobulin genes and the karyotype is typically complex [60]. B-lymphoblastic lymphoma can be easily ruled out by immunohistochemical stain for TDT or CD34, which is negative in DLBCL. The blastoid mantle cell lymphoma can be confirmed by positive stain for cyclin D1 and SOX11.

In DLBCL with blastoid cytology, myeloid sarcoma, blastoid mantle cell lymphoma, and lymphoblastic lymphoma are the main differential diagnosis. Blastoid mantle cell lymphoma and lymphoblastic lymphoma can be ruled out as described above. One of the most useful morphologic features of myeloid sarcoma is the presence of eosinophilic precursors or cytoplasmic eosinophilic granules among the blasts. The blasts in myeloid sarcoma are positive for CD34, CD117, and myeloperoxidase, or CD43, CD68 and lysozyme in cases with monocytic differentiation.

Histiocytic sarcoma should be suspected morphologically by the presence of large cells with abundant eosinophilic cytoplasm. The presence of histiocytic markers such as CD68, CD163 and lysozyme and absence of pan-B cell markers will confirm the diagnosis.

The syncytial variant of nodular sclerosis classical Hodgkin lymphoma (NSCHL) and lymphocyte depleted classical Hodgkin lymphoma can mimic DLBCL. The syncytial variant of NSCHL typically shows areas of coagulation necrosis with adjacent large clusters and sheets of large neoplastic cells. Broad bands of fibrosis and mixed inflammatory cells such as eosinophils and granulocytes would favor NSCHL. The Reed-Sternberg/Hodgkin cells are strongly positive for CD30, and may be positive for CD20, but the CD20 expression is heterogeneous and weak. They are only weakly positive for PAX5 and negative for other B-cell markers CD79a, OCT2 and BOB.1. The strong expression of CD20 and other pan B-cell markers in the absence of strong CD30 and CD15 supports the diagnosis of DLBCL. The uncommon cases, where the neoplastic cells have morphologic features of Reed-Sternberg/Hodgkin cells and strong expression of CD30, CD15 and pan B-cell markers, are best classified as B-cell lymphoma, unclassifiable, with features intermediate between DLBCL and classical Hodgkin lymphoma.

Genetic and Molecular Features

Immunoglobulin heavy (*IgH*) and light chains (*IgK* and *IgL*) are clonally rearranged, and *TCR* genes are in germline configuration. The immunoglobulin heavy chain genes show somatic hypermutations in the variable regions V(H), some with ongoing somatic mutations, evidence of passage of cells through the germinal centers during lymphomagenesis [61].

The t(14;18)(q32;q21) with *BCL2* gene rearrangement is present in approximately 20% cases of DLBCL [62]. Approximately 30% DLBCL have *BCL6* gene rearrangement at chromosomal loci 3q27 [63, 64]. *BCL6* somatic mutations are frequent in approximately 70% cases, and have no relationship with *BCL6* gene rearrangement [65, 66]. BCL6 is a master transcription factor for the development of germinal centers and inhibits differentiation of B-cells to plasma cells [67]. The *BCL6* somatic mutation is another marker indicative of passage of DLBCL cells through the germinal centers. *MYC* (8q24) gene rearrangement, a genetic hallmark of Burkitt lymphoma, is present in up to 10% DLBCL [59, 68-72], and more frequent in HIV-positive DLBCL, immunoblastic variant of DLBCL and plasmablastic lymphoma [73, 74]. *MYC* gene rearrangement is commonly seen in the context of complex karyotype and the partner gene is often located in non-immunoglobulin gene loci [60].

New recurrent translocations, der(14)t(3;14)(q21;q32), t(1;13)(p32;q14), t(1;7)(q21;q22), and der(6)t(6;8)(q11;q11), have been identified by spectral karyotyping [75]. Comparative genomic hybridization (CGH) analysis have identified frequent chromosomal gains in 1q, 2p, 3, 6p, 7, 8q, 9q, 11, 12, 13q, 16p, 18q, 22q, and X, and loss of 1p, 6q, 8p and X [76, 77]. Amplification of individual genes including *REL* (2p12-16), *MYC* (8q24), *BCL2* (18q21), *GLI*, *CDK4*, and *MDM2* (12q13-14) has been demonstrated based on the comparative genomic hybridization (CGH) study [77]. Single nucleotide polymorphism (SNP) array identified five DLBCL clusters with distinct genetic profiles, clinical characteristics and outcomes by unsupervised clustering [78]. Loss of genomic material at 8p23.1 was shown to have the strongest statistical association with worse outcome, and associated with additional aberrations, such as 17p- and 15q- [78].

Gene expression profile studies identified two prognostically significant subgroups of DLBCL with gene expression patterns of different stages of B-cell differentiation [79]. The germinal centre B-like (GCB-like) subgroup in approximately 40-50% DLBCLs expresses genes characteristic of germinal center B-cells, while the activated B-like (ABC-like) subgroup expresses genes in activated peripheral B-cells. The GCB-like subgroup has frequent gains of 12q12, while the ABC-like subgroup shows frequent trisomy 3, gains of 3q, 18q21-q22 and loss of 6q21-q23 [80, 81]. The immunoblastic variant and centroblastic variant with increased immunoblasts are more often the ABC-like DLBCL. t(14;18)(q32;q21) is present in approximately 30% GCB-like and less than 5% ABC-like DLBCL. *BCL2* translocation is characteristically seen in GCB-like subgroup, while *BCL6* translocation is less specific for GCB-like subgroup [82-84]. *MYC* rearrangement and amplification are predominantly seen in GCB-like subgroup as well [85].

TP53 mutations are present in approximately 20% cases and p53 protein expression by immunostain is seen in approximately 40% cases [62, 86]. *TP53* dysfunction is a common occurrence in many neoplasms. There is no causal relationship between p53 protein expression and *TP53* mutation or deletion in DLBCL [87]. Hypermutation in proto-oncogenes *PIM1*, *MYC*, *RhoH/TTF* (*ARHH*) and *PAX5* is seen in more than 50% of DLBCL [88]. Genes regulating chromatin methylation, such as *MLL2*, *MEF2B*, and *EZH2* are frequently mutated in GCB-like DLBCL, while gene mutations in *CARD11*, *CD79B*, *TNFAIP3*, and *MYD88* with subsequent activation of NF-κB and B-cell receptor pathways are seen in ABC-like DLBCL [89, 90]. An interrelationship between *STAT3* activation in JAK-STAT pathway and NF-κB pathways has been demonstrated in ABC-like DLBCL [91].

Mutations in *ARID1B*, *ROBO2* and *MRS1* as potential tumor suppressor genes and *KLHL6*, *IL31* and *LRP1* as oncogenes are identified by combination of SNP array and whole exome/ whole transcriptome sequencing [92].

The DLBCL cells retain the t(14;18)(q32;q21) with strong BCL2 expression in cases transformed from follicular lymphoma [93]. The transformation of DLBCL from low grade B-cell lymphoma is usually accompanied by genetic changes such as *TP53* mutation, *MYC* rearrangement, deletion of p14/16 or mir-17-92 gain/amplification, which may play a role in the pathogenesis of histologic transformation [94]. High-level expression of cyclin D3 (*CCND3*) as a result of t(6;14)(p21.1;q32.3) has been demonstrated in some cases of DLBCL transformed from marginal zone lymphoma [95].

Prognostic Markers

The International Prognostic Index (IPI) based on five clinical and laboratory parameters including age, lactate dehydrogenase (LDH), number of extranodal sites, Ann Arbor stage, and Eastern Cooperative Oncology Group (ECOG) performance status is a powerful prognostic tool for DLBCL in the era of cyclophosphamide, doxorubicin, vincristine, and prednisone (CHOP) chemotherapy [96]. Four discrete risk categories were identified by IPI, with 5-year overall survival (OS) of 26% in the high-risk subgroup (score 4-5), 47% in the intermediate risk group (score 2-3), and 73% in the low-risk subgroup (score 0-1). The predictive power of IPI decreased particularly in the higher-risk DLBCL patients with the introduction of rituximab (R) to CHOP or CHOP-like chemotherapies [97, 98]. A revised IPI (R-IPI) by redistributing the IPI factors shows better prediction of outcomes in in the era of R-CHOP regimen of chemotherapy [98]. Three distinct prognostic groups are identified by the R-IPI with a very good (OS 94%), good (OS 79%), and poor (OS 55%) outcome, respectively. But the IPI (or R-IPI) cannot identify a risk group with <50% overall survival in DLBCL treated by R-CHOP. A recently introduced enhanced International Prognostic Index (NCCN-IPI) uses 5 predictors (age, lactate dehydrogenase (LDH), sites of involvement, Ann Arbor stage, ECOG performance status) to identify 4 prognostic groups: low (0-1), low-intermediate (2-3), high-intermediate (4-5), and high (6-8) [99]. The NCCN-IPI better discriminates low- and high-risk subgroups (5-year OS 96% vs 33%) in the era of Rituximab than the IPI.

The cytological features of DLBCL, based on the presence of immunoblastic variant are unreliable to predict prognosis [100-102]. In patients with bone marrow involvement by DLBCL, the presence of concordant involvement is associated with poor prognosis compared with that of discordant involvement, which shows similar survival to that of DLBCL without bone marrow involvement [11, 103-105].

Despite the successful application of clinical based prognostic model in predicting patients' outcome in DLBCL (IPI and R-IPI), there is still considerably variability of survival in patients with the same prognostic scores, likely due to inherent genetic heterogeneity in each group. Therefore, there are continuing efforts to identify prognostically significant molecular and/or genetic markers. A large number of genes and proteins of the cell cycle regulatory pathways, apoptosis, B-cell differentiation pathways and adhesion molecules have been studied for their prognostic value in DLBCL. The predictive power of these individual genes or proteins is usually variable or contradictory in different studies, likely due to different methodology employed and/or criteria for positive results. For example, *TP53* mutations and/or overexpression, *p27KIP1* overexpression, high proliferation rate by Ki-67, CD5 expression, MUM1 positivity and increased serum level of CD44 have been associated with poor survival in some studies [33, 86, 106-111], but not in others [106, 112-121]. The overexpression of cyclin D3 predicts poor survival and complete remission (CR) rate independent of IPI [122], and the expression of cyclin D2 or survivin is associated with worse outcome [117, 123-126]. p14(*ARF*) abnormal nuclear overexpression is associated with high levels of p53 and HDM2 and more aggressive clinical course [127]. The expression of germinal center proteins BCL6 and HGAL is associated with favorable prognosis [128, 129], while the predictive value of germinal center marker CD10 is contradictory [130, 131]. High level expression of FOXP1, a marker of nongerminal center/activated B-cells, is associated with inferior OS independent of IPI [132]. *BCL2* translocation does not predict survival in DLBCL, but BCL2 expression is associated with inferior OS and disease free survival (DFS) in DLBCL treated with CHOP [43, 114, 133, 134]. The introduction of rituximab to CHOP chemotherapy overcomes the negative effects of BCL2 overexpression on the prognosis [135]. Increased serum levels of proteins in angiogenesis, such as endostatin, vascular endothelial growth factor (VEGF) and fibroblast growth factor (FGF), and expression of matrix metalloproteinases (MMP)-9 but not of MMP-2 are all associated with worse outcomes [136-138].

Due to the often inconclusive and conflicting nature of the individual markers for prognosis in DLBCL, genome-scale gene expression profiling (GEP) studies have been employed to identify genetic signatures useful for prognosis. The GEP study has identified two distinct subgroups of DLBCL, GCB-Like and ABC-like, with significantly different 5 year overall survival independent of IPI (76% of GCB-like vs 16% of ABC-like DLBCL) [79]. A number of the genes in the GCB-like and ABC-like signatures are single prognostic markers identified previously, such as *BCL6*, *HGAL* and *BCL2*. In an effort to simplify the GEP analysis, subsequent studies have identified genetic signatures comprising 17 genes and 6 genes (*LMO2*, *BCL6*, *FN1*, *CCND2*, *SCYA3*, *BCL2*) that are able to predict prognosis in patients treated with R-CHOP [83, 123]. A GEP study also has identified stromal signatures within the microenvironment of DLBCL associated with different outcomes [139]. The prognostically favorable stromal-1 signature reflects extracellular-matrix deposition and histiocytic infiltration, while the prognostically unfavorable stromal-2 signature reflects tumor blood-vessel density. A simple model incorporating the expression of LMO2 in DLBCL cells and tumor necrosis factor receptor superfamily member 9 (TNFRSF9) in infiltrating T cells of the microenvironment has been shown to predict overall survival in DLBCL, independent of "cell-of-origin" classification, "stromal signatures," and IPI, and add to the predictive power of the IPI [140]. As it is often impractical to perform GEP analysis on clinical specimens, a number of immunophenotyping algorithms with antibodies against germinal center and post germinal center antigens have been developed to predict the GCB-like and ABC-like DLBCL. The Hans algorithm with CD10, BCL6 and MUM1 is the most commonly used in practice [110]. However, the Hans algorithm has a relatively low concordance with GEP analysis (approximately 80%). In addition, the Hans algorithm was designed in the era of CHOP therapy and failed to predict survival in patients treated R-CHOP [141]. The new Visco/Young algorithm has a high concordance with GEP analysis (92.6%) and effectively predicts prognosis of DLBCL in patients treated with R-CHOP [142].

The coexpression of MYC/BCL2 detected by immunohistochemical stain predicts poor prognosis in DLBCL patients treated with R-CHOP (Figure 6) [143]. DLBCL with coexpression of MYC/BCL2 occurs more frequently in ABC-like subgroup.

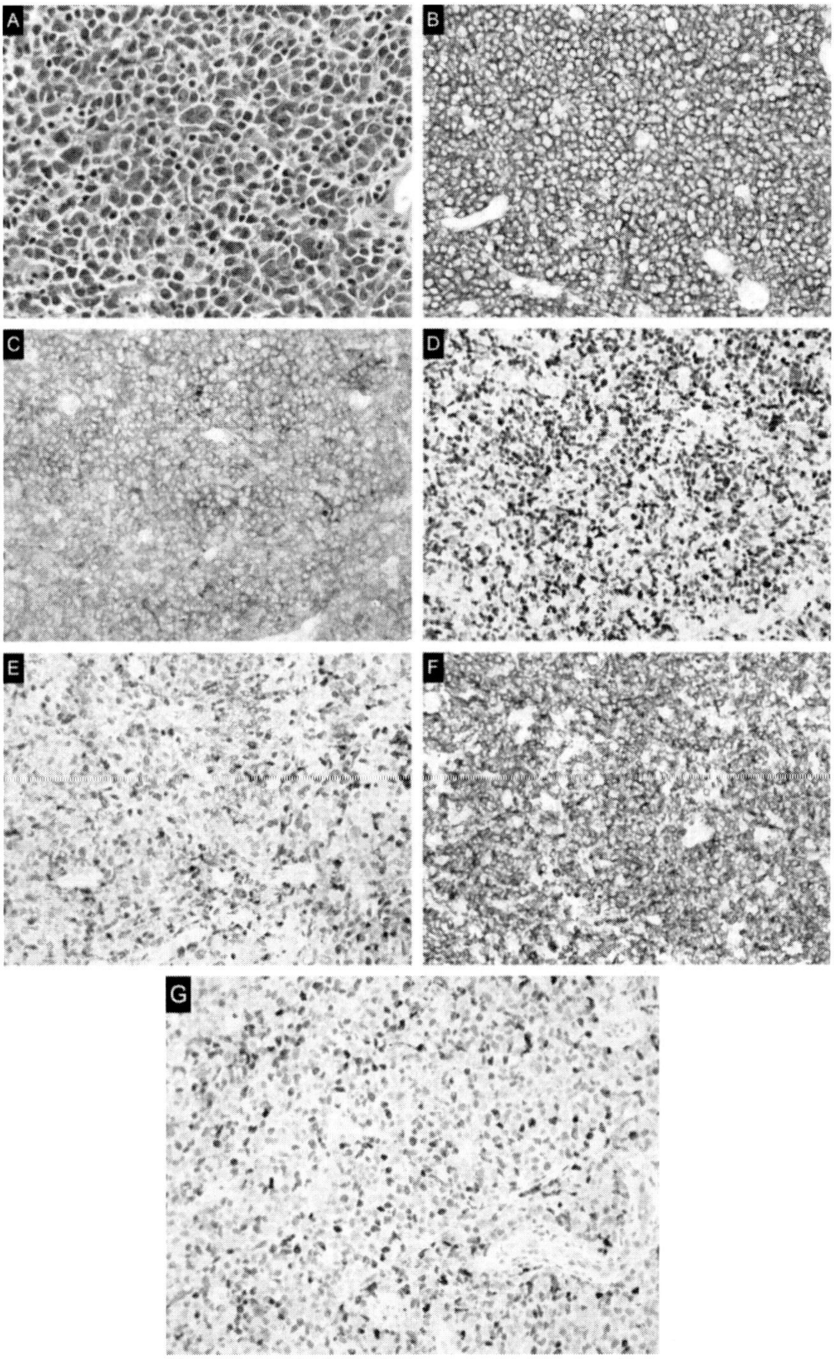

Figure 6. DLBCL with coexpression of BCL2 and MYC. (A). DLBCL cells ((H&E). The DLBCL cells are positive for CD20 (B), CD10 (C), BCL6 (D), MUM1 (E), BCL2 (F) and MYC (G).

The difference in prognosis of GCB-like and ABC-like DLBCL is likely due to the more frequent MYC/BCL2 coexpression in ABC-like DLBCL. MYC/BCL2 coexpression is associated with high risk gene expression signatures. The cutoffs of ≥50%/40% and ≥70%/40% for BCL2 and MYC protein expression respectively by immunohistochemical stain appear to have the same prognostic significance [144].

MORPHOLOGIC SUBTYPES AND OTHER ENTITIES

T-Cell/Histiocyte-Rich Large B-Cell Lymphoma

T-cell/histiocyte-rich large B-cell lymphoma (THRLBCL) is defined by <10% scattered large neoplastic B-cells in a background of abundant T-cells and histiocytes [145-147]. THRLBCL is usually seen in middle aged man with median age of 47 years [145]. It most commonly affects lymph nodes, but extranodal tissues such as liver, spleen and bone marrow are also frequently involved [148]. Patients with THRLBCL usually present with advanced disease (stage III-IV) and more frequent bone marrow involvement than conventional DLBCL. The IPI is the only relevant prognostic factor. THRLBCL is an aggressive disease with poor survival due to advanced stage, but the survival rates are similar to IPI matched conventional DLBCL [145].

Histologically, the lymph node architecture is effaced by diffuse lymphoid infiltrate composed of singly scattered large atypical lymphoid cells in a background rich in small mature lymphocytes and/or histiocytes (Figure 7).

The large atypical lymphoid cells may show uneven distribution with focal loose clustering, but do not form aggregates or sheets. These large atypical lymphoid cells usually show morphologic features of centroblasts, but can be more anaplastic resembling Reed-Sternberg/Hodgkin cells or lymphocyte predominant (LP) cells of the nodular lymphocyte predominant Hodgkin lymphoma [149]. The small mature lymphocytes in the background may show mild cytologic atypia with irregular nuclei.

Variable numbers of histiocytes are present, and large clusters of epithelioid histiocytes can be seen in some cases. Mixed inflammatory cells composed of eosinophils or neutrophils are typically absent. THRLBCL shows a characteristic micronodular pattern of infiltrate in the white pulps of spleen, and portal infiltrate in the liver [149]. Bone marrow is more frequently involved in THRLBCL than conventional DLBCL and usually shows paratrabecular polymorphic lymphoid aggregates with similar cellular composition as that in the lymph nodes [150].

Immunophenotypically, the large atypical lymphoid cells show expression of pan B-cell markers CD20, CD79a, and PAX5, and are usually positive for germinal center marker BCL6 (Figure 7) and variable for BCL2. They are positive for EMA and CD30 in approximately 30-40% cases, especially in cases with LP cell and Reed-Sternberg/Hodgkin cell morphologies, respectively [151]. There are essentially no small mature B-cells in the background. The background small lymphocytes are predominantly CD3 and CD8 positive cytotoxic T-cells. There is no rosetting of large B-cells by PD1/CXCL13 + follicular T-helper cells. Rare cases of THRLBCL with sheets of PD1 positive T-cells have been reported [152]. CD21 shows no follicular dendritic meshworks. EBER is negative for EBV-positive large B-cells. THRLBCL may progress to histologically conventional DLBCL with sheets of large B-cells.

The main differential diagnoses are nodular lymphocyte predominant Hodgkin lymphoma (NLPHL) and lymphocyte-rich classical Hodgkin lymphoma (LRCHL). NLPHL with a diffuse pattern rich in background T-cells closely mimic THRLBCL, and in some cases can be histologically indistinguishable from THRLBCL. Generally, NLPHL has at least focally nodular infiltrate with IgD positive B-cells embedded in CD21 positive follicular dendritic meshworks [148]. The rosetting of PD1/CXCL13 + follicular T-helper cells around the large B-cells is prominent in NLPHL. The distinction from LRCHL is usually straightforward. Although THRLBCL can be CD30 positive, the CD30 expression is usually patchy and variable. The large B-cells in THRLBCL are typically CD15 negative, and positive for CD45 and PAX5. On the other side, Reed-Sternberg/Hodgkin cells are only weakly positive for PAX5, negative for CD45 and usually positive for CD15. Rare cases in which the large B-cells are positive for EBV by EBER are best classified as EBV-positive DLBCL [151].

There is very limited karyotyping study performed on THRLBCL and no recurrent cytogenetic abnormalities identified. Hypermutated *IgVH* gene and ongoing somatic mutations are identified in microdissected lymphoma cells, suggesting passage of lymphoma cells in the germinal centers.

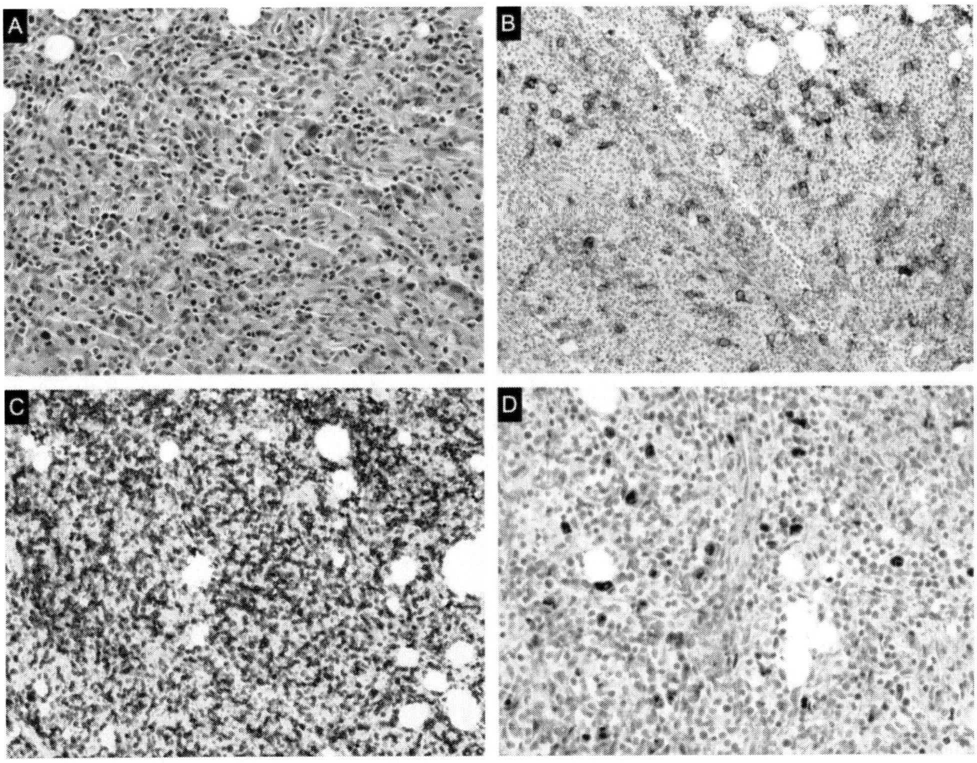

Figure 7. T-cell/histiocyte-rich large B-cell lymphoma. (A). There are scattered large atypical lymphoid cells in a background rich in small mature lymphocytes and histiocytes (H&E). (B). CD20 shows scattered large B-cells. (C). CD3 shows predominance of T-cells in the background. (D). The large lymphoma cells are positive for BCL6.

Gene expression profiling studies have showed clustering of THRLBCL with classical Hodgkin lymphoma and NLPHL [153], and a strong stromal influence of the PD1 pathway in THRLBCL [154, 155]. Array comparative genomic hybridization study has showed gains of 2p16.1 and losses of 2p11.2 and 9p11.2 in both THRLBCL and NLPHL [156], and gene expression profiling studies of microdissected lymphoma cells have showed no clear-cut and consistent differences in the gene expression of the lymphoma cells of NLPHL, THRLBCL-like NLPHL and THRLBCL, but significant differences in the cellular composition in the microenvironment of typical NLPHL and THRLBCL, suggesting that THRLBCL and NLPHL may represent a spectrum of the same disease [157].

Primary DLBCL of the Central Nervous System

Primary DLBCL of the central nervous system (CNS DLBCL) is defined as primary intracerebral or intraocular DLBCL, excluding secondary involvement or immunodeficiency-associated DLBCL. CNS DLBCL comprises approximately 2-3% of brain tumors, and the median age at diagnosis is about 60 years with slight male predominance. CNS DLBCL is located supratentorially in approximately 60% cases, intraocularly in approximately 20% cases and leptomeningeal involvement in 5% cases. Multifocal involvement is seen in approximately 20-40% cases, often in patients with AIDS. Bone marrow is rarely involved. Patients with CNS DLBCL usually present with focal neurologic abnormalities. Increased intracranial pressure and neuropsychiatric symptoms can be seen in a minority of patients. Intraocular involvement is associated with blurred vision or floaters.

Histologically, CNS DLBCL shows a diffuse pattern of infiltrate by large lymphoma cells, which often concentrate in the perivascular space (perivascular pattern of infiltrate) separated by brain parenchyma (Figure 8). The lymphoma cells are most often of the centroblasts type, and mixed with background reactive small mature lymphocytes and histiocytes. Areas of necrosis may be present. At the peripheral of the mass, the predominance of background cells can mask the presence of the large lymphoma cells. Phenotypically, the lymphoma cells are positive for B-cell markers CD20, CD79a, PAX5, and show activated B-cell (ABC) like phenotype with expression of CD10 in approximately 10-20%, BCL6 in approximately 60-100%, MUM1 in approximately 90-100% and FOXP1 in 88% cases [158, 159]. BCL2 is frequently positive. EBV is negative.

BCL6 translocation is present in approximately 30-40% cases, while t(8;14), t(11;14), or t(14;18) are absent [160-162]. CGH analysis has shown frequently losses of genomic material at 6q, and gains involving 12q, 18q and 22q, as well as 1q, 9q, 11q, 12p, 16p and 17q [163]. The most common genetic abnormalities are 18q21 gains including both the *BCL2* and *MALT1* genes [161, 164]. But Southern blot analysis and high-resolution matrix-CGH of the *BCL2* gene have shown no amplification or gene rearrangement [163]. CNS DLBCL cells express MALT1 and BCL10, consistent with activation of the NF-κB pathway and two distinct subgroups can be identified by different transcriptional levels of *BCL10*, *REL* and *IAP1* [165]. CNS DLBCL has high load of ongoing somatic mutations of *IG*, *MYC*, *PAX5*, *PIM1*, *Rho/TTF* and frequent usage of the *V4-34* gene suggesting of antigen stimulation of a shared/super antigen important for pathogenesis [166-168]. While the immunophenotype of CNS DLBCL is typical of non GCB-like DLBCL, gene expression profiling studies have shown close similarity with systemic DLBCL with respect to distribution of cases assigned to both the ABC-like and GCB-like subgroups [169]. The gene expression signature of CNS DLBCL is suggestive of derivation of late GC B cells, reflecting a GC exit phenotype [169]. There is a significant correlation between deletions in 6q and shorter survival in CNS DLBCL [164].

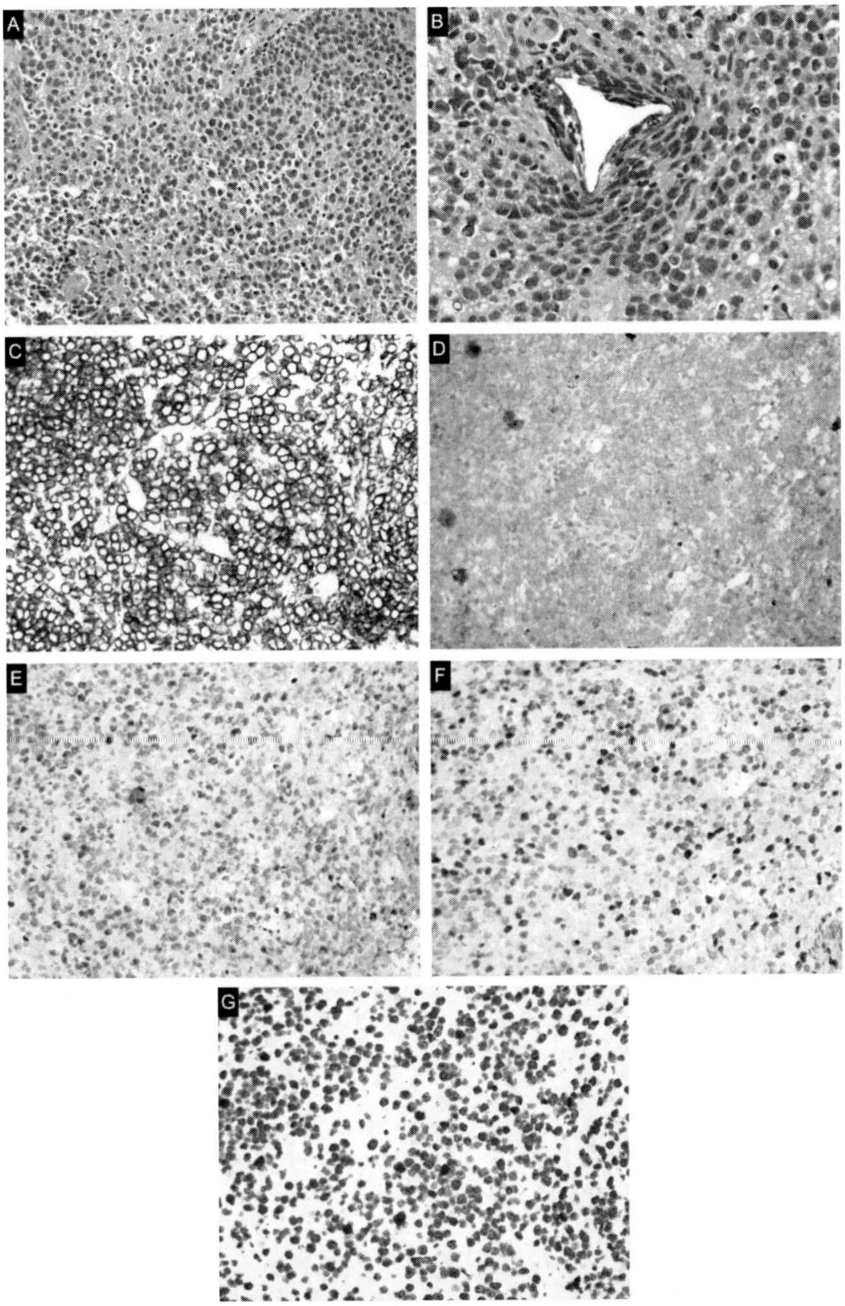

Figure 8. Primary DLBCL of the central nervous system. (A). There is a diffuse infiltrate of brain parenchyma by large lymphoma cells (H&E). (B). Angiocentric growth pattern (H&E). The large lymphoma cells are positive for CD20 (C), BCL6 (E), and MUM1 (F), and negative for CD10 (D). (G). Ki-67 shows high proliferation rate of lymphoma cells.

Primary Cutaneous DLBCL, Leg Type

Primary cutaneous DLBCL, leg type (PCLBCL, leg type) is defined as DLBCL located exclusively in the cutaneous tissue, most commonly in the lower leg. It constitutes approximately 4% of all primary cutaneous lymphomas and 20% of primary cutaneous B-cell lymphoma [170]. It usually occurs in elderly patients with median age at the time of diagnosis of 76 years and with a female predominance [171]. While the lower leg is the most common location, other anatomic sites can also be affected [172-174]. PCLBCL, leg type typically presents with nodules or masses on the lower legs, with frequent secondary dissemination to extracutaneous tissues [172, 174]. The 5 year survival rate is approximately 50% [171, 175]. Multiple skin lesions and inactivation of CDKN2A are associated with adverse prognosis [175, 176].

Histologically, PCLBCL, Leg type shows diffuse infiltrate in the dermis by a monotonous population of large atypical lymphoid cells without epidermotropism. The lymphoma cells show morphologic features of centroblasts or immunoblasts (Figure 9). Mitotic figures are usually easily seen. There are few background small mature lymphocytes. The lymphoma cells are positive for pan B-cell markers, CD20, CD79a and PAX5, and strongly positive for BCL2. It shows phenotypic features of activated B-cell (ABC) type of DLBCL with expression of BCL6, MUM1 and FOXP1, and negative CD10 [177].

The main differential diagnosis is primary cutaneous follicle center lymphoma (PCFCL). This is an important differential diagnosis, as PCFCL is an indolent disease with excellent prognosis, while PCLBCL, leg type is an aggressive lymphoma requiring multi-agent chemotherapy. PCFCL can present with predominance of centroblasts, thus mimicking a PCLBCL, leg type. PCFCL is typically present in the head-neck region, while PCLBCL, leg type is most often seen in the lower leg. The most useful immunostains for this differential diagnosis are BCL2, MUM1 and FOXP1. PCFCL cells are negative or only weakly positive for BCL2, and negative for MUM1 and FOXP1, while PCLBCL, leg type cells are positive for BCL2 (strongly), MUM1 and FOXP1.

The most common genetic abnormalities are high-level DNA amplification of 18q21.31-q21.33 (67%), including the *BCL2* and *MALT1* genes [176].

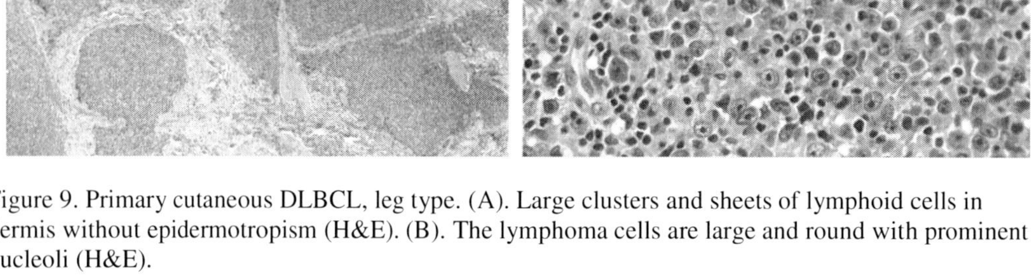

Figure 9. Primary cutaneous DLBCL, leg type. (A). Large clusters and sheets of lymphoid cells in dermis without epidermotropism (H&E). (B). The lymphoma cells are large and round with prominent nucleoli (H&E).

The strong expression of BCL2 is due to amplification of *BCL2* gene, and t(14;18) is absent. Translocations involving *BCL6*, *c-MYC*, and *IgH* genes are seen in approximately 40% cases [178]. Deletions of a small region within 9p21.3 containing the *CDKN2A*, *CDKN2B*, and *NSG-x* genes are present in about two thirds of cases [176]. As suggested by phenotypic analysis, PCLBCL, leg type shows gene expression profiles of ABC-like DLBCL [179].

EBV-Positive DLBCL of the Elderly

EBV-positive DLBCL of the elderly is defined as EBV-positive large B-cell lymphoma in patients >50 years and without any known immunodeficiency or prior lymphoma [180]. Other well defined EBV + lymphoproliferative disorders, such as lymphomatoid granulomatosis, plasmablastic lymphoma, primary effusion lymphoma, DLBCL associated chronic inflammation, and EBV + DLBCL associated with immunodeficiency syndromes are excluded. EBV + DLBCL of the elderly is believed to result from immunosenescence in the aging process. It occurs most frequently in Asian countries and consists of approximately 10% DLBCL in immunocompetent patients [181-183]. In contrast, EBV + DLBCL of the elderly accounts for approximately 3% of DLBCL in the Western countries. The median age at the time of diagnosis is 71 years, and there is a slight male predominance. Most patients present with extranodal disease, with frequent involvement in skin, lung, tonsil and gastrointestinal sites. Primary nodal involvement is seen in approximately 30% cases [180, 184]. The clinical outcome is poor with median survival rate of approximately 2 years. The presence of B symptoms and advanced age >70 years are associated with poor prognosis.

Histologically, the underlying architecture is effaced by atypical lymphoid infiltrate (Figure 10). The lymphoma cells show a variety of cytological features, including centroblasts, immunoblasts, plasmacytoid cells, pleomorphic cells and Reed-Sternberg/ Hodgkin-like cells. Areas of coagulation necrosis are frequent. Two morphologic variants, polymorphous and monomorphic variants, have been described but shown no clinical difference. The monomorphic variant consists of sheets of large lymphoma cells with few background cells. The polymorphic variant resembles classical Hodgkin lymphoma with scattered and clusters of large lymphoma cells in a background rich in small mature lymphocytes, granulocytes, histiocytes and plasma cells. Cases with areas of both monomorphic and polymorphic variants can be seen. Phenotypically, the large lymphoma cells are usually positive for pan B-cell markers CD20, CD79a and PAX5, and of post-germinal center B-cell phenotype with expression of MUM1 and negative CD10 and BCL6. CD20 can be weakly positive or negative in cases with immunoblastic or plasmacytoid cytology. CD30 is often expressed with variable level of expression, and CD15 is typically negative, although rare cases may be positive for CD15. Immunohistochemical stain for kappa and lambda light chain can often show light chain restriction in the lymphoma cells. EBER show large number of EBV positive lymphoma cells (Figure 10), and the EBV positive cells typically show a spectrum of cell sizes.

The main differential diagnosis is classical Hodgkin lymphoma (CHL) with the pleomorphic variant of EBV + DLBCL of the elderly. The Reed-Sternberg/Hodgkin cells are often positive for EBV in CHL, and the lymphoma cells of pleomorphic variant of EBV + DLBCL of the elderly are often CD30 positive and can even be CD15 positive in rare cases.

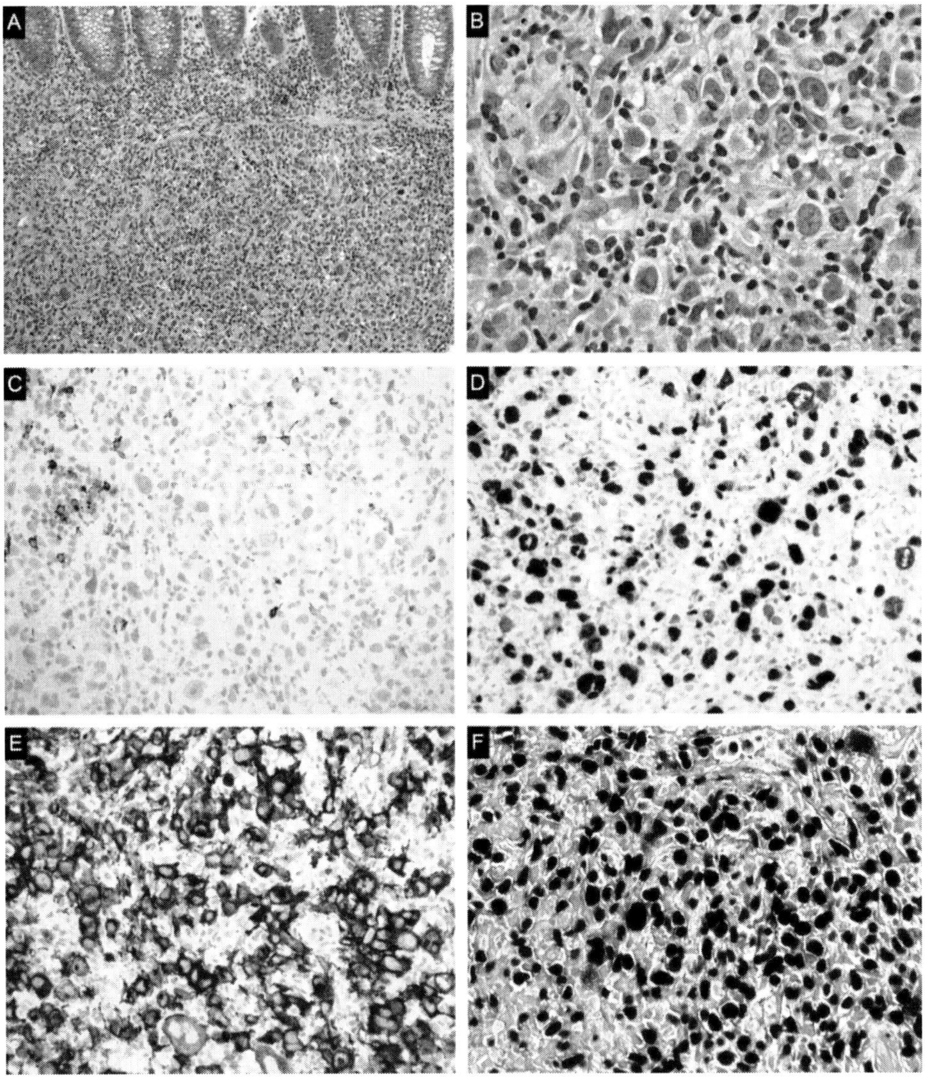

Figure 10. EBV-positive DLBCL of the elderly. Colon mucosa shows extensive lymphoid infiltrate (A, H&E). (B). The lymphoma cells are large and pleomorphic admixed with background small mature lymphocytes and histiocytes. The lymphoma cells are positive for PAX5 (D), CD30 (E), and EBV by EBER (F), and negative for CD20 (C).

The mixed inflammatory background and presence of necrosis are similar in both diseases. The Reed-Sternberg/Hodgkin cells in CHL are usually negative for CD20 and CD79a, and if CD20 is positive, the expression is weak and patchy. There is not much variation in the size of Reed-Sternberg/Hodgkin cells. In contrast, the lymphoma cells of pleomorphic variant of EBV + DLBCL of the elderly are positive for all the B-cell markers and show a spectrum of cell size from small to large pleomorphic cells. The stronger expression of pan B-cell markers and cell size variation are most reliable for this differential diagnosis. Another differential diagnosis is infectious mononucleosis. The infectious mononucleosis shows distorted but not effaced underlying architecture and mixed population of B and T immunoblasts. In addition, infectious mononucleosis shows no clonal *IgH* and *IgK* gene rearrangement.

Clonality analysis shows clonal *IgH* and/or *IgK* gene rearrangements in approximately 64% of cases and clonal T-cell gene rearrangement in 24% of cases [183] *BCL6*, *c-MYC* and *IgH* translocations are present in <20% cases. EBV + DLBCL of the elderly show prominent classical and alternative NF-κB pathway activation in neoplastic cells [183].

Primary Mediastinal (Thymic) Large B-Cell Lymphoma

The primary mediastinal (thymic) large B-cell lymphoma (PMBL) is a large B-cell lymphoma arising from thymus in the mediastinum. This is the few lymphomas for which clinical information is essential for its diagnosis. It accounts for approximately 2-4% of the non-Hodgkin lymphomas and usually occurs in young females with a median age of 35 [1]. The patients usually present with localized anterior superior mediastinal mass, which could be bulky (>10 cm) and aggressive, and frequently causes superior vena cava syndrome. PMBL also frequently invades neighboring structures such as lung, pleura, and pericardium, and could spread to adjacent lymph nodes, such as supraclavicular lymph nodes or cervical lymph nodes. Even though distant spread is infrequent at the outset, PMBL could involve liver, kidney, adrenal, or even central nervous system at the advanced stage. However, involvement of other lymph nodes or bone marrow excludes the diagnosis of PMBL, and is more consistent with systemic diffuse large B-cell lymphoma with mediastinal involvement.

Morphologically, PMBL presents with diffuse infiltrate by large atypical lymphoid cells in a background of characteristic compartmentalizing alveolar fibrosis (Figure 11). Occasional cases show vague nodularity and extensive necrosis. The lymphoma cells are medium to large in size with round or oval nuclei and abundant pale cytoplasm. The number of mitotic figures is generally high. Large pleomorphic or multilobated nuclei could be seen, resembling Reed-Sternberg cells and possibly causing confusion with classical Hodgkin lymphoma (CHL). Immunohistochemical stains will be necessary to confirm the diagnoses. Patients present with features of both PMBL and CHL, should be diagnosed as B-cell lymphoma, unclassifiable, with features intermediate between DLBCL and classical Hodgkin lymphoma, or previously called mediastinal gray zone lymphoma. Composite lymphomas, in which PMBL and cHL coexist in the same specimen, are also possible and have been reported.

Immunophenotypically, PMBL expresses Pan-B cell markers (CD19, CD20, CD22, PAX5, and CD79a), as well as CD23 and IRF4/MUM-1, but characteristically loses the expression of surface or cytoplasmic immunoglobulin. The discordant expression of B cell markers (CD79a positive but sIg negative) is characteristic of PMBL. CD10 is usually negative, and BCL-2 and BCL-6 are variably positive. CD30 is expressed in PMBL in 80% of the cases [185], but is usually weak and heterogeneous as compared with that of CHL. CD15 could occasionally be positive in PMBL. However, the overall morphology and clinically presentation should allow the distinction between these two entities. In addition, PBML are positive for MAL antigen, CD54, CD95, and show co-expression of TRAF1 and nuclear REL.

Conventional metaphase cytogenetics has failed to identify recurrent chromosome abnormalities in PMBL. However, comparative genomic hybridization studies (CGH) have demonstrated gains of chromosome 9p24 (up to 75%), 2p15 (50%), Xp11.4-21 (33%), and Xp24-26 (33%). Candidate genes include *REL*, *BCL11A*, *JAK2*, *PLD1*, and *PLD2*, while constitutively activated pathways include NF-κB pathway and JAK-STAT signaling pathway. Inactivation of *TP53* and *CDKN2A* has been reported [186], but rearrangements of *BCL-2*, *BCL-6*, or *MYC* are rare.

PMBL also shows unique gene expression profile as compared with other diffuse large B cell lymphomas or classical Hodgkin lymphoma even though overlap exists, supporting its existence as a separate entity [185, 187].

Finally, the prognosis of PMBL is reported to be equivalent or superior to conventional DLBCL. It shows good response to intensive chemotherapy. A molecular profile of PMBL has also been reported to be associated with good prognosis, while invasion of adjacent structures or organs is associated with poor prognosis. Some retrospective analyses suggest that it may respond better to third-generation chemotherapy regimens than to CHOP regimen. The addition of rituximab could possibly reduce the difference [188].

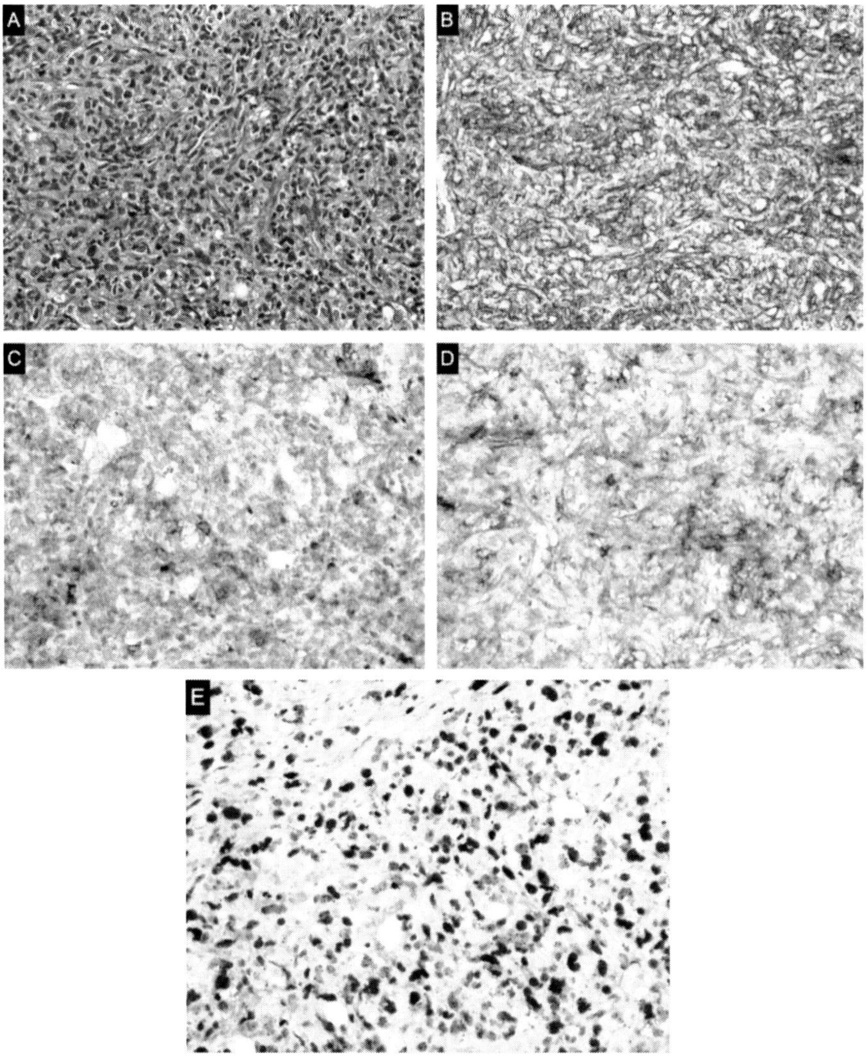

Figure 11. Primary mediastinal (thymic) large B-cell lymphoma. PMBL shows large lymphoma cells with compartmentalizing fibrosis (A, H&E). The lymphoma cells show expression of CD20 (B), partial and weak CD30 (C), partial and weak CD23 (D), and moderately high proliferation rate by Ki-67 (E).

Intravascular Large B-Cell Lymphoma

Intravascular large B-cell lymphoma (IVLBCL) is a rare lymphoma (<1/per million) [189]. It presents with accumulation of large B-cell lymphoma cells selectively in the vascular lumen and not in other locations, presumably due to defect in homing receptors on the lymphoma cells. It occurs in capillary vessels more frequently than in larger arteries or veins. Most of the patients are adults with a median age of 67. It typically involves blood vessels of multiple organs, but involvement of lymph node is rare. The patients commonly present with B symptoms (fever, weight loss, and night sweats). Two forms of symptoms have been described. The patients in Western countries usually present with neurological or cutaneous symptoms, while the patients in Asia, especially Japan, usually present with multi-organ failure, hepatosplenomegaly, pancytopenia, or hemophagocytic syndrome. There have been reports that IVLBCL developed after different lymphoid neoplasm, such as follicular lymphoma or diffuse large B cell lymphoma [190].

Microscopically, intravascular large B-cell lymphoma is characterized by large atypical lymphoid cells confined in the lumen of small or intermediate sized blood vessels (Figure 12), or sinusoids of liver, spleen, or bone marrow. The lymphoma cells might cause fibrin thrombi, and organ hemorrhage or necrosis. Occasionally, the atypical lymphoid cells could be anaplastic. Extravascular presence of lymphoma cells is possible but should be minimal. Peripheral blood involvement is rare.

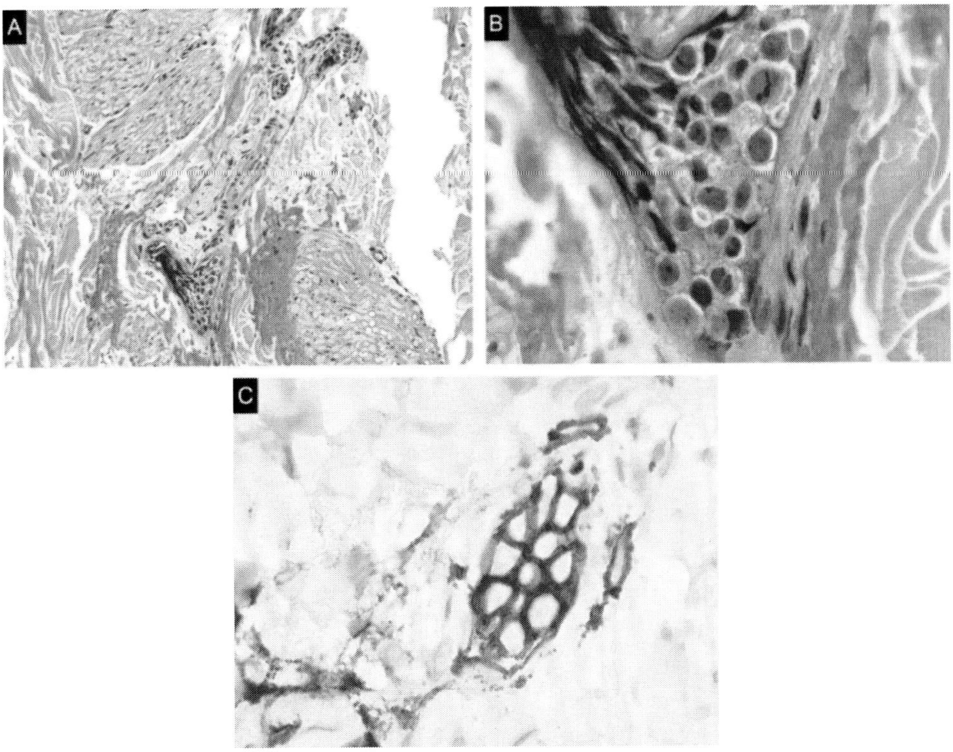

Figure 12. Intravascular large B-cell lymphoma. (A and B). Skin biopsy shows localization of large lymphoma cells within the vascular lumen (H&E). (C). CD20 highlight the large B-cells in vascular space.

The lymphoma cells of IVLBCL are positive for B cells markers (CD19, CD20, and CD79a), as well as MUM-1 and BCL-2. CD5 and CD10 are positive in a small portion of the cases. The lymphoma cells lack surface proteins that are critical to the lymphocyte transvascular migration, including CD29 (β1 integrin) and CD54 (ICAM-1 or CD11a ligand), which contributes to their accumulation within the vascular lumen. There are no specific cytogenetic abnormalities associated with IVLBCL. Cytogenetic alterations reported in other DLBCL can be seen. The most frequent changes include - 6 or 6q -, and + 18, or dup(18q).

Intravascular large B-cell lymphoma is an aggressive and fatal lymphoma with poor response to chemotherapy, and with a mean survival of 13 months [191]. It is usually diagnosed at the advanced or disseminated stage and often at autopsy. Poor predictors include elevated serum lactate dehydrogenase, presence of B symptoms, and thrombocytopenia less than 100 x 10^3/μL. However, limitation of tumor to the skin is associated with better prognosis. In recent years, autologous stem cell transplant and administration of rituximab have been reported to produce positive responses.

Diffuse Large B-Cell Lymphoma Associated with Chronic Inflammation

DLBCL associated with chronic inflammation occurs in patients with long-standing, usually more than 10 years of inflammation. The only significant risk factor is reported to be artificial pneumothorax for pulmonary tuberculosis. Therefore, body cavities, particularly pleural cavity (PAL) of patients with chronic pyothorax, are the most common location for this disease. Chronic osteomyelitis, metallic implant, or chronic skin ulcer, are other conditions associated with the development of diffuse large B-cell lymphoma. The median age of the patients is 65 to 70 years old with a male predominance (male to female ratio of 12.3). In PAL, the tumor is usually a bulky mass and limited to the thoracic cavity, but direct invasion of adjacent structures can be seen. This is in contrast to primary effusion lymphoma, in which no mass is present and only serous effusion is seen. Epstein-Barr virus (EBV) infection is detected in most of the cases [192, 193]. Large B cell lymphoma developed around joints of patients with rheumatoid arthritis is usually EBV negative and should probably not be diagnosed as this lymphoma.

The morphology of DLBCL associated with chronic inflammation is similar to other DLBCL, and more likely to present with centroblasts or immunoblasts with large single or multiple nucleoli. Angiocentric growth and massive necrosis may be present. The lymphoma cells are most likely to be positive for B cells markers, such as CD20 and CD79a. Plasmacytic differentiation and loss of CD20, CD79a, and expression of CD138 and CD30 can be seen. Expression of T cell markers has also been reported. *In-situ* hybridization for EBER (EBV) is typically positive. Cytogenetically, karyotyping is complex and *TP53* mutation is common.

DLBCL associated with chronic inflammation is an aggressive lymphoma with a 5 year survival rate of 20-35% for PAL [194, 195]. Complete tumor resection has been reported to be helpful. Poor prognostic factors include advanced clinical stage, poor performance status, and high serum levels of lactate dehydrogenase.

Lymphomatoid Granulomatosis

Lymphomatoid granulomatosis (LYG) is a rare EBV driven angiocentric and angiodestructive lymphoproliferative disorder. It is usually seen in adults, but can be seen in children with immunodeficiency. Men are affected twice as often as woman [196]. Predisposing conditions include allogeneic organ transplant, human immunodeficiency virus (HIV) infection, Wiskott-Aldrich syndrome, and X-linked lymphoproliferative syndrome. The incidence is higher in Western countries than in Asia. They usually involve extra-nodal sites, especially lungs (90%), kidney (32%), skin (25-50%), and liver (29%). Multiple nodular, usually bilateral, infiltrates in the lungs are seen. Spleen is rarely involved.

LYG most commonly presents with pulmonary nodules with infiltration of Epstein-Barr virus (EBV) positive large B cells admixed with predominant population of reactive T lymphocytes in an angiocentric or angiodestructive pattern. Central necrosis and cavity may be seen. Plasma cells, immunoblasts, and histiocytes are also present. The EBV positive cells are large, and can show immunoblastic morphology, or even multinucleated or pleomorphic morphology resembling Reed-Sternberg/Hodgkin cells. Uniform distribution of large atypical EBV positive lymphoid cells without background of small reactive lymphocytes should be diagnosed as DLBCL instead of LYP. Granulomatous lesions, seen in Wegener granuloma or fungal infections, can be present in skin lesions, and are usually absent in lung or other extra-nodal sites. There is prominent lymphocytic vasculitis, which might cause tissue infarction and necrosis. Notably vasculitis with EBV positive cells can also be seen in extra-nodal NK/T cell lymphoma and should be considered in the differential diagnosis. Inflammatory cells, such as neutrophils, eosinophils, and multinucleated giant cells are generally absent. Posttransplant lymphoproliferative disorder (PTLD) may mimic LYG with EBV-associated lymphoid infiltrate, but differs from LYG in the absence of background T-cell infiltrate. Another mimic of LYP is iatrogenic immunodeficiency-associated lymphoproliferative disorder in patients receiving methotrexate, and age-related EBV positive B-cell lymphoproliferative disorder.

Immunophenotypically, the large lymphoma cells are positive for CD20 and show variable expression of CD30. CD15 is negative, allowing the differentiation from classical Hodgkin lymphoma. The background lymphocytes show more CD4 + T cells than CD8 + T cells.

LYP is graded according to the proportion of EBV positive cells relative to the reactive lymphocytes in the background. In grade 1, large atypical lymphoid cells are absent or rare. Necrosis is focal. EBV positive cells are <5 per high power field. In grade 2, occasional large atypical lymphocytes and clusters are seen. EBV positive cells usually count 5-20, but can be up to 50 per high power field. Necrosis is usually common. Grade 3 shows large clusters of large atypical B lymphoid cells with frequent pleomorphic cells. EBV positive cells are >50 per high power field and may form focal sheets. Extensive necrosis is often present, in which situation in-situ hybridization for EBV might not be reliable due to tumor necrosis. It is especially important to distinguish grade 3 from grade 1 or 2. There is an overlap between grade 2 or 3 of LYP and variants of large B-cell lymphoma. Clonality in grade 1 is inconsistent, and could be due to variation in the number of EBV positive lymphoma cells. However, there is an opinion that the number of EBV positive cells may not consistently correlate with grade, and determining the proportion of large B cells in the infiltrate seems to be a more accurate way to calculate grade [196].

The mortality rate of LYP is high, ranging from 38% to 71%, and most deaths occur within the first two years. Some patients with LYP, including a few with grade 3 LYP, could show spontaneous regression, especially after immunotherapy or after immunodeficiency is corrected. However, grade 3 LYP should be generally treated as diffuse large B-cell lymphoma.

ALK-Positive Large B-Cell Lymphoma

ALK-positive large B-cell lymphoma (ALK + LBCL) is a rare lymphoma of post-germinal center large B cells that are positive for ALK, which is characteristically positive in anaplastic large cell lymphoma, ALK positive. Its incidence is rare (<1% of DLBCL) with a slight preference for male patients (male to female ratio 3:1) and a median age of 36 [197]. ALK + LBCL usually presents as lymphadenopathy, and occasionally as mediastinal mass, or involves other extra-nodal sites, such as nasopharynx, stomach, and duodenum [198].

Morphologically, ALK + LBCL presents with monomorphic large atypical lymphoid cells more often in sinusoidal growth pattern. The large atypical cells mostly show immunoblastic morphology with round pale nuclei, large central located nucleoli, and abundant cytoplasm (Figure 13). Multinucleated giant cells or plasmablastic differentiation can occasionally be seen. ALK + LBCL cells are negative for CD20 and CD79a, and weakly positive or negative for CD45. The B-cell origin of ALK + LBL can be demonstrated by cytoplasmic immunoglobulin expression (usually IgA) with light chain restriction, as well as B-cell gene rearrangement. The lymphoma cells are strongly positive for CD38, CD138 and MUM-1, suggesting plasmacytic differentiation.

Similar to ALK + anaplastic large cell lymphoma, ALK + LBCL are positive for ALK and EMA. However, ALK + LBCL is negative for T cell markers and CD30. Staining for ALK mostly shows strong cytoplasmic pattern (CLTC-ALK fusion protein), and occasionally shows cytoplasmic, nuclear, and nucleolar pattern (NPM-ALK fusion protein). Its weak staining for CD45 and occasional positivity for cytokerain might cause misdiagnosis as carcinoma with limited antibody panel. In the majority of reported cases of ALK + LBCL, monotypic IgA λ is expressed, and EBV was not detected by in-situ hybridization.

Cytogenetically, t(2;17)(p23;q23) associated with *CLTC-ALK* fusion protein is the most frequent abnormality. Less frequently is t(2;5)(p23;35) associated with *NPM-ALK* fusion protein, which is the most common cytogenetic abnormality in ALK + anaplastic T cell lymphoma. A cryptic 3′-*ALK* gene insertion into chromosome 4 has also been reported [199].

ALK + LBCL is usually diagnosed at the late stage and shows poor survival (11 months) in adults [197]. Longer survival has been reported in children [200]. Since CD20 is negative in the majority of ALK + LBCL cases, rituximab is usually not effective.

Plasmablastic Lymphoma

Plasmablastic lymphoma (PBL) is a rare EBV driven B cell lymphoma. It occurs more commonly in the oral cavity of HIV-positive patients or patients with immunodeficiencies, and usually in male adults.

PBL has also been reported in HIV-negative persons, particularly those who have immunosuppression [201]. Rare cases in children with immunodeficiency have also been reported [202].

PBL usually presents as a mass in the oral cavity, and can involve other extra-nodal sites, such as sinonasal cavity, orbit, skin, bone, soft tissue, and gastrointestinal tract. Lymph node involvement is rare, and is more common in HIV negative patients.

Morphologically, PBL shows diffuse infiltrate of large immunonoblast-like cells with prominent central nucleoli and abundant cytoplasm associated with frequent mitotic figures and apoptosis (Figure 14).

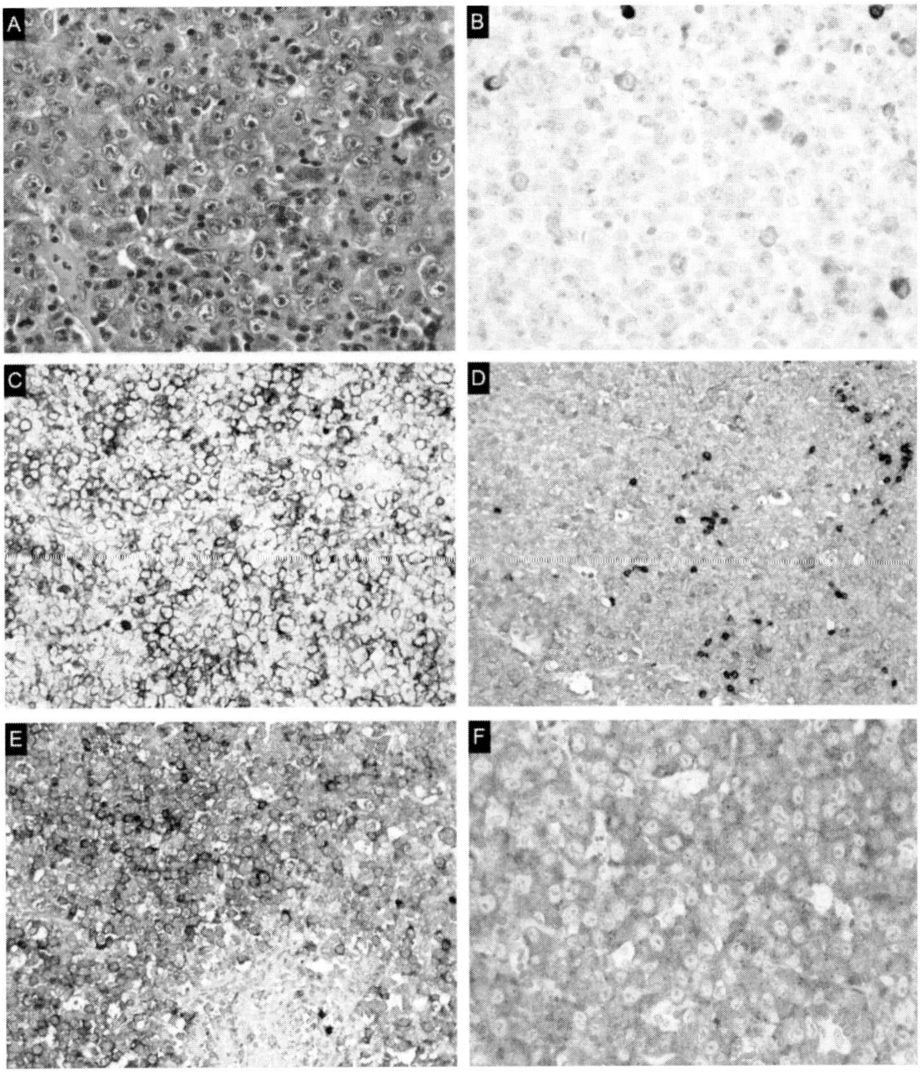

Figure 13. ALK-positive large B-cell lymphoma. The lymph node shows sheets of immunoblasts-like large atypical lymphoid cells (A, H&E). The lymphoma cells are weakly and partially positive for CD79a (B), positive for CD138 (C), ALK with cytoplasmic staining pattern (F), and lambda (E) but not kappa (D) light chain by *in situ* hybridization study.

Prominent plasmablastic cytology is typically seen in the oral cavity lesions of patients with HIV, and needs to be distinguished from plasmablastic plasma cell myeloma. On the other hand, plasmacytic differentiation is more commonly seen in lymph nodes or other exta-nodal sites. Bone marrow involvement has been reported to be 30% in both HIV-positive and HIV-negative patients.

PBL lymphoma cells are positive for CD79a and cytoplasmic immunoglobulin, but negative or only weakly positive for CD20, PAX5, or CD45. They show plasmacytic differentiation with expression of CD38, CD138, and IRF4/MUM1. EMA and CD30 are also commonly positive.

CD56 is usually negative in PBL and is more commonly positive in plasma cell myeloma. EBV EBER is positive in 60-75% of the cases but LMP1 is rarely expressed. Dual infection with EBV and human herpesvirus 8 (HHV8) has been demonstrated in PBL [201]. Recently, BLIMP1 and XBP1, markers of terminal B-cell differentiation, have been reported to be of value in the diagnosis of PBL [203].

MYC gene rearrangement is the most common recurrent cytogenetic abnormality reported in PBL [73], occurring in approximately 50% of the cases. The most common partner for the *MYC* oncogene is the immunoglobulin gene with translocations most often occurring in the context of complex karyotypes. *MYC* rearrangement is more often seen in EBV-positive than in EBV-negative patients.

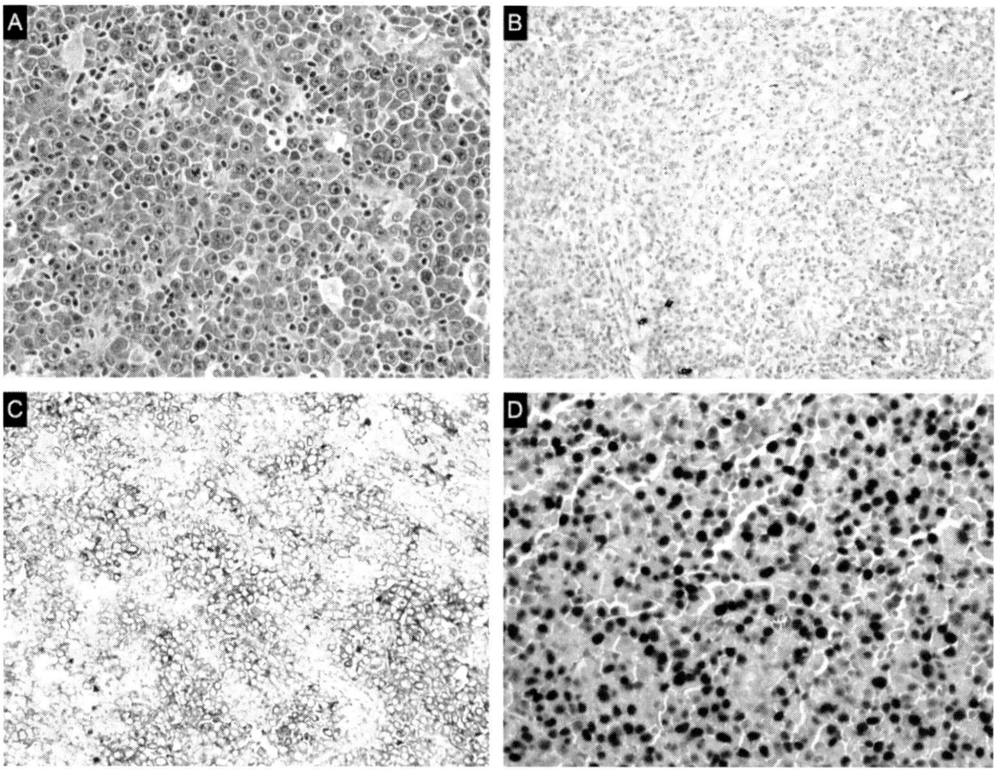

Figure 14. Plasmablastic lymphoma. There are sheets of plasmablasts with prominent central nucleoli (A, H&E). The lymphoma cells are positive for CD138 (C), and EBV by EBER (D), and negative for CD20 (B).

PBL is diagnosed mostly at an advanced stage and shows poor prognosis, with most patients dying in the first year of diagnosis [204]. Due to the lack of CD20 expression, the use of the anti-CD20 monoclonal antibody rituximab is unlikely to be of benefit. Potential value of the proteasome inhibitor bortezomib and thalidomide has been reported [205]. Chimeric antigen receptors (CARs) and CAR-modified T cells targeted to the B cell-specific CD19 antigen have also demonstrated promising results in early clinical trials.

Diffuse Large B-Cell Lymphoma with *IG/IRF4* Translocation

A subset of DLBCL is characterized genetically by recurrent translocations juxtaposing the *IRF4* oncogene to one of the immunoglobulin (IG) loci [206]. The translocations are cytogenetically cryptic, and can only be detected by FISH studies. DLBCL with *IG/IRF4* translocation occurs predominantly in children with a median age of 12 years (range, 4-79 years) and a slight male predominance. There is a preferential involvement in the head and neck region, including Waldeyer's ring and low stage of disease. Patients with *IG/IRF4* translocation have a better prognosis.

Morphologically, there is diffuse infiltrate by large atypical lymphoid cells. The lymphoma cells are positive for pan B-cell markers and strongly positive for MUM1 and BCL6. CD10 and BCL2 are expressed in the majority of cases (approximately 60%). PRDM1/BLIMP1 is negative. CD5 is expressed in a minority of cases (30%), and the expressions of CD5 and CD10 are mutually exclusive. Ki-67 shows overall high proliferation rate. Some lymphomas with IG/IRF4 translocation present histologically as grade 3 follicular lymphoma.

t(14;18)(q32;q21) is absent, while *BCL6* break is common. The gene expression profile of DLBCL with *IG/IRF4* translocation is different from GCB- or ABC-like subtypes. A classifier based on 27 genes can predict the presence of *IG/IRF4* with high accuracy.

Large B-Cell Lymphoma Arising in HHV8-Associated Multicentric Castleman Disease

Large B-cell lymphoma arising in HHV8-associated multicentric Castleman disease is proliferation of HHV8-positive plasmablasts arising in the setting of multicentric Castleman disease. It occurs almost exclusively in HIV-positive adults [207]. The most common sites of involvement are lymph nodes and spleen, but leukemic form can be rarely seen [207, 208]. Patients usually present with marked immunodeficiency, lymphadenopathy and splenomegaly, and often complicated by Kaposi sarcoma. It is a highly aggressive lymphoma with poor response to chemotherapy and a short time of survival.

Morphologically, there are sheets of plasmablasts with round vesicular nuclei, one or two prominent nucleoli and moderate amphophilic cytoplasm. Mitotic figures are usually abundant. The underlying architecture is effaced in the advanced stage. The early stage is the so called "microlymphoma" as microscopic clusters of plasmablasts in a background of HHV8 + multicentric Castleman disease. The plasmablasts are positive for HHV8 antigen LANA-1 (nuclear staining), viral interleukin-6, and strongly positive for cytoplasmic IgM with lambda light chain restriction. The plasmablasts show variable expression of B-cell and plasma cell markers: CD20 –/+, CD79a +, CD138 +/–, CD38 +/–. They are CD30 negative and consistently negative for EBV by EBER. Ki-67 shows extremely high proliferation rate by Ki-67 (approaching 100%).

The main differential diagnosis is KSHV- and EBV-associated germinotropic lymphoproliferative disorder [209], which is a rare indolent disease with favorable response to therapy. KSHV- and EBV-associated germinotropic lymphoproliferative disorder shows partial nodal effacement with clusters or sheets of plasmablasts largely confined to the germinal centers, and the plasmablasts are negative for B-and plasma cell markers (CD20, CD19, CD22, CD79a, CD10, BCL2, BCL6, CD30 and CD138), and positive for both HHV8 and EBV by EBER. These plasmablasts are positive for cytoplasmic IgM and polyclonal for kappa and lambda light chains. In contrast, large B-cell lymphoma arising in HHV8-associated multicentric Castleman disease is negative for EBV and shows lambda light chain restriction.

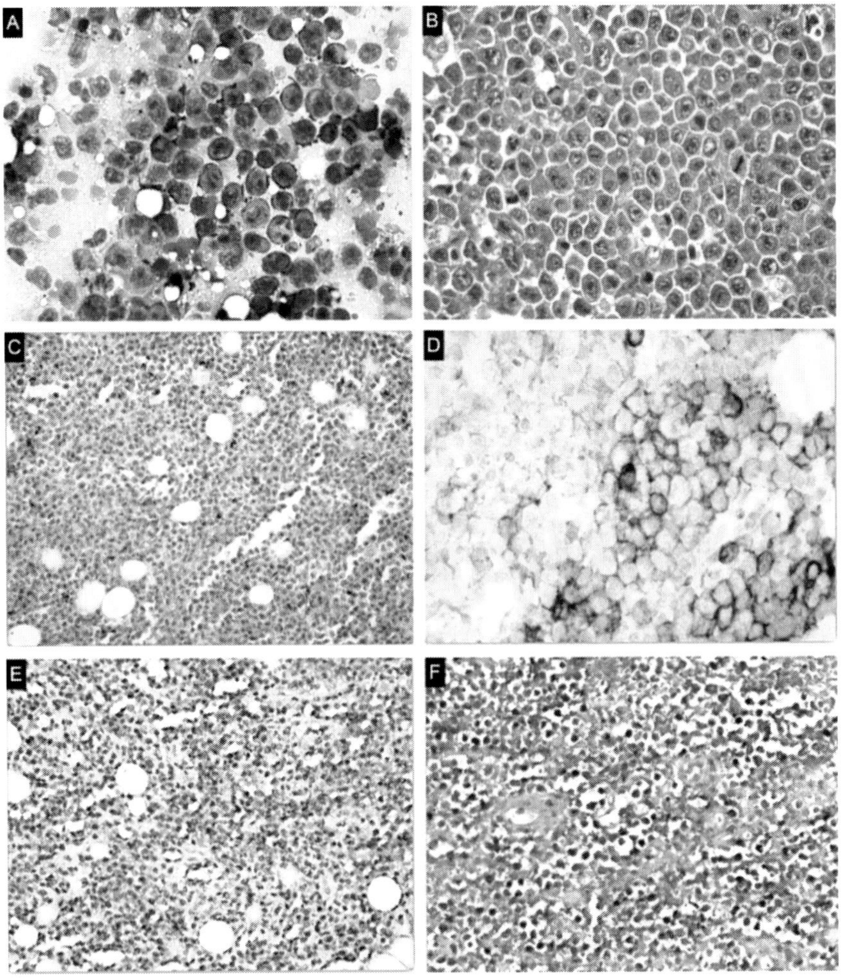

Figure 15. Primary effusion lymphoma. (A), Pleural effusion shows large lymphoma cells with prominent nucleoli and deeply basophilic cytoplasm. (B), Tissue mass shows sheets of large lymphoma cells with immunoblastic morphology and some with plasmacytoid appearance. The lymphoma cells are positive for CD138 (D), HHV8 (E), and EBV by EBER (F), and negative for CD20 (C).

Primary Effusion Lymphoma

Primary effusion lymphoma (PEL) is a rare Non-Hodgkin lymphoma that is associated with HIV-1 and Kaposi Sarcoma Herpes Virus (KSHV)/Human Herpesvirus 8 (HHV8). HIV-1 negative and HHV8 positive PEL has been rarely reported. Co-infection with Epstein-Barr virus (EBV) also occurs. PEL represents only a minor subset (1-4%) of all HIV related NHL with a male predominance (male to female ratio of approximately 15:1) [210, 211]. This could be attributed to the prevalence of male patients diagnosed with HIV/acquired immunodeficiency syndromes (AIDS). A minority of PEL have also been reported in patients that are immunocompromised without HIV infection, such as post solid organ transplantation [212-214] or chronic hepatitis C virus infection [215, 216]. Clinically, PEL is characterized by a unique presentation of serous effusions without detectable tumor masses.

It has a predilection for body cavities, such as pleural, pericardial, or peritoneal cavities. Typically only one body cavity is involved. Solid tumor variant of PEL, namely extracavitary PEL, has also been observed, but is even less common. In some occasions, solid tumor can develop adjacent to a cavity. Lymphadenopathy and organomegaly are usually absent. Approximately half of the patients have pre-existing or subsequent Kaposi sarcoma [211], while some patients have multicentric Castleman disease [217].

Morphologically, PEL exhibits mostly immunoblastic, plasmablastic, or anaplastic morphology with round large nuclei, prominent nucleoli, and abundant basophilic cytoplasm with occasional cytoplasmic vacuoles (Figure 15). Immunophenotypically, PEL lymphoma cells are positive for CD45, but usually lack the expression of B cell markers (CD19, CD20, CD79a, and surface immunoglobulin). They show plasmacytic differentiation (positive for CD138 and MUM-1), and express some activation markers (CD30, CD38, CD71, EMA). The neoplastic cells are positive for HHV8 with nuclear stain of HHV8-associated latent protein LANA [218]. HHV8 must be demonstrated to diagnose PEL. HHV8 viremia is suggestive of PEL, but should not be used solely to diagnose PEL. In-situ hybridization for EBER (EBV) is usually positive, but EBV LMP1 is frequently negative. Solid variants were reported to express B-cell markers more often than the classic form in effusions [219]. No recurrent cytogenetic abnormalities have been identified for PEL. B cell gene rearrangement is positive, while T cell gene rearrangement has also been reported.

PEL should be distinguished from other lymphomas associated with HHV8 or EBV. One differential diagnosis for PEL is pyothorax-associated lymphoma (PAL), which is a rare subtype of body cavity lymphoma after a long standing pyothorax resulting from an artificial pneumothorax following treatment for tuberculosis or tuberculous pleurisy [220, 221]. Similar to PEL, PAL is of B-cell origin, EBV-positive, and shows immunoblastic morphology. All PAL cases express B-cell markers, but it is not associated with HHV8 [222]. Another differential diagnosis is plasmablastic lymphoma, a rare variant of diffuse large B-cell lymphoma that could present with similar morphology and immunophenotype as PEL. It usually occurs in the oral cavities of HIV positive patients. Most of the cases will be positive for CD79a, EBV, but negative for HHV8. Plasmablastic variants of plasma cell myeloma can also show similar morphology and immunophenotypes as PEL, but are often positive for CD56, CD79a, cyclin D1, and negative for HHV8. The other differentials by morphology include primary pleural effusion post-transplant lymphoproliferative disorder, ALK + large B-cell lymphoma, and anaplastic large cell lymphoma, all of which are not associated with HHV8.

PEL has an aggressive clinical course with a median overall survival of less than 6 months and poor response to chemotherapy. Most patients die within 1 year of diagnosis. Treatment with bortezomib-containing regimes has been reported to improve survival [223]. An antiviral combination of interferon-α and azidothymidine has shown dramatic response in a patient [224].

B-Cell Lymphoma, Unclassifiable, with Features Intermediate between DLBCL and Classical Hodgkin Lymphoma

B-cell lymphoma, unclassifiable, with features intermediate between DLBCL and classical Hodgkin lymphoma, also known as mediastinal gray zone lymphoma (GZL), shows histological, biological and clinical overlap between primary mediastinal large B-cell lymphoma (PMBL) and nodular sclerosis classical Hodgkin lymphoma (NS-CHL). PMBL and NS-CHL share some clinical, morphologic and genetic features. Both present with anterior mediastinal masses involving the thymus and with a female preference. Reed-Sternberg-like cells may be seen in PMBL [225]. CD30 is positive in both except a small percentage of PMBLs. Both PBML and CHL show similar cytogenetic abnormalities including gains at 2p15 (*REL* locus) and 9p24 (*JAK2* locus) and breaks at CIITA in subset of cases [226-228].

Gene expression profiling studies show similarities between PMBL and CHL with activation of the NF-κB, JAK-STAT and P13K/AKT pathways, downregulation of BCR signaling pathway, overexpression of TNF family proteins and extracellular matrix [187, 229-232]. The gene expression signature of PMBL is different from the GCB-like and ABC-like DLBCL [187]. As lymphoma cells of PMBL and CHL are both believed to derive from thymic B-cells [233], it is evident that PMBL and CHL are histogenetically related. GZL has features intermediate between PMBL and CHL-NS but does not fit into either classification.

Clinically, GZL predominantly affects young patients with median age of 31 years and a male predominance [234]. Patients most commonly present with a large anterior mediastinal mass, and may have superior vena cava syndrome. The masses may spread into adjacent structures such as the lungs and chest wall by direct extension.

Occasional cases may have peripheral lymph nodes as primary site of involvement. GZL is more aggressive with poorer clinical outcome than both CHL and PMBCL [234, 235].

Morphologically, GZL typically shows sheet-like confluent infiltrate by pleomorphic lymphoma cells in a diffusely fibrotic stroma (Figure 16).

The lymphoma cells may resemble lacunar cells and Hodgkin cells or PMBL cells, and there is usually wide spectrum of cytological features in different areas of the specimen. A few mixed inflammatory cells such as eosinophils, neutrophils, lymphocytes, and histiocytes may be present. Phenotypically, the lymphoma cells show preservation of the B-cell program with expression of the transcription factors PAX5, OCT-2, BOB.1 and PU.1, as well as strong CD20 and CD79a.

In addition, the lymphoma cells show expression of CHL markers CD30 and CD15. They are positive for CD45 and negative for surface immunoglobulin expression. MAL, a marker for PMBL, is also present in the majority of cases of GZL. In cases resembling CHL but with increased RS/Hodgkin-like cells, the strong expression of CD20 and other pan B-cell markers is consistent with GZL.

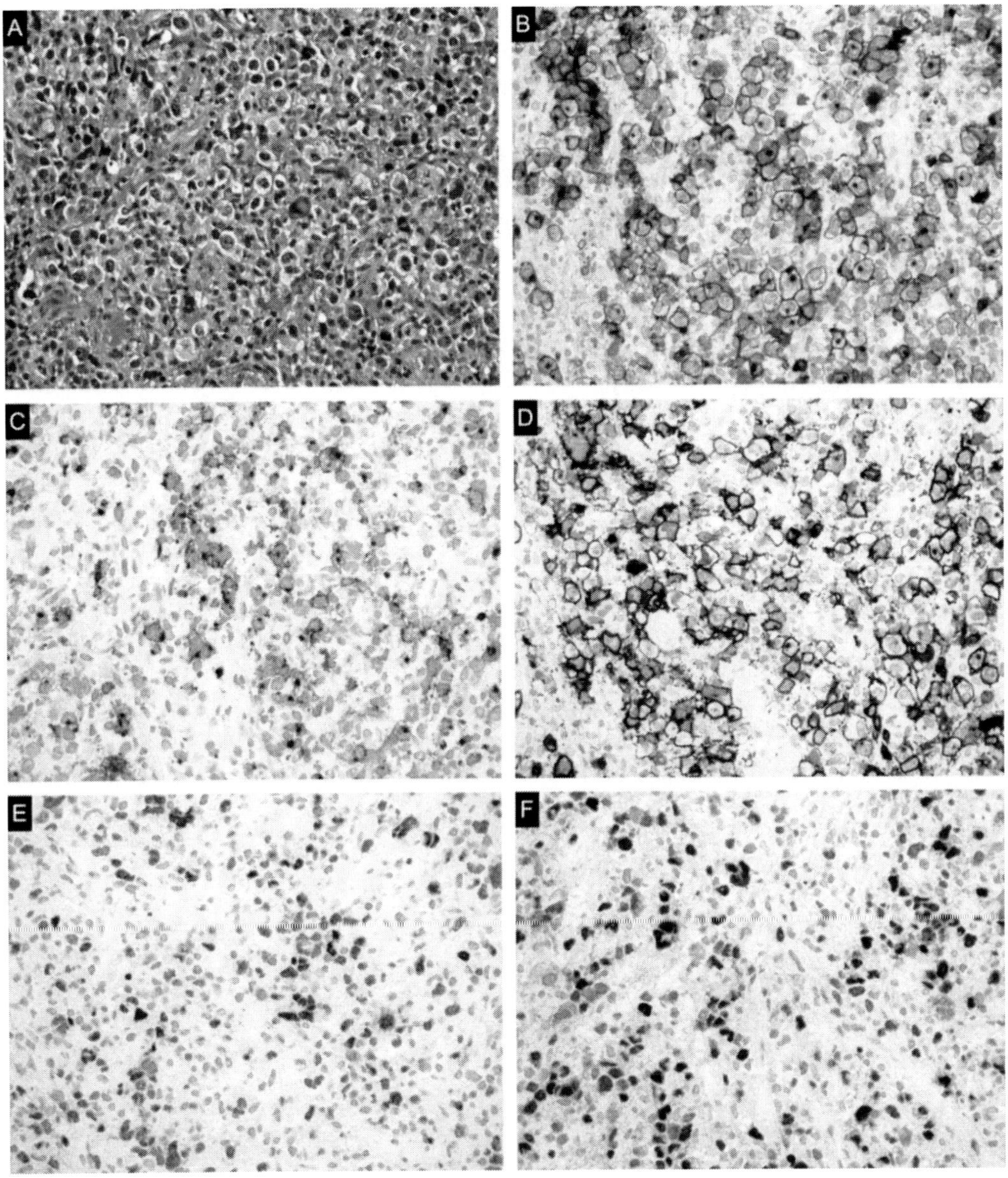

Figure 16. Mediastinal gray zone lymphoma. There are clusters of large lymphoid cells with moderate to abundant pale cytoplasm. (A, H&E). The lymphoma cells are positive for CD30 (B), CD15 (C), strong CD20 (D), strong PAX5 (E), and OCT2 (F).

In cases resembling PMBL, the expression of CD30 and CD15 in lymphoma cells will fit the diagnosis of GZL. EBER is negative.

A large-scale DNA methylation analysis has demonstrated distinct epigenetic profile intermediate between CHL and PMBL and different from that of DLBCL [236]. Class prediction models with genes like *HOXA5*, *MMP9*, *EPHA7* and *DAPK1* are able to reliably distinguish between GZL, CHL and PML. The distinct methylation pattern from both CHL and PMBL confirms that the GZL is a biologically distinct entity.

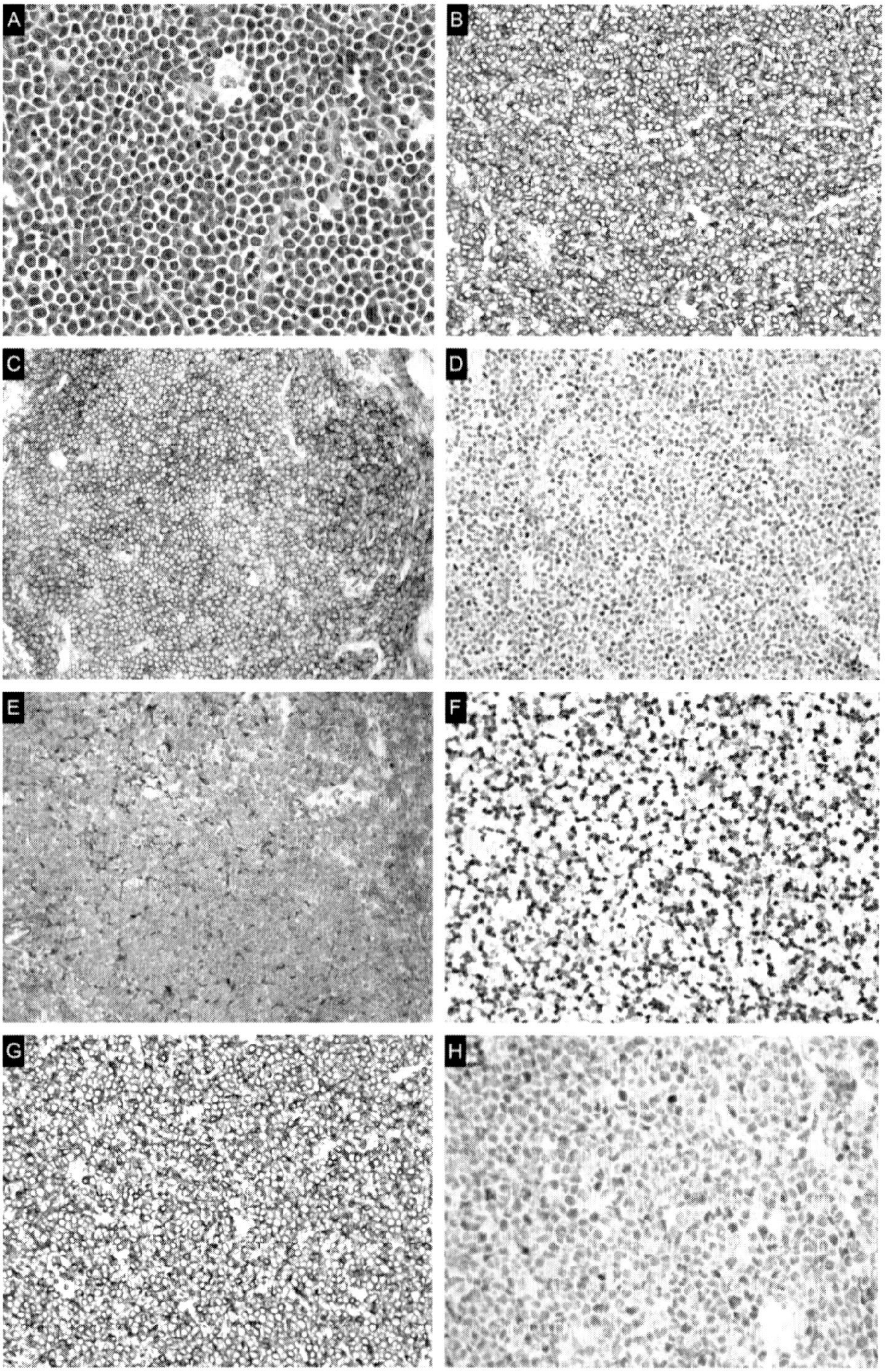

Figure 17. Double hit lymphoma. There are sheets of medium sized lymphoid cells with round nuclei, fine chromatin and scant cytoplasm admixed with scattered tingible body macrophages (A, H&E). The lymphoma cells are positive for CD79a (B), CD10 (C), BCL6 (D), BCL2 (G) and MYC (H), and negative for MUM1 (E). Ki-67 shows moderate to high proliferation rate with approximately 60% positive cells.

B-Cell Lymphoma, Unclassifiable, with Features Intermediate between DLBCL and Burkitt Lymphoma

It is clinically important to distinguish between DLBCL and Burkitt lymphoma (BL) due to different regimens of chemotherapy. A subset of aggressive B-cell lymphoma cannot be classified into either DLBCL or BL, but rather shows overlapping morphologic and phenotypic features of both, and therefore is designated as B-cell lymphoma, unclassifiable, with features intermediate between DLBCL and BL (BCLU) by the 2008 WHO classification [1]. BCLU occurs mainly in adults, and in lymph nodes or extranodal sites. Bone marrow and peripheral blood may be involved. BCLU is clinically highly aggressive with high stage of disease and resistant to current chemotherapy [237].

Morphologically, there is diffuse proliferation of medium to large atypical lymphoid cells with few background small mature lymphocytes. Starry sky pattern with scattered tingible body macrophages is usually present. Mitotic figures and apoptotic bodies are abundant.

Rare cases show small lymphoid cells with fine chromatin resembling lymphoblastic lymphoma. Cases with cells resembling BL cells but with marked variable cell sizes and nuclear irregularity are classified as BCLU. Phenotypically, the lymphoma cells are positive for pan B-cell markers, CD19, CD20, CD79, and PAX5, and with surface immunoglobulin light chain restriction. The proliferation rate by Ki-67 is variable, but usually high [238, 239]. Cases otherwise typical of BL with expression of germinal center markers CD10 and BCL6, negative MUM1, but with strong BCL2 expression are classified as BCLU, and many of these cases are the so-called "double hit" lymphoma (Figure 17). These cases typically show diffuse and strong expression MYC protein by immunohistochemical stain. However, MYC immunostain is nonspecific and should not be used to diagnose BCLU *per se*. Occasional cases of DLBCL have extremely high proliferation rate by Ki-67, but should not be classified as BCLU.

MYC translocation is the most frequent cytogenetic abnormality, occurring in approximately 35-50% cases [237, 240]. In contrast to BL, *MYC* in BCLU is typically rearranged to a non-*IG* partner gene, or in the context of complex karyotype. Many have concurrent rearrangement of *BCL2* and/or *BCL6* along *MYC* rearrangement, and these cases are termed "double hit" lymphomas. The double hit lymphomas are typically of GCB-like immunophenotype with expression of CD10 and BCL6, negative MUM1 and strong expression of BCL2. Some of the double hit lymphoma represents transformation from low grade follicular lymphoma with acquisition of *MYC* translocation during clonal evolution. Gene expression profiling studies show genetic signature of BCLU similar to that of FL [241] or intermediate between DLBCL and BL [60].

References

[1] Swerdlow, S. H., Campo, E., Harris, N. L., Jaffe, E. S., Pileri, S. A., Stein, H. 2008; *WHO classification of tumours of haematopoietic and lymphoid tissues*. IARC, Lyon.

[2] Lennert, K., Feller, A. C. 1990; *High Grade Malignant Lymphoma of B-Cell Type. Histopathology of Non-Hodgkin's Lymphoma*. 2nd ed.; Springer-Verlag Berlin.

[3] 1982. "National Cancer Institute sponsored study of classifications of non-Hodgkin's lymphomas: summary and description of a working formulation for clinical usage. The Non-Hodgkin's Lymphoma Pathologic Classification Project." *Cancer* 49:2112-2135.

[4] Harris, N. L., Jaffe, E. S., Stein, H., Banks, P. M., Chan, J. K., Cleary, M. L., Delsol, G. et al. 1994. "A revised European-American classification of lymphoid neoplasms: a proposal from the International Lymphoma Study Group." *Blood* 84:1361-1392.

[5] Gatter, K. C., Warnke, R. A. 2001; *Diffuse large B-cell lymphoma. Jaffe ES Harris NL Stein H Vardiman JW Pathology and Genetics: Tumours of Haematopoietic and Lymphoid Tissues. World Health Organization Classification of Tumours.* IARC, Lyon.

[6] 1997. "A clinical evaluation of the International Lymphoma Study Group classification of non-Hodgkin's lymphoma. The Non-Hodgkin's Lymphoma Classification Project." *Blood* 89:3909-3918.

[7] Armitage, J. O., Weisenburger, D. D. 1998. "New approach to classifying non-Hodgkin's lymphomas: clinical features of the major histologic subtypes. Non-Hodgkin's Lymphoma Classification Project." *J. Clin. Oncol.* 16:2780-2795.

[8] Hutchison, R. E., Berard, C. W., Shuster, J. J., Link, M. P., Pick, T. E., Murphy, S. B. 1995. "B-cell lineage confers a favorable outcome among children and adolescents with large-cell lymphoma: a Pediatric Oncology Group study." *J. Clin. Oncol.* 13:2023-2032.

[9] Mora, J., Filippa, D. A., Thaler, H. T., Polyak, T., Cranor, M. L., Wollner, N. 2000. "Large cell non-Hodgkin lymphoma of childhood: Analysis of 78 consecutive patients enrolled in 2 consecutive protocols at the Memorial Sloan-Kettering Cancer Center." *Cancer* 88:186-197.

[10] Campbell, J., Seymour, J. F., Matthews, J., Wolf, M., Stone, J., Juneja, S. 2006. "The prognostic impact of bone marrow involvement in patients with diffuse large cell lymphoma varies according to the degree of infiltration and presence of discordant marrow involvement." *Eur. J. Haematol.* 76:473-480.

[11] Chung, R., Lai, R., Wei, P., Lee, J., Hanson, J., Belch, A. R., Turner, A. R., Reiman, T. 2007. "Concordant but not discordant bone marrow involvement in diffuse large B-cell lymphoma predicts a poor clinical outcome independent of the International Prognostic Index." *Blood* 110:1278-1282.

[12] Arber, D. A., George, T. I. 2005. "Bone marrow biopsy involvement by non-Hodgkin's lymphoma: frequency of lymphoma types, patterns, blood involvement, and discordance with other sites in 450 specimens." *Am. J. Surg. Pathol.* 29:1549-1557.

[13] Casey, T. T., Cousar, J. B., Mangum, M., Williams, M. E., Lee, J. T., Greer, J. P., Collins, R. D. 1990. "Monomorphic lymphomas arising in patients with Hodgkin's disease. Correlation of morphologic, immunophenotypic, and molecular genetic findings in 12 cases." *Am. J. Pathol.* 136:81-94.

[14] Kamel, O. W. 1997. "Iatrogenic lymphoproliferative disorders in nontransplantation settings." *Semin. Diagn. Pathol.* 14:27-34.

[15] Abruzzo, L. V., Rosales, C. M., Medeiros, L. J., Vega, F., Luthra, R., Manning, J. T., Keating, M. J., Jones, D. 2002. "Epstein-Barr virus-positive B-cell lymphoproliferative disorders arising in immunodeficient patients previously treated with fludarabine for low-grade B-cell neoplasms." *Am. J. Surg. Pathol.* 26:630-636.

[16] Oyama, T., Ichimura, K., Suzuki, R., Suzumiya, J., Ohshima, K., Yatabe, Y., Yokoi, T. et al. 2003. "Senile EBV + B-cell lymphoproliferative disorders: a clinicopathologic study of 22 patients." *Am. J. Surg. Pathol.* 27:16-26.

[17] Attygalle, A. D., Kyriakou, C., Dupuis, J., Grogg, K. L., Diss, T. C., Wotherspoon, A. C., Chuang, S. S. et al. 2007. "Histologic evolution of angioimmunoblastic T-cell lymphoma in consecutive biopsies: clinical correlation and insights into natural history and disease progression." *Am. J. Surg. Pathol.* 31:1077-1088.

[18] Johnson, L. R., Nalesnik, M. A., Swerdlow, S. H. 2006. "Impact of Epstein-Barr virus in monomorphic B-cell posttransplant lymphoproliferative disorders: a histogenetic study." *Am. J. Surg. Pathol.* 30:1604-1612.

[19] Noy, A. 2007. "Update on HIV lymphoma." *Curr. Oncol. Rep.* 9:384-390.

[20] Chan, J. K. C., Aozasa, K., Gaulard, P. 2001; *DLBCL associated with chronic inflammation. Jaffe ES Harris NL Stein H Vardiman JW Pathology and Genetics: Tumours of Haematopoietic and Lymphoid Tissues. World Health Organization Classification of Tumours.* IARC, Lyon.

[21] Maurer, R., Schmid, U., Davies, J. D., Mahy, N. J., Stansfeld, A. G., Lukes, R. J. 1986. "Lymph-node infarction and malignant lymphoma: a multicentre survey of European, English and American cases." *Histopathology* 10:571-588.

[22] Strauchen, J. A., Miller, L. K. 2003. "Lymph node infarction. An immunohistochemical study of 11 cases." *Arch. Pathol. Lab. Med.* 127:60-63.

[23] Cleary, K. R., Osborne, B. M., Butler, J. J. 1982. "Lymph node infarction foreshadowing malignant lymphoma." *Am. J. Surg. Pathol.* 6:435-442.

[24] Yamauchi, A., Ikeda, J., Nakamichi, I., Kohara, M., Fukuhara, S., Hino, M., Kanakura, Y. et al. 2008. "Diffuse large B-cell lymphoma showing an interfollicular pattern of proliferation: a study of the Osaka Lymphoma Study Group." *Histopathology* 52:731-737.

[25] Miller, J. B., Variakojis, D., Bitran, J. D., Sweet, D. L., Kinzie, J. J., Golomb, H. M., Ultmann, J. E. 1981. "Diffuse histiocytic lymphoma with sclerosis: a clinicopathologic entity frequently causing superior venacaval obstruction." *Cancer* 47:748-756.

[26] Pileri, S. A., Zinzani, P. L., Ascani, S., Orcioni, G. F., Gamberi, B., Piccioli, M., Sabattini, E. et al. 2001. "Diffuse large B-cell lymphoma with primary retroperitoneal presentation: clinico-pathologic study of nine cases." *Ann. Oncol.* 12:1445-1453.

[27] Chuang, S. S., Ye, H., Du, M. Q., Lu, C. L., Dogan, A., Hsieh, P. P., Huang, W. T., Jung, Y. C. 2007. "Histopathology and immunohistochemistry in distinguishing Burkitt lymphoma from diffuse large B-cell lymphoma with very high proliferation index and with or without a starry-sky pattern: a comparative study with EBER and FISH." *Am. J. Clin. Pathol.* 128:558-564.

[28] Kanagal-Shamanna, R., Medeiros, L. J., Lu, G., Wang, S. A., Manning, J. T., Lin, P., Penn, G. M. et al. 2012. "High-grade B cell lymphoma, unclassifiable, with blastoid features: an unusual morphological subgroup associated frequently with BCL2 and/or MYC gene rearrangements and a poor prognosis." *Histopathology* 61:945-954.

[29] Kennedy, G. A., Tey, S. K., Cobcroft, R., Marlton, P., Cull, G., Grimmett, K., Thomson, D., Gill, D. 2002. "Incidence and nature of CD20-negative relapses following rituximab therapy in aggressive B-cell non-Hodgkin's lymphoma: a retrospective review." *Br. J. Haematol.* 119:412-416.

[30] Li, S., Eshleman, J. R., Borowitz, M. J. 2002. "Lack of surface immunoglobulin light chain expression by flow cytometric immunophenotyping can help diagnose peripheral B-cell lymphoma." *Am. J. Clin. Pathol.* 118:229-234.

[31] Wang, J., Chen, C., Lau, S., Raghavan, R. I., Rowsell, E. H., Said, J., Weiss, L. M., Huang, Q. 2009. "CD3-positive large B-cell lymphoma." *Am. J. Surg. Pathol.* 33:505-512.

[32] Suzuki, Y., Yoshida, T., Wang, G., Aoki, T., Katayama, T., Miyamoto, S., Miyazaki, K. et al. 2013. "Incidence and clinical significance of aberrant T-cell marker expression on diffuse large B-cell lymphoma cells." *Acta Haematol.* 130:230-237.

[33] Yamaguchi, M., Seto, M., Okamoto, M., Ichinohasama, R., Nakamura, N., Yoshino, T., Suzumiya, J. et al. 2002. "De novo CD5 + diffuse large B-cell lymphoma: a clinicopathologic study of 109 patients." *Blood* 99:815-821.

[34] Dogan, A., Bagdi, E., Munson, P., Isaacson, P. G. 2000. "CD10 and BCL-6 expression in paraffin sections of normal lymphoid tissue and B-cell lymphomas." *Am. J. Surg. Pathol.* 24:846-852.

[35] Uherova, P., Ross, C. W., Schnitzer, B., Singleton, T. P., Finn, W. G. 2001. "The clinical significance of CD10 antigen expression in diffuse large B-cell lymphoma." *Am. J. Clin. Pathol.* 115:582-588.

[36] King, B. E., Chen, C., Locker, J., Kant, J., Okuyama, K., Falini, B., Swerdlow, S. H. 2000. "Immunophenotypic and genotypic markers of follicular center cell neoplasia in diffuse large B-cell lymphomas." *Mod. Pathol.* 13:1219-1231.

[37] Fang, J. M., Finn, W. G., Hussong, J. W., Goolsby, C. L., Cubbon, A. R., Variakojis, D. 1999. "CD10 antigen expression correlates with the t(14;18)(q32;q21) major breakpoint region in diffuse large B-cell lymphoma." *Mod. Pathol.* 12:295-300.

[38] Huang, J. Z., Sanger, W. G., Greiner, T. C., Staudt, L. M., Weisenburger, D. D., Pickering, D. L., Lynch, J. C. et al. 2002. "The t(14;18) defines a unique subset of diffuse large B-cell lymphoma with a germinal center B-cell gene expression profile." *Blood* 99:2285-2290.

[39] Barrans, S. L., O'Connor, S. J., Evans, P. A., Davies, F. E., Owen, R. G., Haynes, A. P., Morgan, G. J., Jack, A. S. 2002. "Rearrangement of the BCL6 locus at 3q27 is an independent poor prognostic factor in nodal diffuse large B-cell lymphoma." *Br. J. Haematol.* 117:322-332.

[40] Onizuka, T., Moriyama, M., Yamochi, T., Kuroda, T., Kazama, A., Kanazawa, N., Sato, K. et al. 1995. "BCL-6 gene product, a 92- to 98-kD nuclear phosphoprotein, is highly expressed in germinal center B cells and their neoplastic counterparts." *Blood* 86:28-37.

[41] Ree, H. J., Yang, W. I., Kim, C. W., Huh, J., Lee, S. S., Cho, E. Y., Ko, Y. H., Charney, D. 2001. "Coexpression of Bcl-6 and CD10 in diffuse large B-cell lymphomas: significance of Bcl-6 expression patterns in identifying germinal center B-cell lymphoma." *Hum. Pathol.* 32:954-962.

[42] Barrans, S. L., Carter, I., Owen, R. G., Davies, F. E., Patmore, R. D., Haynes, A. P., Morgan, G. J., Jack, A. S. 2002. "Germinal center phenotype and bcl-2 expression combined with the International Prognostic Index improves patient risk stratification in diffuse large B-cell lymphoma." *Blood* 99:1136-1143.

[43] Hill, M. E., MacLennan, K. A., Cunningham, D. C., Vaughan Hudson, B., Burke, M., Clarke, P., Di Stefano, F. et al. 1996. "Prognostic significance of BCL-2 expression and

bcl-2 major breakpoint region rearrangement in diffuse large cell non-Hodgkin's lymphoma: a British National Lymphoma Investigation Study." *Blood* 88:1046-1051.

[44] Rantanen, S., Monni, O., Joensuu, H., Franssila, K., Knuutila, S. 2001. "Causes and consequences of BCL2 overexpression in diffuse large B-cell lymphoma." *Leuk. Lymphoma* 42:1089-1098.

[45] Falini, B., Fizzotti, M., Pucciarini, A., Bigerna, B., Marafioti, T., Gambacorta, M., Pacini, R. et al. 2000. "A monoclonal antibody (MUM1p) detects expression of the MUM1/IRF4 protein in a subset of germinal center B cells, plasma cells, and activated T cells." *Blood* 95:2084-2092.

[46] Hu, S., Xu-Monette, Z. Y., Balasubramanyam, A., Manyam, G. C., Visco, C., Tzankov, A., Liu, W. M. et al. 2013. "CD30 expression defines a novel subgroup of diffuse large B-cell lymphoma with favorable prognosis and distinct gene expression signature: a report from the International DLBCL Rituximab-CHOP Consortium Program Study." *Blood* 121:2715-2724.

[47] Gerdes, J., Dallenbach, F., Lennert, K., Lemke, H., Stein, H. 1984. "Growth fractions in malignant non-Hodgkin's lymphomas (NHL) as determined *in situ* with the monoclonal antibody Ki-67." *Hematol. Oncol.* 2:365-371.

[48] Weiss, L. M., Strickler, J. G., Medeiros, L. J., Gerdes, J., Stein, H., Warnke, R. A. 1987. "Proliferative rates of non-Hodgkin's lymphomas as assessed by Ki-67 antibody." *Hum. Pathol.* 18:1155-1159.

[49] Hall, P. A., Richards, M. A., Gregory, W. M., d'Ardenne, A. J., Lister, T. A., Stansfeld, A. G. 1988. "The prognostic value of Ki67 immunostaining in non-Hodgkin's lymphoma." *J. Pathol.* 154:223-235.

[50] Miller, T. P., Grogan, T. M., Dahlberg, S., Spier, C. M., Braziel, R. M., Banks, P. M., Foucar, K. et al. 1994. "Prognostic significance of the Ki-67-associated proliferative antigen in aggressive non-Hodgkin's lymphomas: a prospective Southwest Oncology Group trial." *Blood* 83:1460-1466.

[51] Horn, H., Ziepert, M., Becher, C., Barth, T. F., Bernd, H. W., Feller, A. C., Klapper, W. et al. 2013. "MYC status in concert with BCL2 and BCL6 expression predicts outcome in diffuse large B-cell lymphoma." *Blood* 121:2253-2263.

[52] Ok, C. Y., Papathomas, T. G., Medeiros, L. J., Young, K. H. 2013. "EBV-positive diffuse large B-cell lymphoma of the elderly." *Blood* 122:328-340.

[53] Segal, G. H., Kjeldsberg, C. R., Smith, G. P., Perkins, S. L. 1994. "CD30 antigen expression in florid immunoblastic proliferations. A clinicopathologic study of 14 cases." *Am. J. Clin. Pathol.* 102:292-298.

[54] Childs, C. C., Parham, D. M., Berard, C. W. 1987. "Infectious mononucleosis. The spectrum of morphologic changes simulating lymphoma in lymph nodes and tonsils." *Am. J. Surg. Pathol.* 11:122-132.

[55] Strickler, J. G., Fedeli, F., Horwitz, C. A., Copenhaver, C. M., Frizzera, G. 1993. "Infectious mononucleosis in lymphoid tissue. Histopathology, *in situ* hybridization, and differential diagnosis." *Arch. Pathol. Lab. Med.* 117:269-278.

[56] Bosch, X., Guilabert, A., Miquel, R., Campo, E. 2004. "Enigmatic Kikuchi-Fujimoto disease: a comprehensive review." *Am. J. Clin. Pathol.* 122:141-152.

[57] Plumbley, J. A., Fan, H., Eagan, P. A., Ehsan, A., Schnitzer, B., Gulley, M. L. 2002. "Lymphoid tissues from patients with infectious mononucleosis lack monoclonal B and T cells." *J. Mol. Diagn.* 4:37-43.

[58] Hsiao, S. C., Cortada, I. R., Colomo, L., Ye, H., Liu, H., Kuo, S. Y., Lin, S. H. et al. 2012. "SOX11 is useful in differentiating cyclin D1-positive diffuse large B-cell lymphoma from mantle cell lymphoma." *Histopathology* 61:685-693.

[59] Akasaka, T., Akasaka, H., Ueda, C., Yonetani, N., Maesako, Y., Shimizu, A., Yamabe, H. et al. 2000. "Molecular and clinical features of non-Burkitt's, diffuse large-cell lymphoma of B-cell type associated with the c-MYC/immunoglobulin heavy-chain fusion gene." *J. Clin. Oncol.* 18:510-518.

[60] Hummel, M., Bentink, S., Berger, H., Klapper, W., Wessendorf, S., Barth, T. F., Bernd, H. W. et al. 2006. "A biologic definition of Burkitt's lymphoma from transcriptional and genomic profiling." *N. Engl. J. Med.* 354:2419-2430.

[61] Lossos, I. S., Okada, C. Y., Tibshirani, R., Warnke, R., Vose, J. M., Greiner, T. C., Levy, R. 2000. "Molecular analysis of immunoglobulin genes in diffuse large B-cell lymphomas." *Blood* 95:1797-1803.

[62] Gascoyne, R. D. 1997. "Pathologic prognostic factors in diffuse aggressive non-Hodgkin's lymphoma." *Hematol. Oncol. Clin. North Am.* 11:847-862.

[63] Lo Coco, F., Ye, B. H., Lista, F., Corradini, P., Offit, K., Knowles, D. M., Chaganti, R. S., Dalla-Favera, R. 1994. "Rearrangements of the BCL6 gene in diffuse large cell non-Hodgkin's lymphoma." *Blood* 83:1757-1759.

[64] Otsuki, T., Yano, T., Clark, H. M., Bastard, C., Kerckaert, J. P., Jaffe, E. S., Raffeld, M. 1995. "Analysis of LAZ3 (BCL-6) status in B-cell non-Hodgkin's lymphomas: results of rearrangement and gene expression studies and a mutational analysis of coding region sequences." *Blood* 85:2877-2884.

[65] Migliazza, A., Martinotti, S., Chen, W., Fusco, C., Ye, B. H., Knowles, D. M., Offit, K., Chaganti, R. S., Dalla-Favera, R. 1995. "Frequent somatic hypermutation of the 5' noncoding region of the BCL6 gene in B-cell lymphoma." *Proc. Natl. Acad. Sci. US* 92: 12520-12524.

[66] Capello, D., Vitolo, U., Pasqualucci, L., Quattrone, S., Migliaretti, G., Fassone, L., Ariatti, C. et al. 2000. "Distribution and pattern of BCL-6 mutations throughout the spectrum of B-cell neoplasia." *Blood* 95:651-659.

[67] Ye, B. H., Cattoretti, G., Shen, Q., Zhang, J., Hawe, N., de Waard, R., Leung, C. et al. 1997. "The BCL-6 proto-oncogene controls germinal-centre formation and Th2-type inflammation." *Nat. Genet.* 16:161-170.

[68] Ladanyi, M., Offit, K., Jhanwar, S. C., Filippa, D. A., Chaganti, R. S. 1991. "MYC rearrangement and translocations involving band 8q24 in diffuse large cell lymphomas." *Blood* 77:1057-1063.

[69] Kramer, M. H., Hermans, J., Wijburg, E., Philippo, K., Geelen, E., van Krieken, J. H., de Jong, D. et al. 1998. "Clinical relevance of BCL2, BCL6, and MYC rearrangements in diffuse large B-cell lymphoma." *Blood* 92:3152-3162.

[70] Vitolo, U., Gaidano, G., Botto, B., Volpe, G., Audisio, E., Bertini, M., Calvi, R. et al. 1998. "Rearrangements of bcl-6, bcl-2, c-myc and 6q deletion in B-diffuse large-cell lymphoma: clinical relevance in 71 patients." *Ann. Oncol.* 9:55-61.

[71] Kawasaki, C., Ohshim, K., Suzumiya, J., Kanda, M., Tsuchiya, T., Tamura, K., Kikuchi, M. 2001. "Rearrangements of bcl-1, bcl-2, bcl-6, and c-myc in diffuse large B-cell lymphomas." *Leuk. Lymphoma* 42:1099-1106.

[72] Cigudosa, J. C., Parsa, N. Z., Louie, D. C., Filippa, D. A., Jhanwar, S. C., Johansson, B., Mitelman, F., Chaganti, R. S. 1999. "Cytogenetic analysis of 363 consecutively ascertained diffuse large B-cell lymphomas." *Genes Chromosomes Cancer* 25:123-133.

[73] Valera, A., Balague, O., Colomo, L., Martinez, A., Delabie, J., Taddesse-Heath, L., Jaffe, E. S., Campo, E. 2010. "IG/MYC rearrangements are the main cytogenetic alteration in plasmablastic lymphomas." *Am. J. Surg. Pathol.* 34:1686-1694.

[74] Horn, H., Staiger, A. M., Vohringer, M., Hay, U., Campo, E., Rosenwald, A., Ott, G., Ott, M. M. 2015. "Diffuse large B-cell lymphomas of immunoblastic type are a major reservoir for MYC-IGH translocations." *Am. J. Surg. Pathol.* 39:61-66.

[75] Nanjangud, G., Rao, P. H., Hegde, A., Teruya-Feldstein, J., Donnelly, G., Qin, J., Jhanwar, S. C., Zelenetz, A. D., Chaganti, R. S. 2002. "Spectral karyotyping identifies new rearrangements, translocations, and clinical associations in diffuse large B-cell lymphoma." *Blood* 99:2554-2561.

[76] Monni, O., Joensuu, H., Franssila, K., Knuutila, S. 1996. "DNA copy number changes in diffuse large B-cell lymphoma--comparative genomic hybridization study." *Blood* 87:5269-5278.

[77] Rao, P. H., Houldsworth, J., Dyomina, K., Parsa, N. Z., Cigudosa, J. C., Louie, D. C., Popplewell, L. et al. 1998. "Chromosomal and gene amplification in diffuse large B-cell lymphoma." *Blood* 92:234-240.

[78] Scandurra, M., Mian, M., Greiner, T. C., Rancoita, P. M., De Campos, C. P., Chan, W. C., Vose, J. M. et al. 2010. "Genomic lesions associated with a different clinical outcome in diffuse large B-Cell lymphoma treated with R-CHOP-21." *Br. J. Haematol.* 151:221-231.

[79] Alizadeh, A. A., Eisen, M. B., Davis, R. E., Ma, C., Lossos, I. S., Rosenwald, A., Boldrick, J. C. et al. 2000. "Distinct types of diffuse large B-cell lymphoma identified by gene expression profiling." *Nature* 403:503-511.

[80] Bea, S., Zettl, A., Wright, G., Salaverria, I., Jehn, P., Moreno, V., Burek, C. et al. 2005. "Diffuse large B-cell lymphoma subgroups have distinct genetic profiles that influence tumor biology and improve gene-expression-based survival prediction." *Blood* 106: 3183-3190.

[81] Tagawa, H., Suguro, M., Tsuzuki, S., Matsuo, K., Karnan, S., Ohshima, K., Okamoto, M. et al. 2005. "Comparison of genome profiles for identification of distinct subgroups of diffuse large B-cell lymphoma." *Blood* 106:1770-1777.

[82] Visco, C., Tzankov, A., Xu-Monette, Z. Y., Miranda, R. N., Tai, Y. C., Li, Y., Liu, W. M. et al. 2013. "Patients with diffuse large B-cell lymphoma of germinal center origin with BCL2 translocations have poor outcome, irrespective of MYC status: a report from an International DLBCL rituximab-CHOP Consortium Program Study." *Haematologica* 98:255-263.

[83] Rosenwald, A., Wright, G., Chan, W. C., Connors, J. M., Campo, E., Fisher, R. I., Gascoyne, R. D. et al. 2002. "The use of molecular profiling to predict survival after chemotherapy for diffuse large-B-cell lymphoma." *N. Engl. J. Med.* 346:1937-1947.

[84] Lossos, I. S., Alizadeh, A. A., Eisen, M. B., Chan, W. C., Brown, P. O., Botstein, D., Staudt, L. M., Levy, R. 2000. "Ongoing immunoglobulin somatic mutation in germinal center B cell-like but not in activated B cell-like diffuse large cell lymphomas." *Proc. Natl. Acad. Sci. US* 97:10209-10213.

[85] Yoon, S. O., Jeon, Y. K., Paik, J. H., Kim, W. Y., Kim, Y. A., Kim, J. E., Kim, C. W. 2008. "MYC translocation and an increased copy number predict poor prognosis in adult diffuse large B-cell lymphoma (DLBCL), especially in germinal centre-like B cell (GCB) type." *Histopathology* 53:205-217.
[86] Ichikawa, A., Kinoshita, T., Watanabe, T., Kato, H., Nagai, H., Tsushita, K., Saito, H., Hotta, T. 1997. "Mutations of the p53 gene as a prognostic factor in aggressive B-cell lymphoma." *N. Engl. J. Med.* 337:529-534.
[87] Xu-Monette, Z. Y., Medeiros, L. J., Li, Y., Orlowski, R. Z., Andreeff, M., Bueso-Ramos, C. E., Greiner, T. C., McDonnell, T. J., Young, K. H. 2012. "Dysfunction of the TP53 tumor suppressor gene in lymphoid malignancies." *Blood* 119:3668-3683.
[88] Pasqualucci, L., Neumeister, P., Goossens, T., Nanjangud, G., Chaganti, R. S., Kuppers, R., Dalla-Favera, R. 2001. "Hypermutation of multiple proto-oncogenes in B-cell diffuse large-cell lymphomas." *Nature* 412:341-346.
[89] Pasqualucci, L., Trifonov, V., Fabbri, G., Ma, J., Rossi, D., Chiarenza, A., Wells, V. A. et al. 2011. "Analysis of the coding genome of diffuse large B-cell lymphoma." *Nat. Genet.* 43:830-837.
[90] Morin, R. D., Mendez-Lago, M., Mungall, A. J., Goya, R., Mungall, K. L., Corbett, R. D., Johnson, N. A. et al. 2011. "Frequent mutation of histone-modifying genes in non-Hodgkin lymphoma." *Nature* 476:298-303.
[91] Lam, L. T., Wright, G., Davis, R. E., Lenz, G., Farinha, P., Dang, L., Chan, J. W. et al. 2008. "Cooperative signaling through the signal transducer and activator of transcription 3 and nuclear factor-{kappa}B pathways in subtypes of diffuse large B-cell lymphoma." *Blood* 111: 3701-3713.
[92] Trifonov, V., Pasqualucci, L., Dalla Favera, R., Rabadan, R. 2013. "MutComFocal: an integrative approach to identifying recurrent and focal genomic alterations in tumor samples." *BMC Syst. Biol.* 7:25.
[93] Maeshima, A. M., Omatsu, M., Nomoto, J., Maruyama, D., Kim, S. W., Watanabe, T., Kobayashi, Y., Tobinai, K., Matsuno, Y. 2008. "Diffuse large B-cell lymphoma after transformation from low-grade follicular lymphoma: morphological, immunohistochemical, and FISH analyses." *Cancer Sci.* 99:1760-1768.
[94] Di Lisio, L., Martinez, N., Montes-Moreno, S., Piris-Villaespesa, M., Sanchez-Beato, M., Piris, M. A. 2012. "The role of miRNAs in the pathogenesis and diagnosis of B-cell lymphomas." *Blood* 120:1782-1790.
[95] Sonoki, T., Harder, L., Horsman, D. E., Karran, L., Taniguchi, I., Willis, T. G., Gesk, S. et al. 2001. "Cyclin D3 is a target gene of t(6;14) (p21.1;q32.3) of mature B-cell malignancies." *Blood* 98:2837-2844.
[96] 1993. "A predictive model for aggressive non-Hodgkin's lymphoma. The International Non-Hodgkin's Lymphoma Prognostic Factors Project." *N. Engl. J. Med.* 329:987-994.
[97] Ziepert, M., Hasenclever, D., Kuhnt, E., Glass, B., Schmitz, N., Pfreundschuh, M., Loeffler, M. 2010. "Standard International prognostic index remains a valid predictor of outcome for patients with aggressive CD20 + B-cell lymphoma in the rituximab era." *J. Clin. Oncol.* 28:2373-2380.
[98] Sehn, L. H., Berry, B., Chhanabhai, M., Fitzgerald, C., Gill, K., Hoskins, P., Klasa, R. et al. 2007. "The revised International Prognostic Index (R-IPI) is a better predictor of outcome than the standard IPI for patients with diffuse large B-cell lymphoma treated with R-CHOP." *Blood* 109:1857-1861.

[99] Zhou, Z., Sehn, L. H., Rademaker, A. W., Gordon, L. I., Lacasce, A. S., Crosby-Thompson, A., Vanderplas, A. et al. 2014. "An enhanced International Prognostic Index (NCCN-IPI) for patients with diffuse large B-cell lymphoma treated in the rituximab era." *Blood* 123:837-842.

[100] Nakamine, H., Bagin, R. G., Vose, J. M., Bast, M. A., Bierman, P. J., Armitage, J. O., Weisenburger, D. D. 1993. "Prognostic significance of clinical and pathologic features in diffuse large B-cell lymphoma." *Cancer* 71:3130-3137.

[101] Salar, A., Fernandez de Sevilla, A., Romagosa, V., Domingo-Claros, A., Gonzalez-Barca, E., Pera, J., Climent, J., Granena, A. 1998. "Diffuse large B-cell lymphoma: is morphologic subdivision useful in clinical management?" *Eur. J. Haematol.* 60:202-208.

[102] Kwak, L. W., Wilson, M., Weiss, L. M., Horning, S. J., Warnke, R. A., Dorfman, R. F. 1991. "Clinical significance of morphologic subdivision in diffuse large cell lymphoma." *Cancer* 68:1988-1993.

[103] Fisher, D. E., Jacobson, J. O., Ault, K. A., Harris, N. L. 1989. "Diffuse large cell lymphoma with discordant bone marrow histology. Clinical features and biological implications." *Cancer* 64:1879-1887.

[104] Conlan, M. G., Bast, M., Armitage, J. O., Weisenburger, D. D. 1990. "Bone marrow involvement by non-Hodgkin's lymphoma: the clinical significance of morphologic discordance between the lymph node and bone marrow. Nebraska Lymphoma Study Group." *J. Clin. Oncol.* 8:1163-1172.

[105] Hodges, G. F., Lenhardt, T. M., Cotelingam, J. D. 1994. "Bone marrow involvement in large-cell lymphoma. Prognostic implications of discordant disease." *Am. J. Clin. Pathol.* 101:305-311.

[106] Zhang, A., Ohshima, K., Sato, K., Kanda, M., Suzumiya, J., Shimazaki, K., Kawasaki, C., Kikuchi, M. 1999. "Prognostic clinicopathologic factors, including immunologic expression in diffuse large B-cell lymphomas." *Pathol. Int.* 49:1043-1052.

[107] Leroy, K., Haioun, C., Lepage, E., Le Metayer, N., Berger, F., Labouyrie, E., Meignin, V. et al. 2002. "p53 gene mutations are associated with poor survival in low and low-intermediate risk diffuse large B-cell lymphomas." *Ann. Oncol.* 13:1108-1115.

[108] Saez, A., Sanchez, E., Sanchez-Beato, M., Cruz, M. A., Chacon, I., Munoz, E., Camacho, F. I. et al. 1999. "p27KIP1 is abnormally expressed in Diffuse Large B-cell Lymphomas and is associated with an adverse clinical outcome." *Br. J. Cancer* 80: 1427-1434.

[109] Grogan, T. M., Lippman, S. M., Spier, C. M., Slymen, D. J., Rybski, J. A., Rangel, C. S., Richter, L. C., Miller, T. P. 1988. "Independent prognostic significance of a nuclear proliferation antigen in diffuse large cell lymphomas as determined by the monoclonal antibody Ki-67." *Blood* 71:1157-1160.

[110] Hans, C. P., Weisenburger, D. D., Greiner, T. C., Gascoyne, R. D., Delabie, J., Ott, G., Muller-Hermelink, H. K. et al. 2004. "Confirmation of the molecular classification of diffuse large B-cell lymphoma by immunohistochemistry using a tissue microarray." *Blood* 103:275-282.

[111] Chang, C. C., McClintock, S., Cleveland, R. P., Trzpuc, T., Vesole, D. H., Logan, B., Kajdacsy-Balla, A., Perkins, S. L. 2004. "Immunohistochemical expression patterns of germinal center and activation B-cell markers correlate with prognosis in diffuse large B-cell lymphoma." *Am. J. Surg. Pathol.* 28:464-470.

[112] Sohn, S. K., Jung, J. T., Kim, D. H., Kim, J. G., Kwak, E. K., Park, Ti, Shin, D. G., Sohn, K. R., Lee, K. B. 2003. "Prognostic significance of bcl-2, bax, and p53 expression in diffuse large B-cell lymphoma." *Am. J. Hematol.* 73:101-107.

[113] Maartense, E., Kramer, M. H., le Cessie, S., Kluin-Nelemans, J. C., Kluin, P. M., Snijder, S., Noordijk, E. M. 2004. "Lack of prognostic significance of BCL2 and p53 protein overexpression in elderly patients with diffuse large B-cell non-Hodgkin's lymphoma: results from a population-based non-Hodgkin's lymphoma registry." *Leuk. Lymphoma* 45:101-107.

[114] Kramer, M. H., Hermans, J., Parker, J., Krol, A. D., Kluin-Nelemans, J. C., Haak, H. L., van Groningen, K. et al. 1996. "Clinical significance of bcl2 and p53 protein expression in diffuse large B-cell lymphoma: a population-based study." *J. Clin. Oncol.* 14:2131-2138.

[115] Seki, R., Okamura, T., Koga, H., Yakushiji, K., Hashiguchi, M., Yoshimoto, K., Ogata, H. et al. 2003. "Prognostic significance of the F-box protein Skp2 expression in diffuse large B-cell lymphoma." *Am. J. Hematol.* 73:230-235.

[116] Jerkeman, M., Anderson, H., Dictor, M., Kvaloy, S., Akerman, M., Cavallin-Stahl, E., Nordic Lymphoma Group, study. 2004. "Assessment of biological prognostic factors provides clinically relevant information in patients with diffuse large B-cell lymphoma--a Nordic Lymphoma Group study." *Ann. Hematol.* 83:414-419.

[117] Saez, A. I., Saez, A. J., Artiga, M. J., Perez-Rosado, A., Camacho, F. I., Diez, A., Garcia, J. F. et al. 2004. "Building an outcome predictor model for diffuse large B-cell lymphoma." *Am. J. Pathol.* 164:613-622.

[118] Colomo, L., Lopez-Guillermo, A., Perales, M., Rives, S., Martinez, A., Bosch, F., Colomer, D. et al. 2003. "Clinical impact of the differentiation profile assessed by immunophenotyping in patients with diffuse large B-cell lymphoma." *Blood* 101:78-84.

[119] Bauer, K. D., Merkel, D. E., Winter, J. N., Marder, R. J., Hauck, W. W., Wallemark, C. B., Williams, T. J., Variakojis, D. 1986. "Prognostic implications of ploidy and proliferative activity in diffuse large cell lymphomas." *Cancer Res.* 46:3173-3178.

[120] Katzenberger, T., Lohr, A., Schwarz, S., Dreyling, M., Schoof, J., Nickenig, C., Stilgenbauer, S. et al. 2003. "Genetic analysis of de novo CD5 + diffuse large B-cell lymphomas suggests an origin from a somatically mutated CD5 + progenitor B cell." *Blood* 101:699-702.

[121] Berglund, M., Thunberg, U., Amini, R. M., Book, M., Roos, G., Erlanson, M., Linderoth, J. et al. 2005. "Evaluation of immunophenotype in diffuse large B-cell lymphoma and its impact on prognosis." *Mod. Pathol.* 18:1113-1120.

[122] Filipits, M., Jaeger, U., Pohl, G., Stranzl, T., Simonitsch, I., Kaider, A., Skrabs, C., Pirker, R. 2002. "Cyclin D3 is a predictive and prognostic factor in diffuse large B-cell lymphoma." *Clin. Cancer Res.* 8:729-733.

[123] Lossos, I. S., Czerwinski, D. K., Alizadeh, A. A., Wechser, M. A., Tibshirani, R., Botstein, D., Levy, R. 2004. "Prediction of survival in diffuse large-B-cell lymphoma based on the expression of six genes." *N. Engl. J. Med.* 350:1828-1837.

[124] Hans, C. P., Weisenburger, D. D., Greiner, T. C., Chan, W. C., Aoun, P., Cochran, G. T., Pan, Z. et al. 2005. "Expression of PKC-beta or cyclin D2 predicts for inferior survival in diffuse large B-cell lymphoma." *Mod. Pathol.* 18:1377-1384.

[125] Adida, C., Haioun, C., Gaulard, P., Lepage, E., Morel, P., Briere, J., Dombret, H. et al. 2000. "Prognostic significance of survivin expression in diffuse large B-cell lymphomas." *Blood* 96:1921-1925.
[126] Watanuki-Miyauchi, R., Kojima, Y., Tsurumi, H., Hara, T., Goto, N., Kasahara, S., Saio, M., Moriwaki, H., Takami, T. 2005. "Expression of survivin and of antigen detected by a novel monoclonal antibody, T332, is associated with outcome of diffuse large B-cell lymphoma and its subtypes." *Pathol. Int.* 55:324-330.
[127] Sanchez-Aguilera, A., Sanchez-Beato, M., Garcia, J. F., Prieto, I., Pollan, M., Piris, M. A. 2002. "p14(ARF) nuclear overexpression in aggressive B-cell lymphomas is a sensor of malfunction of the common tumor suppressor pathways." *Blood* 99:1411-1418.
[128] Lossos, I. S., Jones, C. D., Warnke, R., Natkunam, Y., Kaizer, H., Zehnder, J. L., Tibshirani, R., Levy, R. 2001. "Expression of a single gene, BCL-6, strongly predicts survival in patients with diffuse large B-cell lymphoma." *Blood* 98:945-951.
[129] Lossos, I. S., Alizadeh, A. A., Rajapaksa, R., Tibshirani, R., Levy, R. 2003. "HGAL is a novel interleukin-4-inducible gene that strongly predicts survival in diffuse large B-cell lymphoma." *Blood* 101:433-440.
[130] Ohshima, K., Kawasaki, C., Muta, H., Muta, K., Deyev, V., Haraoka, S., Suzumiya, J., Podack, E. R., Kikuchi, M. 2001. "CD10 and Bcl10 expression in diffuse large B-cell lymphoma: CD10 is a marker of improved prognosis." *Histopathology* 39:156-162.
[131] Fabiani, B., Delmer, A., Lepage, E., Guettier, C., Petrella, T., Briere, J., Penny, A. M. et al. 2004. "CD10 expression in diffuse large B-cell lymphomas does not influence survival." *Virchows Arch.* 445:545-551.
[132] Barrans, S. L., Fenton, J. A., Banham, A., Owen, R. G., Jack, A. S. 2004. "Strong expression of FOXP1 identifies a distinct subset of diffuse large B-cell lymphoma (DLBCL) patients with poor outcome." *Blood* 104:2933-2935.
[133] Hermine, O., Haioun, C., Lepage, E., d'Agay, M. F., Briere, J., Lavignac, C., Fillet, G. et al. 1996. "Prognostic significance of bcl-2 protein expression in aggressive non-Hodgkin's lymphoma. Groupe d'Etude des Lymphomes de l'Adulte (GELA)." *Blood* 87:265-272.
[134] Gascoyne, R. D., Adomat, S. A., Krajewski, S., Krajewska, M., Horsman, D. E., Tolcher, A. W., O'Reilly, S. E. et al. 1997. "Prognostic significance of Bcl-2 protein expression and Bcl-2 gene rearrangement in diffuse aggressive non-Hodgkin's lymphoma." *Blood* 90:244-251.
[135] Mounier, N., Briere, J., Gisselbrecht, C., Emile, J. F., Lederlin, P., Sebban, C., Berger, F. et al. 2003. "Rituximab plus CHOP (R-CHOP) overcomes bcl-2--associated resistance to chemotherapy in elderly patients with diffuse large B-cell lymphoma (DLBCL)." *Blood* 101:4279-4284.
[136] Bono, P., Teerenhovi, L., Joensuu, H. 2003. "Elevated serum endostatin is associated with poor outcome in patients with non-Hodgkin lymphoma." *Cancer* 97:2767-2775.
[137] Salven, P., Orpana, A., Teerenhovi, L., Joensuu, H. 2000. "Simultaneous elevation in the serum concentrations of the angiogenic growth factors VEGF and bFGF is an independent predictor of poor prognosis in non-Hodgkin lymphoma: a single-institution study of 200 patients." *Blood* 96:3712-3718.
[138] Sakata, K., Satoh, M., Someya, M., Asanuma, H., Nagakura, H., Oouchi, A., Nakata, K. et al. 2004. "Expression of matrix metalloproteinase 9 is a prognostic factor in patients with non-Hodgkin lymphoma." *Cancer* 100:356-365.

[139] Lenz, G., Wright, G., Dave, S. S., Xiao, W., Powell, J., Zhao, H., Xu, W. et al. 2008. "Stromal gene signatures in large-B-cell lymphomas." *N. Engl. J. Med.* 359:2313-2323.

[140] Alizadeh, A. A., Gentles, A. J., Alencar, A. J., Liu, C. L., Kohrt, H. E., Houot, R., Goldstein, M. J. et al. 2011. "Prediction of survival in diffuse large B-cell lymphoma based on the expression of 2 genes reflecting tumor and microenvironment." *Blood* 118:1350-1358.

[141] Benesova, K., Forsterova, K., Votavova, H., Campr, V., Stritesky, J., Velenska, Z., Prochazka, B., Pytlik, R., Trneny, M. 2013. "The Hans algorithm failed to predict outcome in patients with diffuse large B-cell lymphoma treated with rituximab." *Neoplasma* 60:68-73.

[142] Visco, C., Li, Y., Xu-Monette, Z. Y., Miranda, R. N., Green, T. M., Li, Y., Tzankov, A. et al. 2012. "Comprehensive gene expression profiling and immunohistochemical studies support application of immunophenotypic algorithm for molecular subtype classification in diffuse large B-cell lymphoma: a report from the International DLBCL Rituximab-CHOP Consortium Program Study." *Leukemia* 26:2103-2113.

[143] Hu, S., Xu-Monette, Z. Y., Tzankov, A., Green, T., Wu, L., Balasubramanyam, A., Liu, W. M. et al. 2013. "MYC/BCL2 protein coexpression contributes to the inferior survival of activated B-cell subtype of diffuse large B-cell lymphoma and demonstrates high-risk gene expression signatures: a report from The International DLBCL Rituximab-CHOP Consortium Program." *Blood* 121:4021-4031; quiz 4250.

[144] Schneider, K. M., Banks, P. M., Collie, A. M., Lanigan, C. P., Manilich, E., Durkin, L. M., Hill, B. T., Hsi, E. D. 2015. "Dual Expression of MYC and BCL2 Proteins Predicts Worse Outcomes in Diffuse Large B-Cell Lymphoma." *Leuk. Lymphoma* 1-23.

[145] Bouabdallah, R., Mounier, N., Guettier, C., Molina, T., Ribrag, V., Thieblemont, C., Sonet, A. et al. 2003. "T-cell/histiocyte-rich large B-cell lymphomas and classical diffuse large B-cell lymphomas have similar outcome after chemotherapy: a matched-control analysis." *J. Clin. Oncol.* 21:1271-1277.

[146] Rodriguez, J., Pugh, W. C., Cabanillas, F. 1993. "T-cell-rich B-cell lymphoma." *Blood* 82:1586-1589.

[147] Greer, J. P., Macon, W. R., Lamar, R. E., Wolff, S. N., Stein, R. S., Flexner, J. M., Collins, R. D., Cousar, J. B. 1995. "T-cell-rich B-cell lymphomas: diagnosis and response to therapy of 44 patients." *J. Clin. Oncol.* 13:1742-1750.

[148] Fraga, M., Sanchez-Verde, L., Forteza, J., Garcia-Rivero, A., Piris, M. A. 2002. "T-cell/histiocyte-rich large B-cell lymphoma is a disseminated aggressive neoplasm: differential diagnosis from Hodgkin's lymphoma." *Histopathology* 41:216-229.

[149] Dogan, A., Burke, J. S., Goteri, G., Stitson, R. N., Wotherspoon, A. C., Isaacson, P. G. 2003. "Micronodular T-cell/histiocyte-rich large B-cell lymphoma of the spleen: histology, immunophenotype, and differential diagnosis." *Am. J. Surg. Pathol.* 27:903-911.

[150] Skinnider, B. F., Connors, J. M., Gascoyne, R. D. 1997. "Bone marrow involvement in T-cell-rich B-cell lymphoma." *Am. J. Clin. Pathol.* 108:570-578.

[151] Lim, M. S., Beaty, M., Sorbara, L., Cheng, R. Z., Pittaluga, S., Raffeld, M., Jaffe, E. S. 2002. "T-cell/histiocyte-rich large B-cell lymphoma: a heterogeneous entity with derivation from germinal center B cells." *Am. J. Surg. Pathol.* 26:1458-1466.

[152] Ohgami, R. S., Zhao, S., Natkunam, Y. 2014. "Large B-cell lymphomas poor in B cells and rich in PD-1+ T cells can mimic T-cell lymphomas." *Am. J. Clin. Pathol.* 142:150-156.

[153] Brune, V., Tiacci, E., Pfeil, I., Doring, C., Eckerle, S., van Noesel, C. J., Klapper, W. et al. 2008. "Origin and pathogenesis of nodular lymphocyte-predominant Hodgkin lymphoma as revealed by global gene expression analysis." *J. Exp. Med.* 205:2251-2268.

[154] Chetaille, B., Bertucci, F., Finetti, P., Esterni, B., Stamatoullas, A., Picquenot, J. M., Copin, M. C. et al. 2009. "Molecular profiling of classical Hodgkin lymphoma tissues uncovers variations in the tumor microenvironment and correlations with EBV infection and outcome." *Blood* 113:2765-3775.

[155] Hodges, E., Hamid, Y., Quin, C. T., Angus, B., Wilkins, B. S., Wright, D. H., Smith, J. L. 2000. "Molecular analysis reveals somatically mutated and unmutated clonal and oligoclonal B cells in T-cell-rich B-cell lymphoma." *J. Pathol.* 192:479-487.

[156] Hartmann, S., Doring, C., Vucic, E., Chan, F. C., Ennishi, D., Tousseyn, T., de Wolf-Peeters, C. et al. 2015. "Array comparative genomic hybridization reveals similarities between nodular lymphocyte predominant Hodgkin lymphoma and T cell/histiocyte rich large B cell lymphoma." *Br. J. Haematol.* 169:415-422.

[157] Hartmann, S., Doring, C., Jakobus, C., Rengstl, B., Newrzela, S., Tousseyn, T., Sagaert, X. et al. 2013. "Nodular lymphocyte predominant Hodgkin lymphoma and T cell/ histiocyte rich large B cell lymphoma--endpoints of a spectrum of one disease?" *PLoS One* 8:e78812.

[158] Camilleri-Broet, S., Criniere, E., Broet, P., Delwail, V., Mokhtari, K., Moreau, A., Kujas, M. et al. 2006. "A uniform activated B-cell-like immunophenotype might explain the poor prognosis of primary central nervous system lymphomas: analysis of 83 cases." *Blood* 107:190 196.

[159] Courts, C., Brunn, A., Montesinos-Rongen, M., Siemer, D., Hans, V., Paulus, W., Wiestler, O. D. et al. 2009. "Preferential expression of truncated isoforms of FOXP1 in primary central nervous system lymphoma." *J. Neuropathol. Exp. Neurol.* 68:972-976.

[160] Montesinos-Rongen, M., Akasaka, T., Zuhlke-Jenisch, R., Schaller, C., Van Roost, D., Wiestler, O. D., Siebert, R., Deckert, M. 2003. "Molecular characterization of BCL6 breakpoints in primary diffuse large B-cell lymphomas of the central nervous system identifies GAPD as novel translocation partner." *Brain Pathol.* 13:534-538.

[161] Montesinos-Rongen, M., Zuhlke-Jenisch, R., Gesk, S., Martin-Subero, J. I., Schaller, C., Van Roost, D., Wiestler, O. D., Deckert, M., Siebert, R. 2002. "Interphase cytogenetic analysis of lymphoma-associated chromosomal breakpoints in primary diffuse large B-cell lymphomas of the central nervous system." *J. Neuropathol. Exp. Neurol.* 61:926-933.

[162] Schwindt, H., Akasaka, T., Zuhlke-Jenisch, R., Hans, V., Schaller, C., Klapper, W., Dyer, M. J., Siebert, R., Deckert, M. 2006. "Chromosomal translocations fusing the BCL6 gene to different partner loci are recurrent in primary central nervous system lymphoma and may be associated with aberrant somatic hypermutation or defective class switch recombination." *J. Neuropathol. Exp. Neurol.* 65:776-782.

[163] Weber, T., Weber, R. G., Kaulich, K., Actor, B., Meyer-Puttlitz, B., Lampel, S., Buschges, R. et al. 2000. "Characteristic chromosomal imbalances in primary central nervous system lymphomas of the diffuse large B-cell type." *Brain Pathol.* 10:73-84.

[164] Rickert, C. H., Dockhorn-Dworniczak, B., Simon, R., Paulus, W. 1999. "Chromosomal imbalances in primary lymphomas of the central nervous system." *Am. J. Pathol.* 155: 1445-1451.

[165] Courts, C., Montesinos-Rongen, M., Martin-Subero, J. I., Brunn, A., Siemer, D., Zuhlke-Jenisch, R., Pels, H. et al. 2007. "Transcriptional profiling of the nuclear factor-kappaB pathway identifies a subgroup of primary lymphoma of the central nervous system with low BCL10 expression." *J. Neuropathol. Exp. Neurol.* 66:230-237.

[166] Montesinos-Rongen, M., Kuppers, R., Schluter, D., Spieker, T., Van Roost, D., Schaller, C., Reifenberger, G., Wiestler, O. D., Deckert-Schluter, M. 1999. "Primary central nervous system lymphomas are derived from germinal-center B cells and show a preferential usage of the V4-34 gene segment." *Am. J. Pathol.* 155:2077-2086.

[167] Thompsett, A. R., Ellison, D. W., Stevenson, F. K., Zhu, D. 1999. "V(H) gene sequences from primary central nervous system lymphomas indicate derivation from highly mutated germinal center B cells with ongoing mutational activity." *Blood* 94: 1738-1746.

[168] Montesinos-Rongen, M., Van Roost, D., Schaller, C., Wiestler, O. D., Deckert, M. 2004. "Primary diffuse large B-cell lymphomas of the central nervous system are targeted by aberrant somatic hypermutation." *Blood* 103:1869-1875.

[169] Montesinos-Rongen, M., Brunn, A., Bentink, S., Basso, K., Lim, W. K., Klapper, W., Schaller, C. et al. 2008. "Gene expression profiling suggests primary central nervous system lymphomas to be derived from a late germinal center B cell." *Leukemia* 22:400-405.

[170] Willemze, R., Jaffe, E. S., Burg, G., Cerroni, L., Berti, E., Swerdlow, S. H., Ralfkiaer, E. et al. 2005. "WHO-EORTC classification for cutaneous lymphomas." *Blood* 105: 3768-3785.

[171] Vermeer, M. H., Geelen, F. A., van Haselen, C. W., van Voorst Vader, P. C., Geerts, M. L., van Vloten, W. A., Willemze, R. 1996. "Primary cutaneous large B-cell lymphomas of the legs. A distinct type of cutaneous B-cell lymphoma with an intermediate prognosis. Dutch Cutaneous Lymphoma Working Group." *Arch. Dermatol.* 132:1304-1308.

[172] Kodama, K., Massone, C., Chott, A., Metze, D., Kerl, H., Cerroni, L. 2005. "Primary cutaneous large B-cell lymphomas: clinicopathologic features, classification, and prognostic factors in a large series of patients." *Blood* 106:2491-2497.

[173] Senff, N. J., Hoefnagel, J. J., Jansen, P. M., Vermeer, M. H., van Baarlen, J., Blokx, W. A., Canninga-van Dijk, M. R. et al. 2007. "Reclassification of 300 primary cutaneous B-Cell lymphomas according to the new WHO-EORTC classification for cutaneous lymphomas: comparison with previous classifications and identification of prognostic markers." *J. Clin. Oncol.* 25:1581-1587.

[174] Zinzani, P. L., Quaglino, P., Pimpinelli, N., Berti, E., Baliva, G., Rupoli, S., Martelli, M. et al. 2006. "Prognostic factors in primary cutaneous B-cell lymphoma: the Italian Study Group for Cutaneous Lymphomas." *J. Clin. Oncol.* 24:1376-1382.

[175] Grange, F., Bekkenk, M. W., Wechsler, J., Meijer, C. J., Cerroni, L., Bernengo, M., Bosq, J. et al. 2001. "Prognostic factors in primary cutaneous large B-cell lymphomas: a European multicenter study." *J. Clin. Oncol.* 19:3602-3610.

[176] Dijkman, R., Tensen, C. P., Jordanova, E. S., Knijnenburg, J., Hoefnagel, J. J., Mulder, A. A., Rosenberg, C. et al. 2006. "Array-based comparative genomic hybridization

analysis reveals recurrent chromosomal alterations and prognostic parameters in primary cutaneous large B-cell lymphoma." *J. Clin. Oncol.* 24:296-305.
[177] Hoefnagel, J. J., Vermeer, M. H., Jansen, P. M., Fleuren, G. J., Meijer, C. J., Willemze, R. 2003. "Bcl-2, Bcl-6 and CD10 expression in cutaneous B-cell lymphoma: further support for a follicle centre cell origin and differential diagnostic significance." *Br. J. Dermatol.* 149:1183-1191.
[178] Hallermann, C., Kaune, K. M., Gesk, S., Martin-Subero, J. I., Gunawan, B., Griesinger, F., Vermeer, M. H. et al. 2004. "Molecular cytogenetic analysis of chromosomal breakpoints in the IGH, MYC, BCL6, and MALT1 gene loci in primary cutaneous B-cell lymphomas." *J. Invest. Dermatol.* 123:213-219.
[179] Hoefnagel, J. J., Dijkman, R., Basso, K., Jansen, P. M., Hallermann, C., Willemze, R., Tensen, C. P., Vermeer, M. H. 2005. "Distinct types of primary cutaneous large B-cell lymphoma identified by gene expression profiling." *Blood* 105:3671-3678.
[180] Oyama, T., Yamamoto, K., Asano, N., Oshiro, A., Suzuki, R., Kagami, Y., Morishima, Y. et al. 2007. "Age-related EBV-associated B-cell lymphoproliferative disorders constitute a distinct clinicopathologic group: a study of 96 patients." *Clin. Cancer Res.* 13:5124-5132.
[181] Park, S., Lee, J., Ko, Y. H., Han, A., Jun, H. J., Lee, S. C., Hwang, I. G. et al. 2007. "The impact of Epstein-Barr virus status on clinical outcome in diffuse large B-cell lymphoma." *Blood* 110:972-978.
[182] Shimoyama, Y., Yamamoto, K., Asano, N., Oyama, T., Kinoshita, T., Nakamura, S. 2008. "Age-related Epstein-Barr virus-associated B-cell lymphoproliferative disorders: special references to lymphomas surrounding this newly recognized clinicopathologic disease." *Cancer Sci.* 99:1085-1091.
[183] Montes-Moreno, S., Odqvist, L., Diaz-Perez, J. A., Lopez, A. B., de Villambrosia, S. G., Mazorra, F., Castillo, M. E. et al. 2012. "EBV-positive diffuse large B-cell lymphoma of the elderly is an aggressive post-germinal center B-cell neoplasm characterized by prominent nuclear factor-kB activation." *Mod. Pathol.* 25:968-982.
[184] Kuze, T., Nakamura, N., Hashimoto, Y., Sasaki, Y., Abe, M. 2000. "The characteristics of Epstein-Barr virus (EBV)-positive diffuse large B-cell lymphoma: comparison between EBV(+) and EBV(-) cases in Japanese population." *Jpn. J. Cancer Res.* 91: 1233-1240.
[185] Higgins, J. P., Warnke, R. A. 1999. "CD30 expression is common in mediastinal large B-cell lymphoma." *Am. J. Clin. Pathol.* 112:241-247.
[186] Scarpa, A., Moore, P. S., Rigaud, G., Inghirami, G., Montresor, M., Menegazzi, M., Todeschini, G., Menestrina, F. 1999. "Molecular features of primary mediastinal B-cell lymphoma: involvement of p16INK4A, p53 and c-myc." *Br. J. Haematol.* 107:106-113.
[187] Savage, K. J., Monti, S., Kutok, J. L., Cattoretti, G., Neuberg, D., De Leval, L., Kurtin, P. et al. 2003. "The molecular signature of mediastinal large B-cell lymphoma differs from that of other diffuse large B-cell lymphomas and shares features with classical Hodgkin lymphoma." *Blood* 102:3871-3879.
[188] Zinzani, P. L., Piccaluga, P. P. 2011. "Primary mediastinal DLBCL: evolving biologic understanding and therapeutic strategies." *Curr. Oncol. Rep.* 13:407-415.
[189] Orwat, D. E., Batalis, N. I. 2012. "Intravascular large B-cell lymphoma." *Arch. Pathol. Lab. Med.* 136:333-338.

[190] Carter, D. K., Batts, K. P., de Groen, P. C., Kurtin, P. J. 1996. "Angiotropic large cell lymphoma (intravascular lymphomatosis) occurring after follicular small cleaved cell lymphoma." *Mayo Clin. Proc.* 71:869-873.

[191] Murase, T., Yamaguchi, M., Suzuki, R., Okamoto, M., Sato, Y., Tamaru, J., Kojima, M. et al. 2007. "Intravascular large B-cell lymphoma (IVLBCL): a clinicopathologic study of 96 cases with special reference to the immunophenotypic heterogeneity of CD5." *Blood* 109:478-485.

[192] Cheuk, W., Chan, A. C., Chan, J. K., Lau, G. T., Chan, V. N., Yiu, H. H. 2005. "Metallic implant-associated lymphoma: a distinct subgroup of large B-cell lymphoma related to pyothorax-associated lymphoma?" *Am. J. Surg. Pathol.* 29:832-836.

[193] Copie-Bergman, C., Niedobitek, G., Mangham, D. C., Selves, J., Baloch, K., Diss, T. C., Knowles, D. N., Delsol, G., Isaacson, P. G. 1997. "Epstein-Barr virus in B-cell lymphomas associated with chronic suppurative inflammation." *J. Pathol.* 183:287-292.

[194] Nakatsuka, S., Yao, M., Hoshida, Y., Yamamoto, S., Iuchi, K., Aozasa, K. 2002. "Pyothorax-associated lymphoma: a review of 106 cases." *J. Clin. Oncol.* 20:4255-4260.

[195] Narimatsu, H., Ota, Y., Kami, M., Takeuchi, K., Suzuki, R., Matsuo, K., Matsumura, T. et al. 2007. "Clinicopathological features of pyothorax-associated lymphoma; a retrospective survey involving 98 patients." *Ann. Oncol.* 18:122-128.

[196] Katzenstein, A. L., Doxtader, E., Narendra, S. 2010. "Lymphomatoid granulomatosis: insights gained over 4 decades." *Am. J. Surg. Pathol.* 34:e35-48.

[197] Reichard, K. K., McKenna, R. W., Kroft, S. H. 2007. "ALK-positive diffuse large B-cell lymphoma: report of four cases and review of the literature." *Mod. Pathol.* 20:310-319.

[198] Xing, X., Lin, D., Ran, W., Liu, H. 2014. "ALK-positive diffuse large B-cell lymphoma of the duodenum: A case report and review of the literature." *Exp. Ther. Med.* 8:409-412.

[199] Stachurski, D., Miron, P. M., Al-Homsi, S., Hutchinson, L., Harris, N. L., Woda, B., Wang, S. A. 2007. "Anaplastic lymphoma kinase-positive diffuse large B-cell lymphoma with a complex karyotype and cryptic 3' ALK gene insertion to chromosome 4 q22-24." *Hum. Pathol.* 38:940-945.

[200] Onciu, M., Behm, F. G., Raimondi, S. C., Moore, S., Harwood, E. L., Pui, C. H., Sandlund, J. T. 2003. "ALK-positive anaplastic large cell lymphoma with leukemic peripheral blood involvement is a clinicopathologic entity with an unfavorable prognosis. Report of three cases and review of the literature." *Am. J. Clin. Pathol.* 120: 617-625.

[201] Lee, O. J., Kim, K. W., Lee, G. K. 2006. "Epstein-Barr virus and human immunodeficiency virus-negative oral plasmablastic lymphoma." *J. Oral Pathol. Med.* 35:382-384.

[202] Delecluse, H. J., Anagnostopoulos, I., Dallenbach, F., Hummel, M., Marafioti, T., Schneider, U., Huhn, D. et al. 1997. "Plasmablastic lymphomas of the oral cavity: a new entity associated with the human immunodeficiency virus infection." *Blood* 89: 1413-1420.

[203] Montes-Moreno, S., Gonzalez-Medina, A. R., Rodriguez-Pinilla, S. M., Maestre, L., Sanchez-Verde, L., Roncador, G., Mollejo, M. et al. 2010. "Aggressive large B-cell lymphoma with plasma cell differentiation: immunohistochemical characterization of

plasmablastic lymphoma and diffuse large B-cell lymphoma with partial plasmablastic phenotype." *Haematologica* 95:1342-1349.

[204] Dong, H. Y., Scadden, D. T., de Leval, L., Tang, Z., Isaacson, P. G., Harris, N. L. 2005. "Plasmablastic lymphoma in HIV-positive patients: an aggressive Epstein-Barr virus-associated extramedullary plasmacytic neoplasm." *Am. J. Surg. Pathol.* 29:1633-1641.

[205] Elyamany, G., Al Mussaed, E., Alzahrani, A. M. 2015. "Plasmablastic Lymphoma: A Review of Current Knowledge and Future Directions." *Adv. Hematol.* 2015:315289.

[206] Salaverria, I., Philipp, C., Oschlies, I., Kohler, C. W., Kreuz, M., Szczepanowski, M., Burkhardt, B. et al. 2011. "Translocations activating IRF4 identify a subtype of germinal center-derived B-cell lymphoma affecting predominantly children and young adults." *Blood* 118:139-147.

[207] Oksenhendler, E., Boulanger, E., Galicier, L., Du, M. Q., Dupin, N., Diss, T. C., Hamoudi, R. et al. 2002. "High incidence of Kaposi sarcoma-associated herpesvirus-related non-Hodgkin lymphoma in patients with HIV infection and multicentric Castleman disease." *Blood* 99:2331-2336.

[208] Dupin, N., Diss, T. L., Kellam, P., Tulliez, M., Du, M. Q., Sicard, D., Weiss, R. A., Isaacson, P. G., Boshoff, C. 2000. "HHV-8 is associated with a plasmablastic variant of Castleman disease that is linked to HHV-8-positive plasmablastic lymphoma." *Blood* 95:1406-1412.

[209] D'Antonio, A., Boscaino, A., Addesso, M., Piris, M. A., Nappi, O. 2007. "KSHV- and EBV-associated germinotropic lymphoproliferative disorder: a rare lymphoproliferative disease of HIV patient with plasmablastic morphology, indolent course and favourable response to therapy." *Leuk. Lymphoma* 48:1444-1447.

[210] Simonelli, C., Spina, M., Cinelli, R., Talamini, R., Tedeschi, R., Gloghini, A., Vaccher, E., Carbone, A., Tirelli, U. 2003. "Clinical features and outcome of primary effusion lymphoma in HIV-infected patients: a single-institution study." *J. Clin. Oncol.* 21: 3948-3954.

[211] Nador, R. G., Cesarman, E., Chadburn, A., Dawson, D. B., Ansari, M. Q., Sald, J., Knowles, D. M. 1996. "Primary effusion lymphoma: a distinct clinicopathologic entity associated with the Kaposi's sarcoma-associated herpes virus." *Blood* 88:645-656.

[212] Jones, D., Ballestas, M. E., Kaye, K. M., Gulizia, J. M., Winters, G. L., Fletcher, J., Scadden, D. T., Aster, J. C. 1998. "Primary-effusion lymphoma and Kaposi's sarcoma in a cardiac-transplant recipient." *N. Engl. J. Med.* 339:444-449.

[213] Dotti, G., Fiocchi, R., Motta, T., Facchinetti, B., Chiodini, B., Borleri, G. M., Gavazzeni, G., Barbui, T., Rambaldi, A. 1999. "Primary effusion lymphoma after heart transplantation: a new entity associated with human herpesvirus-8." *Leukemia* 13:664-670.

[214] Melo, N. C., Sales, M. M., Santana, A. N., Costalonga, E. C., Pedreira, A. B., Ianhez, L. E. 2008. "Pleural primary effusion lymphoma in a renal transplant recipient." *Am. J. Transplant.* 8:906-907.

[215] Makis, W., Stern, J. "Hepatitis C-related primary effusion lymphoma of the pleura and peritoneum, imaged with F-18 FDG PET/CT." *Clin. Nucl. Med.* 35:797-799.

[216] Nakayama-Ichiyama, S., Yokote, T., Kobayashi, K., Hirata, Y., Hiraoka, N., Iwaki, K., Takayama, A. et al. "Primary effusion lymphoma of T-cell origin with t(7;8)(q32;q13) in an HIV-negative patient with HCV-related liver cirrhosis and hepatocellular carcinoma positive for HHV6 and HHV8." *Ann. Hematol.* 90:1229-1231.

[217] Teruya-Feldstein, J., Zauber, P., Setsuda, J. E., Berman, E. L., Sorbara, L., Raffeld, M., Tosato, G., Jaffe, E. S. 1998. “Expression of human herpesvirus-8 oncogene and cytokine homologues in an HIV-seronegative patient with multicentric Castleman's disease and primary effusion lymphoma.” *Lab. Invest.* 78:1637-1642.
[218] Dupin, N., Fisher, C., Kellam, P., Ariad, S., Tulliez, M., Franck, N., van Marck, E. et al. 1999. “Distribution of human herpesvirus-8 latently infected cells in Kaposi’s sarcoma, multicentric Castleman’s disease, and primary effusion lymphoma.” *Proc. Natl. Acad. Sci. US* 96:4546-4551.
[219] Chadburn, A., Hyjek, E., Mathew, S., Cesarman, E., Said, J., Knowles, D. M. 2004. “KSHV-positive solid lymphomas represent an extra-cavitary variant of primary effusion lymphoma.” *Am. J. Surg. Pathol.* 28:1401-1416.
[220] Iuchi, K., Aozasa, K., Yamamoto, S., Mori, T., Tajima, K., Minato, K., Mukai, K. et al. 1989. “Non-Hodgkin's lymphoma of the pleural cavity developing from long-standing pyothorax. Summary of clinical and pathological findings in thirty-seven cases.” *Jpn. J. Clin. Oncol.* 19:249-257.
[221] Iuchi, K., Ichimiya, A., Akashi, A., Mizuta, T., Lee, Y. E., Tada, H., Mori, T. et al. 1987. “Non-Hodgkin’s lymphoma of the pleural cavity developing from long-standing pyothorax.” *Cancer* 60:1771-1775.
[222] Cesarman, E., Nador, R. G., Bai, F., Bohenzky, R. A., Russo, J. J., Moore, P. S., Chang, Y., Knowles, D. M. 1996. “Kaposi’s sarcoma-associated herpesvirus contains G protein-coupled receptor and cyclin D homologs which are expressed in Kaposi’s sarcoma and malignant lymphoma.” *J. Virol.* 70:8218-8223.
[223] Siddiqi, T., Joyce, R. M. 2008. “A case of HIV-negative primary effusion lymphoma treated with bortezomib, pegylated liposomal doxorubicin, and rituximab.” *Clin. Lymphoma Myeloma* 8:300-304.
[224] Ghosh, S. K., Wood, C., Boise, L. H., Mian, A. M., Deyev, V. V., Feuer, G., Toomey, N. L. et al. 2003. “Potentiation of TRAIL-induced apoptosis in primary effusion lymphoma through azidothymidine-mediated inhibition of NF-kappa B.” *Blood* 101: 2321-2327.
[225] Lamarre, L., Jacobson, J. O., Aisenberg, A. C., Harris, N. L. 1989. “Primary large cell lymphoma of the mediastinum. A histologic and immunophenotypic study of 29 cases.” *Am. J. Surg. Pathol.* 13:730-739.
[226] Joos, S., Otano-Joos, M. I., Ziegler, S., Bruderlein, S., du Manoir, S., Bentz, M., Moller, P., Lichter, P. 1996. “Primary mediastinal (thymic) B-cell lymphoma is characterized by gains of chromosomal material including 9p and amplification of the REL gene.” *Blood* 87:1571-1578.
[227] Wessendorf, S., Barth, T. F., Viardot, A., Mueller, A., Kestler, H. A., Kohlhammer, H., Lichter, P. et al. 2007. “Further delineation of chromosomal consensus regions in primary mediastinal B-cell lymphomas: an analysis of 37 tumor samples using high-resolution genomic profiling (array-CGH).” *Leukemia* 21:2463-2469.
[228] Steidl, C., Shah, S. P., Woolcock, B. W., Rui, L., Kawahara, M., Farinha, P., Johnson, N. A. et al. 2011. “MHC class II transactivator CIITA is a recurrent gene fusion partner in lymphoid cancers.” *Nature* 471:377-381.
[229] Rosenwald, A., Wright, G., Leroy, K., Yu, X., Gaulard, P., Gascoyne, R. D., Chan, W. C. et al. 2003. “Molecular diagnosis of primary mediastinal B cell lymphoma identifies

a clinically favorable subgroup of diffuse large B cell lymphoma related to Hodgkin lymphoma." *J. Exp. Med.* 198:851-862.

[230] Feuerhake, F., Kutok, J. L., Monti, S., Chen, W., LaCasce, A. S., Cattoretti, G., Kurtin, P. et al. 2005. "NFkappaB activity, function, and target-gene signatures in primary mediastinal large B-cell lymphoma and diffuse large B-cell lymphoma subtypes." *Blood* 106:1392-1399.

[231] Guiter, C., Dusanter-Fourt, I., Copie-Bergman, C., Boulland, M. L., Le Gouvello, S., Gaulard, P., Leroy, K., Castellano, F. 2004. "Constitutive STAT6 activation in primary mediastinal large B-cell lymphoma." *Blood* 104:543-549.

[232] Renne, C., Willenbrock, K., Martin-Subero, J. I., Hinsch, N., Doring, C., Tiacci, E., Klapper, W. et al. 2007. "High expression of several tyrosine kinases and activation of the PI3K/AKT pathway in mediastinal large B cell lymphoma reveals further similarities to Hodgkin lymphoma." *Leukemia* 21:780-787.

[233] Copie-Bergman, C., Plonquet, A., Alonso, M. A., Boulland, M. L., Marquet, J., Divine, M., Moller, P., Leroy, K., Gaulard, P. 2002. "MAL expression in lymphoid cells: further evidence for MAL as a distinct molecular marker of primary mediastinal large B-cell lymphomas." *Mod. Pathol.* 15:1172-1180.

[234] Traverse-Glehen, A., Pittaluga, S., Gaulard, P., Sorbara, L., Alonso, M. A., Raffeld, M., Jaffe, E. S. 2005. "Mediastinal gray zone lymphoma: the missing link between classic Hodgkin's lymphoma and mediastinal large B-cell lymphoma." *Am. J. Surg. Pathol.* 29:1411-1421.

[235] Garcia, J. F., Mollejo, M., Fraga, M., Forteza, J., Muniesa, J. A., Perez-Guillermo, M., Perez-Seoane, C. et al. 2005. "Large B-cell lymphoma with Hodgkin's features." *Histopathology* 47:101-110.

[236] Eberle, F. C., Rodriguez-Canales, J., Wei, L., Hanson, J. C., Killian, J. K., Sun, H. W., Adams, L. G. et al. 2011. "Methylation profiling of mediastinal gray zone lymphoma reveals a distinctive signature with elements shared by classical Hodgkin's lymphoma and primary mediastinal large B-cell lymphoma." *Haematologica* 96:558-566.

[237] McClure, R. F., Remstein, E. D., Macon, W. R., Dewald, G. W., Habermann, T. M., Hoering, A., Kurtin, P. J. 2005. "Adult B-cell lymphomas with burkitt-like morphology are phenotypically and genotypically heterogeneous with aggressive clinical behavior." *Am. J. Surg. Pathol.* 29:1652-1660.

[238] Mationg-Kalaw, E., Tan, L. H., Tay, K., Lim, S. T., Tang, T., Lee, Y. Y., Tan, S. Y. 2012. "Does the proliferation fraction help identify mature B cell lymphomas with double- and triple-hit translocations?" *Histopathology* 61:1214-1218.

[239] Li, S., Lin, P., Young, K. H., Kanagal-Shamanna, R., Yin, C. C., Medeiros, L. J. 2013. "MYC/BCL2 double-hit high-grade B-cell lymphoma." *Adv. Anat. Pathol.* 20:315-326.

[240] Haralambieva, E., Boerma, E. J., van Imhoff, G. W., Rosati, S., Schuuring, E., Muller-Hermelink, H. K., Kluin, P. M., Ott, G. 2005. "Clinical, immunophenotypic, and genetic analysis of adult lymphomas with morphologic features of Burkitt lymphoma." *Am. J. Surg. Pathol.* 29:1086-1094.

[241] Dave, S. S., Fu, K., Wright, G. W., Lam, L. T., Kluin, P., Boerma, E. J., Greiner, T. C. et al. 2006. "Molecular diagnosis of Burkitt's lymphoma." *N. Engl. J. Med.* 354:2431-2442.

In: Diffuse Large B-Cell Lymphoma (DLBCL)
Editor: Haipeng Shao
ISBN: 978-1-63484-402-4

Chapter 2

DIFFUSE LARGE B-CELL LYMPHOMA: DIAGNOSIS, TREATMENT AND PROGNOSIS

Ashley T. Freeman and Steven I. Park*
School of Medicine, Lineberger Comprehensive Cancer Center,
University of North Carolina at Chapel Hill, Chapel Hill, NC, US

ABSTRACT

Diffuse large B-Cell lymphoma (DLBCL) is the most common type of non-Hodgkin lymphoma (NHL) accounting for approximately one third of NHL cases. This chapter will provide an overview of the diagnosis, prognosis, and treatment of DLBCL. The clinical presentation and diagnostic workup will be reviewed with emphasis on the morphologic, molecular, immunophenotypic, and clinical features that divide DLBCL into prognostically significant subtypes. We will review the history of DLBCL treatment including the development of CHOP chemotherapy, the trend toward more aggressive regimens, and the randomized clinical trials re-establishing CHOP as the regimen of choice in the 1990s. We will describe the current standard of care for limited and advanced stage DLBCL with R-CHOP and evaluate alternatives in challenging patient populations such as the elderly or those with relapsed/refractory disease. Emerging therapies and ongoing clinical trials will be reviewed. Salvage chemotherapy for relapsed DLBCL and the role of hematopoietic stem cell transplant will also be discussed.

INTRODUCTION

There will be an estimated 71, 850 cases of non-Hodgkin lymphoma (NHL) diagnosed in the United States in 2015 [1]. Diffuse large B-cell lymphoma (DLBCL) is the most common subtype of NHL accounting for 30 to 40% of NHL diagnoses [2]. Incidence increases with age and is slightly higher in males (55%) and Caucasians [3]. This group of lymphomas was named for the characteristic appearance of large, abnormal lymphoid cells. However, we now

* Corresponding author: Email: sipark@med.unc.edu; Phone: (919)-843-6616.

understand that the term DLBCL represents a group of clinically and biologically diverse lymphomas [4].

In this chapter we will review the presentation, diagnosis, and prognosis of DLBCL. The current World Health Organization (WHO) classification [2] of DLBCL will be discussed with emphasis on the more recently discovered genetic characteristics that provide prognostic significance. We will then review the management of DLBCL and consider how this can be modified in certain patient populations. Finally, we will discuss targeted therapies currently in development as a result of our recent appreciation of the molecular aberrations driving tumorigenesis in DLBCL.

Clinical Presentation of DLBCL

DLBCL often presents with symptoms of rapidly enlarging lymphadenopathy or a mass that may invade into adjacent structures. Systemic B symptoms (fever, night sweats, weight loss) are present in approximately 30% of cases. Extranodal disease occurs in 40% of cases and can occur in nearly every part of the body, with the most frequent site of involvement being the gastrointestinal tract [5]. Laboratory studies may reveal evidence of rapid cell turnover including elevated serum lactate dehydrogenase (LDH) and uric acid. There may also be signs of organ failure due to infiltration by DLBCL or mechanical obstruction. In order to make the diagnosis, an excisional lymph node biopsy should be performed whenever possible to allow adequate morphologic evaluation and immunophenotyping.

DLBCL is staged using the Lugano staging system, which is based on the Ann-Arbor staging system [6]. This system broadly divides DLBCL into limited (stage I and II) or advanced disease (stage III and IV) based on disease site (nodal vs extranodal) and extent. Positron emission tomography/computed tomography (PET/CT) is used to determine the extent of disease and monitor response to therapy. Since PET/CT is sensitive for detection of bone marrow involvement, a bone marrow biopsy could be avoided for staging if PET/CT scan demonstrates bone marrow uptake. However, a bone marrow biopsy may still be required if the PET/CT does not show bone involvement and if this would impact treatment decisions.

Prognosis of DLBCL

The factors associated with prognosis in DLBCL are the International Prognostic Index (IPI) score, molecular subtype and initial response to chemotherapy.

The IPI is the main prognostic scoring tool used for DLBCL. It was initially developed in 1993 to distinguish patients with aggressive NHL that might benefit from more aggressive chemotherapeutic regimens. The age-adjusted IPI (aaIPI) is now the most commonly used prognostic score for DLBCL in clinical trials and divides patients into 4 risk categories based on serum LDH, performance status and Ann-Arbor stage for 2 different age groups (greater than or less than 60 years). Five-year survival for patients less than 60 years of age with an aaIPI score of 0, 1, 2 and 3 was 83, 69, 46, and 32 percent respectively [7]. The most recent scoring system put forth by the National Comprehensive Cancer Network (NCCN) requires more detailed information about age, LDH value, and site of extranodal disease. When compared to the original IPI, the NCCN-IPI allowed better discrimination for risk groups [8].

As we will discuss in more detail in the following section, the molecular subtype of DLBCL has significant implication for prognosis. The activated B-cell (ABC) subtype of DLBCL has been associated with a worse outcome and poor response to chemotherapy. Five-year survival for ABC-type DLBCL was 35% compared to 60% for other subtypes [9]. Tumors that have "double-hit" genetics (translocations involving *MYC* and *BCL*-2 or *BCL*-6) are also known to have a worse prognosis [10]. It is possible to measure circulating tumor DNA in the plasma and this has been shown to correlate with burden and stage of disease [11, 12]. The role of this technology in predicting prognosis and monitoring for relapse has yet to be elucidated.

Pathologic Characteristics and Classification of DLBCL

Histologically, DLBCL is characterized by total effacement of the normal lymph node architecture and diffuse growth of large neoplastic B-lymphoid cells [13]. The current WHO classification categorizes DLBCL according to morphology, immunophenotype and anatomic site. Despite these groupings, a significant heterogeneity is observed within groups in terms of response to chemotherapy and survival. The application of advanced molecular techniques to the study of DLBCL has led to the identification of 3 distinct molecular subtypes arising from different stages of B-cell development: germinal center B-cell (GCB) type, activated B-cell type and primary mediastinal B-cell lymphoma (PMBCL), which already comprises its own subtype under the WHO classification [9, 14]. An additional 15-30% of DLBCL remain unclassified [14-16]. Here we will review the current WHO classification with a focused discussion of thcsc 3 molccular subtypcs.

DLBCL, Not Otherwise Specified (NOS)

DLCBCL NOS is the most commonly diagnosed subtype of DLBCL. It can arise de novo or following transformation from an indolent lymphoma such as follicular lymphoma or chronic lymphocytic leukemia. Three main morphologic subtypes have been described (centroblastic, immunoblastic, and anaplastic), but these have not been reliably shown to predict prognosis.

As previously mentioned, gene-expressing profiling (GEP) studies have identified 2 important molecular subtypes of DLBCL that fall under this classification, named for their presumed cell-of-origin: GCB-type and ABC-type DLBCL [14, 17]. It is an important distinction as the ABC subtype is associated with a worse prognosis and poor response to therapy [9, 18, 19]. Molecular studies have revealed that uncontrolled cellular proliferation in ABC type DLBCLs is driven by mutations causing chronic activity of B-cell receptor (BCR) signaling and constitutive activation of the NF-κB pathway [18, 20, 21].

Unfortunately, the molecular techniques used to identify these subtypes in the initial GEP studies were carried out on fresh frozen tissue, which is not how biopsy samples are typically obtained in practice. Assays are currently underdevelopment that use surrogate immunohistochemistry (IHC) markers, but there is some concern about the validity of this approach given heterogeneity in specimen handling, IHC antibody performance and interpretation of stains [22-24]. Despite these concerns, there are several IHC algorithms available to delineate GCB from non-GCB DLBCLs using antibodies against CD10, BCL6, and MUM-1 [25, 26]. GCB-type DLBCLs typically express CD-10 or are CD-10 negative/BCL-6 positive with negative MUM-1. Non-GCB types are MUM-1 positive.

In addition to cell-of-origin, translocation and overexpression of certain genes are associated with poor prognosis. MYC is a transcription factor involved in cell survival and proliferation. MYC expression is closely regulated by BCL6 acting to repress MYC expression in normal germinal centers. BCL-2 functions as an antiapoptotic protein. DLBCLs with translocations of both *MYC* and *BCL-2* or *BCL-6* are termed double-hit lymphomas (DHLs) and carry a poor prognosis as previously mentioned [27-29]. Even in the absence of translocation, MYC and BCL-2 overexpression is associated with worse outcomes [10, 27].

Primary Mediastinal Large B-Cell Lymphoma (PMBCL)

PMBCL is a distinct clinicopathologic entity that usually affects young adults in the third or fourth decade of life with a female predominance [30, 31]. Patients present with a bulky mediastinal mass that may infiltrate into the lung, chest wall and pericardium. Distant spread is less common on presentation, but frequent sites of later dissemination include the adrenals, liver, kidneys, and CNS. Bone marrow involvement is less common. It is thought to arise from a thymic post-germinal center B-cell or a germinal center B-cell that has migrated to the thymus [15, 16]. The malignant cells express CD20, CD79a, lack surface immunoglobulin and may weakly express CD30. GEP reveals activation of the NF-κB pathway [15, 16, 32], similar to nodular classical Hodgkin's lymphoma and sometimes the distinction between these two entities can be difficult as discussed below.

T-Cell/Histiocyte-Rich Large B-Cell Lymphoma

This is a morphologic variant of DLBCL accounting for approximately 10% of DLBCL in which the malignant cells occur in a background of T-cells/histiocytes. It most often affects middle-aged men and commonly presents in advanced stage with bone marrow, spleen and liver involvement [33]. The malignant large B cells stain positive for CD20, CD79a and Pax-5 on a background of CD3 and CD8 positive T cells [34].

EBV-Positive DLBCL

EBV-positive DLBCL is defined as a clonal proliferation of EBV positive B-cells that occur in patients over the age of 50 with no known history of immunodeficiency or lymphoma. It is thought to be related to immunosenescence causing inadequate surveillance of EBV-infected B cells [35], but rarely does occur in younger individuals [36]. Patients often present in late stage and tend to have a poor prognosis [35]. The morphologic appearance of the malignant cells can resemble Reed-Sternberg/Hodgkin cells. IHC may demonstrate negative or weak CD20 expression, CD30 expression, positive EBV-related latent membrane protein, but negative CD15. In addition they demonstrate an ABC immunophenotype, which is associated with poor prognosis [35].

DLBCL in Specific Anatomic Sites

This category includes primary central nervous system (PCNS) DLBCL, primary cutaneous DLBCL, leg-type, and intravascular DLBCL.

PCNS DLBCL arises from and is contained within the CNS or intraocular region, but the histologic and IHC profiles are similar to DLBCL NOS. The molecular profile is similar to that of DLBCL arising from the testis and this may implicate the relative immune privilege in these sites as a driver of tumorigenesis [37-40].

Primary cutaneous DLBCL, leg type typically presents in elderly women and generally hasan indolent course although the prognosis is inferior to that of other B-cell cutaneous lymphoma types, such as primary cutaneous follicular center lymphoma and primary cutaneous marginal zone lymphoma. The molecular profile resembles the ABC subtype of nodal DLBCL. IHC will usually demonstrate expression of BCL-2, MUM1 and FOXP1 [41].

Intravascular large B-cell lymphoma is rare and occurs within the lumina of small or intermediate blood vessels [42]. It can present with neurocutaneous manifestations or as a disseminated syndrome including pancytopenia, hepatomegaly, multiorgan failure and hemophagocytosis [42]. IHC reveals an ABC-like phenotype often with co-expression of CD5 [43].

DLBCL with Plasma Cell Immunophenotype

This refers to the following DLBCLs that have weak B-cell staining, but have acquired positive staining for plasma cell markers: ALK-positive large B-cell lymphoma, plasmablastic lymphoma, and primary effusion lymphoma.

ALK-positive large B-cell lymphoma is a rare subtype of DLBCL that has a male predominance. The malignant cells have a plasmablastic immunophenotype expressing CD138, EMA andcytoplasmic IgA lambda immunoglobulin in addition to the overexpression of ALK. The cells are CD30 negative unlike anaplastic large cell lymphoma. The prognosis is very poor [44].

Plasmablastic lymphoma is aggressive and occurs in the setting of immunodeficiency, usually AIDS [45]. This also has a marked male predominance and tends to present in extranodal sites with a mucosal or cutaneous component. In addition to the plasma cell markers (CD138, CD38), these malignant cells are usually EBV positive and HHV8 negative. There seems to be a close relationship between plasmablastic lymphoma and the plasmablastic variant of multiple myeloma as evidenced by common cytogenetic changes and high incidence of *MYC* translocations in both [46, 47].

Primary effusion lymphoma also occurs in the setting of immunodeficiency, most often AIDS, and is associated with HHV8/EBV co-infection. The malignant cells express plasma cell markers (CD138, CD38), EMA, and CD30, lack routine B-cell markers (CD20, CD19,

CD79a and surface immunoglobulin) and may aberrantly express T-cell antigens. Staining for HHV8 will be positive. Prognosis is also very poor with a median survival of less than 6 months [48, 49].

B-Cell Lymphoma, Unclassifiable, with Features Intermediate between DLBCL and Burkitt Lymphoma

This subtype encompasses lymphomas with morphologic, immunophenotypic and cytogenetic characteristics that overlap between DLBCL and Bukitt lymphoma [50]. It often presents with an advanced stage in middle-aged to elderly adults [51] and have poor prognosis with poor response to chemotherapy [52]. Morphologically they often resemble Burkitt lymphoma, but have an atypical immunophenotype, such as strong BCL-2 expression and lower than expected Ki-67 proliferative index (<95%). Gene expression profiling studies have found that many of these tumors have double hit genetics with translocations involving *MYC* and *BCL-2* or *BCL-6* [53].

B-Cell Lymphoma, Unclassifiable, with Features Intermediate between DLBCL and Hodgkin Lymphoma

This subtype is commonly referred to as "mediastinal grey-zone lymphoma" and is most often diagnosed when there are features intermediate between PMBCL and classical Hodgkin's lymphoma. While PMBCL and classical Hodgkin's lymphoma are more likely to occur in young women, mediastinal grey-zone lymphomas are more common in young men [54]. Morphologically, these tumors have features of both classical Hodgkin's lymphoma and PMBCL. IHC commonly demonstrates expression of B-cell markers (CD20, CD79a, PAX5 and OCT2), CD15 and CD30 [55]. GEP studies are not yet available for this category, but epigenetic studies have demonstrated that mediastinal grey-zone lymphoma has a unique profile from both classical Hodgkin and PMBCL [56].

Treatment of DLBCL

While many patients with DLBCL are cured with standard chemotherapy, up to 40% either do not respond or relapse and ultimately die from their disease. It is clear that a single chemotherapy regimen will not be optimal for all cases of DLBCL given the molecular heterogeneity discussed above. Here we will review the clinical trials that lead to the current standard of care for DLBCL, discuss areas of uncertainty, and introduce targeted therapies currently in development for DLBCL.

Current Standard of Care: Rituximab, Cyclophosphamide, Doxorubicin, Vincristine and Prednisone (R-CHOP)

Since the 1970s CHOP chemotherapy has comprised the backbone of DLBCL treatment. Several other anthracycline-based regimens were compared to CHOP in prospective trials, but were largely associated with increased toxicity and no improvement in outcomes [57-60]. It was not until the addition of rituximab in the early 2000s that overall survival (OS) for DLBCL was significantly improved. The superiority of R-CHOP was first demonstrated in a landmark phase III trial conducted by the Groupe d'Etude des Lymphomes de l'Adulte (GELA) in which R-CHOP was compared to CHOP in patients aged 60-80 years. Improvement in progression free survival (PFS) and OS was demonstrated in that study and confirmed in follow up. The 10-year OS for the R-CHOP group was 43.5% compared to 27.6% for the CHOP group [61, 62]. The improvement in OS and PFS was confirmed in patients of all ages by subsequent studies including a large phase III US-intergroup trial [63], the MabThera International (MInT) trial [64], and a Canadian retrospective, population-based analysis [65].

Prior to the advent of rituximab, there were attempts to improve upon CHOP by reducing the cycle length and adding growth factor support (CHOP-14) with mixed results [65-67]. After the addition of rituximab, the controversy about the optimal cycle length continued. There have been 3 prospective trials that compared CHOP-like regimens plus rituximab given every 21 days to the same regimen given every 14 days and no clear benefit was demonstrated with a shorter cycle length [68, 69]. Furthermore, a higher incidence of febrile neutropenia occurred in older adults in one of the studies [69]. Thus, R-CHOP-21 has remained the standard front line therapy for patients with both limited and advanced stage disease.

Thc optimal number of R CHOP cycles required for treatment of DLBCL is a matter of debate and has not been specifically addressed in randomized clinical trial for R-CHOP-21. One prospective trial compared 6 to 8 cycles of CHOP-14 with and without rituximab and found no difference in survival [70]. It is unclear whether these results can be applied to R-CHOP-21, but it is generally accepted that 6 cycles of R-CHOP are adequate. Two strategies for determining number of cycles are currently used in practice. The first is to use a defined number of cycles (6-8) for each patient and the second is to administer 2 cycles after the patient achieves a complete response by PET/CT scan.

In order to address the high rate of disease relapse or progression despite treatment with R-CHOP, more intensive regimens have been studied including R-ACVBP (rituximab, doxorubicin, cyclophosphamide, vindesine, bleomycin, prednisone), DA-EPOCH-R (dose-adjusted etoposide, prednisone, vincristine, cyclophosphamide, doxorubicin plus rituximab), and consolidative autologous stem cell transplant (ASCT). GELA compared R-CHOP-21 to R-ACVBP plus consolidation with high dose methotrexate, etoposide, ifosfamide and cytarabine [71]. The patients selected for this trial were less than 60 years of age with advanced disease. While toxicity was significantly increased, OS was superior in the R-ACVBP arm (92 versus 84%). Subsequent analysis revealed that the improvement in survival was limited to tumors with a non-GCB immunophenotype [72]. Of note, vindesine is currently not available in the United States. DA-EPOCH-R has previously been shown to have efficacy in DLBCL [73, 74] and PMBCL [75]. A phase III Cancer and Leukemia Group B (CALGB) trial comparing R-CHOP to DA-EPOCH-Rfor stage II-IV DLBCL has been completed, but the results are pending at the time of this publication (clinicaltrial.gov identifier NCT00118209). This regimen will be evaluated for ABC subtypes as well as for tumors with double hit genetics and MYC over-expression. The benefit of consolidative ASCT remains unclear. For patients with low risk disease, the risk of morbidity likely outweighs the potential benefit. For patients with high-risk disease (aaIPI≥ 2) ASCT may still be considered [76], but the benefit is uncertain given the conflicting results of 4 different phase III trials [77-80]. Two of these studies demonstrated improvement in PFS but not OS [77, 78] and the other 2 trials failed to show any benefit [79, 80]. The Lymphoma Study Association is currently conducting a trial to evaluate the role of consolidative ASCT in patients with a positive PET/CT scan after the first 2 cycles of chemotherapy (clinicaltrials.gov identifier NCT01285765).

Treatment of Older Adults

The management of DLBCL in older adults (>60 years of age) is complicated by the presence of medical comorbidities and increased treatment-related toxicities. Since DLBCL is a potentially curable disease and OS is associated with the dose of initial chemotherapy [81], dose reductions are avoided if possible. In patients with significant co-morbidities or those over the age of 80, reduced doses of CHOP with standard dose rituximab, termed R-miniCHOP, may be considered [82]. In addition, pre-phase treatment with vincristine and corticosteroids for elderly patients with a high burden of disease may reduce early mortality [65].

Treatment of Patients with Cardiac Dysfunction

For patients with cardiac disease precluding the use of anthracyclines (ejection fraction <30%), alternative regimens can be considered including R-GCVP (rituximab, gemcitabine, cyclophosphamide, vincristine, prednisolone) [83], R-CEPP (rituximab, cyclophosphamide, etoposide, prednisone, procarbazine) [84], and R-CEOP (rituximab, cyclophosphamide, etoposide, vincristine, prednisolone) [85]. These regimens have not been evaluated in randomized clinical trials and cannot be directly compared. As such, the appropriate regimen should be selected by the clinician based on toxicity profile.

HIV-Associated Lymphomas

Systemic DLBCLs associated with HIV are aggressive and usually present in advanced stage. Treatment is complicated by the underlying immunodeficiency and the potential for further reductions in CD4 count. Additionally, antiretroviral medications may have interactions or overlapping side effects with chemotherapy. Despite the potential for interactions, antiretroviral therapy should be incorporated into the treatment in order to decrease risk of opportunistic infections and improve outcomes [86]. The best initial chemotherapeutic regimen has not been established, but both R-CHOP and DA-EPOCH-R are reasonable options. Of note, rituximab should only be used in the case of CD-20 positive disease and when the CD4 count is greater than 50 per microliter [86]. DA-EPOCH-R should be considered if the patient has high-risk disease or plasmablastic histology.

Primary Mediastinal Large B-Cell Lymphoma

As previously mentioned, PMBCL is a distinct clinicopathologicentitiy with features similar to nodular sclerosing classical Hodgkin lymphoma. There are few randomized trials specifically evaluating the treatment of PMBCL due to its rarity. Radiation therapy remains a part of standard therapy due to early studies showing improved outcomes [87]. As this condition occurs primarily in young women, there is an interest in avoiding radiation to prevent long-term complications including second malignancies. The current approach is to treat limited stage disease with either 6 cycles of R-CHOP plus radiation or 6-8 cycles of DA-EPOCH-R without radiation. This is based on a National Cancer Institute study of 51 patients treated with DA-EPOCH-R without radiation that demonstrated an OS of 97% at 5 years [75]. A large multicenter clinical study by the International Extranodal Study Group is currently investigating whether patients with a negative PET/CT at the end of therapy can go without radiation (clinicaltrials.gov identifier NCT01599559). Additional agents under investigation for the treatment of PMBCL include Brentuximab-vedotin in combination with R-CHOP and PD-1 inhibitors· In the future, therapies targeted to the JAK-STAT and NF-κB pathways may prove beneficial for PMBCL [88]. Of note, mediastinal grey-zone lymphomas have a poor prognosis with limited response to chemotherapy. DA-EPOCH-R potentially in combination with radiation should be considered until effective targeted therapies are defined [88].

Relapsed/Refractory DLBCL

For patients who are refractory to or relapse following frontline therapy, high-dose chemotherapy followed by ASCT is considered the standard. While it can be difficult to achieve a complete remission (CR) in primary refractory patients, a proportion of relapsed patients will achieve a second CR and approximately half of these will maintain a durable response after ASCT [89]. There are several induction regimens used to achieve a CR prior to ASCT. The Intergroup Collaborative Trial in Relapsed Aggressive Lymphoma (CORAL) conducted a randomized clinical trial of R-ICE (rituximab, ifosfamide, carboplatin, etoposide) vs R-DHAP (rituximab, dexamethasone, high dose cytarabine, cisplatin) in relapsed/ refractory patients and found no difference in 3-year EFS and OS although R-DHAP was associated with improved clinical outcomes compared to R-ICE in GCB subtype [90]. Either of these regimens would be reasonable to use in the setting of relapse prior to ASCT. Allogeneic stem cell transplant can be considered in the setting of a second relapse [91].

Future Directions in the Treatment of DLBCL

Targeted Therapies for Surface Markers in DLBCL

Building on the successful addition of rituximab to CHOP chemotherapy, 2 new anti-CD20 monoclonal antibodies, Ofatumumab and Obinutuzumab, have been studied. Obinutuzumab has been shown to be more effective than rituximab for patients with chronic lymphocytic leukemia [92] and we are currently awaiting results of a phase III trial of Obinutuzumab plus CHOP chemotherapy for DLBCL (clinicaltrials.gov identifier NCT01287741). In addition, multiple antibody-drug conjugates are under development. Brentuximab-vedotin, directed towards CD30 was initially approved for Hodgkin's disease and is currently being evaluated as monotherapy for relapsed/refractory DLBCL (clinicaltrials.gov identifier NCT01421667) and as frontline therapy in combination with R-CHOP (clinicaltrials.gov identifier NCT01925612). Polatuzumab is an antibody-drug conjugate that targets CD79b, which is universally expressed in DLBCL. A phase II trial demonstrated a response rate of up to 48% in relapsed/refractory patients and there are ongoing trials looking at this agent in combination with chemotherapy [93]. Inotuzumabozogamicin (INO) consists of an anti-CD22 antibody conjugated to calicheamicin. A phase I/II study of INO in combination with rituximab for relapsed DLBCL showed an overall response rate of 74% [94]. However, a phase III trial was halted after an independent data monitoring committee determined that the experimental arm would not meet the primary objective of improved OS.

Targeted Therapies for GCB-Type DLBCL

Potential therapies under development for GCB-type DLBCLs target the abnormal epigenome and products of mutated oncogenes, such as *BCL6*. Epigenetic abnormalities are strongly associated with tumorigenesis in DLBCL and greater epigenetic heterogeneity has been associated with worse clinical outcomes [95]. Abnormal methylation leads to uncontrolled cell proliferation via activation of EZH2, which leads to decreased expression of tumor suppression genes. In addition, somatic activating mutations of EZH2 occur in up to 22% of GCB-type DLBCLs [95]. EZH2 inhibitors have shown encouraging pre-clinical results [96] and early phase clinical trials have begun (clinicaltrials.gov identifiers NCT01897571 and NCT02082977). Likewise, pre-clinical studies of BCL6 inhibitors have shown promising results [97].

Targeted therapies for ABC-Type DLBCL

Emerging therapies for the treatment of ABC-type DLBCLs include those targeted against abnormal NF-κB and BCR signaling. Since signaling through the NF-κB pathway requires proteasome degradation of IκB-alpha, proteasome inhibitors are currently under study. A phase I clinical trial demonstrated an acceptable toxicity profile for bortezomib plus R-CHOP in the front-line setting [98]. A phase II clinical trial evaluated proteasome inhibitors as monotherapy for relapsed/refractory DLBCL, but yielded disappointing results [99]. However, the addition of bortezomib to DA-EPOCH-R for relapsed/refractory DLBCL significantly improved outcomes for ABC-type DLBCLs (OS 10.8 months versus 3.4 months for GCB-type) [20]. Another study found that addition of bortezomib to R-CHOP in front-line treatment of non-GCB resulted in ORR of 100% with CR in 86% [100] and this overcame the poor outcome normally associated with this subtype. Several other clinical trials evaluating bortezomib as front-line therapy for non-GCB type DLBCLs are ongoing (clinicaltrial.gov identifiers NCT01324596 and BCT01848132). Similarly, lenalidomide, which is thought to inhibit NF-κB signaling, may improve the outcome for ABC-type DLBCL when added to front-line chemotherapy [101].

As a downstream regulator in the BCR signaling pathway, Bruton's Tyrosine Kinase (BTK) is another attractive target for ABC-type DLBCLs. Use of ibrutinib, a BTK inhibitor, as a single-agent in relapsed/refractory ABC-type DLBCL showed an overall response rate of 51% compared to 5% in the GCB subtype [88]. Furthermore, the addition of ibrutinib to R-CHOP was safe in phase I trial [102]. There are ongoing clinical trials evaluating ibrutinib in combination with chemotherapy in the upfront setting ClinicalTrial.gov identifiers NCT01855750 and NCT01569750). Numerous other potential targets in the BCR signaling pathway are under investigation.

Chimeric Antigen Receptor T (CAR T)-Cell Therapy

T cells can be modified to express chimeric antigen receptors for specific antigens present on tumor cells resulting in T-cell binding and tumor cell lysis. Recent success using anti-CD19 CAR T-cells in mature B-cell malignancies has been reported [103] Kochenderfer et al. reported a series of 15 patients with advanced B-cell malignancies treated with anti-CD19 CAR T-cells. Of the 7 evaluable patients with chemotherapy-refractory DLBCL, 4 achieved a CR durable up to 23 months at the time of most recent analysis [104].

Conclusion

The term DLBCL encompasses a broad range of clinically and biologically diverse lymphomas. DLBCLs are classified according to morphology, immunophenotype and anatomic location. However, recent gene expression profiling studies have revealed distinct molecular subtypes that have greater clinical significance. The current standard of care for DLBCL continues to change as targeted therapies are developed and as we determine how to incorporate these into front-line therapy.

References

[1] Siegel, R. L., Miller, K. D., Jemal, A. 2015. "Cancer statistics." *CA Cancer J. Clin.* 65: 5-29.

[2] Swerdlow SH, Campo E, Harris NL, Jaffe ES, Pileri SA, Stein H. 2008; *WHO classification of tumours of haematopoietic and lymphoid tissues*. IARC, Lyon.

[3] Morton, L. M., Wang, S. S., Devesa, S. S., Hartge, P., Weisenburger, D. D., Linet, M. S. 2006. "Lymphoma incidence patterns by WHO subtype in the United States, 1992-2001." *Blood* 107: 265-276.

[4] Sehn, L. H., Gascoyne, R. D. 2015. "Diffuse large B-cell lymphoma: optimizing outcome in the context of clinical and biologic heterogeneity." *Blood* 125: 22-32.

[5] Armitage, J. O., Weisenburger, D. D. 1998. "New approach to classifying non-Hodgkin's lymphomas: clinical features of the major histologic subtypes. Non-Hodgkin's Lymphoma Classification Project." *J. Clin. Oncol.* 16: 2780-2795.

[6] Cheson, B. D., Fisher, R. I., Barrington, S. F., Cavalli, F., Schwartz, L. H., Zucca, E., Lister, T. A. 2014. "Recommendations for initial evaluation, staging, and response assessment of Hodgkin and non-Hodgkin lymphoma: the Lugano classification." *J. Clin. Oncol.* 32: 3059-3068.

[7] 1993. "A predictive model for aggressive non-Hodgkin's lymphoma. The International Non-Hodgkin's Lymphoma Prognostic Factors Project." *N Engl. J. Med.* 329: 987-994.

[8] Zhou, Z., Sehn, L. H., Rademaker, A. W., Gordon, L. I., Lacasce, A. S., Crosby-Thompson, A., Vanderplas, A., et al. 2014. "An enhanced International Prognostic Index (NCCN-IPI) for patients with diffuse large B-cell lymphoma treated in the rituximab era." *Blood* 123: 837-842.

[9] Rosenwald, A., Wright, G., Chan, W. C., Connors, J. M., Campo, E., Fisher, R. I., Gascoyne, R. D., et al. 2002. "The use of molecular profiling to predict survival after chemotherapy for diffuse large-B-cell lymphoma." *N. Engl. J. Med.* 346: 1937-1947.

[10] Johnson, N. A., Slack, G. W., Savage, K. J., Connors, J. M., Ben-Neriah, S., Rogic, S., Scott, D. W., et al. 2012. "Concurrent expression of MYC and BCL2 in diffuse large B-cell lymphoma treated with rituximab plus cyclophosphamide, doxorubicin, vincristine, and prednisone." *J. Clin. Oncol.* 30: 3452-3459.

[11] Kurtz, D. M., Green, M. R., Bratman, S. V., Scherer, F., Liu, C. L., Kunder, C. A., Takahashi, K., et al. 2015. "Noninvasive monitoring of diffuse large B-cell lymphoma by immunoglobulin high-throughput sequencing." *Blood* 125: 3679-3687.

[12] Armand, P., Oki, Y., Neuberg, D. S., Faham, M., Cummings, C., Klinger, M., Weng, L., et al. 2013. "Detection of circulating tumour DNA in patients with aggressive B-cell non-Hodgkin lymphoma." *Br. J. Haematol.* 163: 123-126.

[13] Campo, E., Swerdlow, S. H., Harris, N. L., Pileri, S., Stein, H., Jaffe, E. S. 2011. "The 2008 WHO classification of lymphoid neoplasms and beyond: evolving concepts and practical applications." *Blood* 117: 5019-5032.

[14] Alizadeh, A. A., Eisen, M. B., Davis, R. E., Ma, C., Lossos, I. S., Rosenwald, A., Boldrick, J. C., et al. 2000. "Distinct types of diffuse large B-cell lymphoma identified by gene expression profiling." *Nature* 403: 503-511.

[15] Rosenwald, A., Wright, G., Leroy, K., Yu, X., Gaulard, P., Gascoyne, R. D., Chan, W. C., et al. 2003. "Molecular diagnosis of primary mediastinal B cell lymphoma identifies

a clinically favorable subgroup of diffuse large B cell lymphoma related to Hodgkin lymphoma." *J. Exp. Med.* 198: 851-862.

[16] Savage, K. J., Monti, S., Kutok, J. L., Cattoretti, G., Neuberg, D., De Leval, L., Kurtin, P., et al. 2003. "The molecular signature of mediastinal large B-cell lymphoma differs from that of other diffuse large B-cell lymphomas and shares features with classical Hodgkin lymphoma." *Blood* 102: 3871-3879.

[17] Pasqualucci, L., Trifonov, V., Fabbri, G., Ma, J., Rossi, D., Chiarenza, A., Wells, V. A., et al. 2011. "Analysis of the coding genome of diffuse large B-cell lymphoma." *Nat. Genet.* 43: 830-837.

[18] Wright, G., Tan, B., Rosenwald, A., Hurt, E. H., Wiestner, A., Staudt, L. M. 2003. "A gene expression-based method to diagnose clinically distinct subgroups of diffuse large B cell lymphoma." *Proc. Natl. Acad. Sci. U S A* 100: 9991-9996.

[19] Lenz, G., Wright, G., Dave, S. S., Xiao, W., Powell, J., Zhao, H., Xu, W., et al. 2008. "Stromal gene signatures in large-B-cell lymphomas." *N. Engl. J. Med.* 359: 2313-2323.

[20] Dunleavy, K., Pittaluga, S., Czuczman, M. S., Dave, S. S., Wright, G., Grant, N., Shovlin, M., et al. 2009. "Differential efficacy of bortezomib plus chemotherapy within molecular subtypes of diffuse large B-cell lymphoma." *Blood* 113: 6069-6076.

[21] Sweetenham, J. W. 2011. "Molecular signatures in the diagnosis and management of diffuse large B-cell lymphoma." *Curr. Opin. Hematol.* 18: 288-292.

[22] Gutierrez-Garcia, G., Cardesa-Salzmann, T., Climent, F., Gonzalez-Barca, E., Mercadal, S., Mate, J. L., Sancho, J. M., et al. 2011. "Gene-expression profiling and not immunophenotypic algorithms predicts prognosis in patients with diffuse large B-cell lymphoma treated with immunochemotherapy." *Blood* 117: 4836-4843.

[23] Zu, Y., Steinberg, S. M., Campo, E., Hans, C. P., Weisenburger, D. D., Braziel, R. M., Delabie, J., et al. 2005. "Validation of tissue microarray immunohistochemistry staining and interpretation in diffuse large B-cell lymphoma." *Leuk. Lymphoma.* 46: 693-701.

[24] de Jong, D., Xie, W., Rosenwald, A., Chhanabhai, M., Gaulard, P., Klapper, W., Lee, A., et al. 2009. "Immunohistochemical prognostic markers in diffuse large B-cell lymphoma: validation of tissue microarray as a prerequisite for broad clinical applications (a study from the Lunenburg Lymphoma Biomarker Consortium)." *J. Clin. Pathol.* 62: 128-138.

[25] Hans, C. P., Weisenburger, D. D., Greiner, T. C., Gascoyne, R. D., Delabie, J., Ott, G., Muller-Hermelink, H. K., et al. 2004. "Confirmation of the molecular classification of diffuse large B-cell lymphoma by immunohistochemistry using a tissue microarray." *Blood* 103: 275-282.

[26] Visco, C., Li, Y., Xu-Monette, Z. Y., Miranda, R. N., Green, T. M., Tzankov, A., Wen, W., et al. 2012. "Comprehensive gene expression profiling and immunohistochemical studies support application of immunophenotypic algorithm for molecular subtype classification in diffuse large B-cell lymphoma: a report from the International DLBCL Rituximab-CHOP Consortium Program Study." *Leukemia* 26: 2103-2113.

[27] Barrans, S., Crouch, S., Smith, A., Turner, K., Owen, R., Patmore, R., Roman, E., Jack, A. 2010. "Rearrangement of MYC is associated with poor prognosis in patients with diffuse large B-cell lymphoma treated in the era of rituximab." *J. Clin. Oncol.* 28: 3360-3365.

[28] Savage, K. J., Johnson, N. A., Ben-Neriah, S., Connors, J. M., Sehn, L. H., Farinha, P., Horsman, D. E., Gascoyne, R. D. 2009. "MYC gene rearrangements are associated with a poor prognosis in diffuse large B-cell lymphoma patients treated with R-CHOP chemotherapy." *Blood* 114: 3533-3537.

[29] Snuderl, M., Kolman, O. K., Chen, Y. B., Hsu, J. J., Ackerman, A. M., Dal Cin, P., Ferry, J. A., et al. 2010. "B-cell lymphomas with concurrent IGH-BCL2 and MYC rearrangements are aggressive neoplasms with clinical and pathologic features distinct from Burkitt lymphoma and diffuse large B-cell lymphoma." *Am. J. Surg. Pathol.* 34: 327-340.

[30] Barth, T. F., Leithauser, F., Joos, S., Bentz, M., Moller, P. 2002. "Mediastinal (thymic) large B-cell lymphoma: where do we stand?" *Lancet Oncol.* 3: 229-234.

[31] Oschlies, I., Burkhardt, B., Salaverria, I., Rosenwald, A., d'Amore, E. S., Szczepanowski, M., Koch, K., et al. 2011. "Clinical, pathological and genetic features of primary mediastinal large B-cell lymphomas and mediastinal gray zone lymphomas in children." *Haematologica* 96: 262-268.

[32] Feuerhake, F., Kutok, J. L., Monti, S., Chen, W., LaCasce, A. S., Cattoretti, G., Kurtin, P., et al. 2005. "NFkappaB activity, function, and target-gene signatures in primary mediastinal large B-cell lymphoma and diffuse large B-cell lymphoma subtypes." *Blood* 106: 1392-1399.

[33] Achten, R., Verhoef, G., Vanuytsel, L., De Wolf-Peeters, C. 2002. "Histiocyte-rich, T-cell-rich B-cell lymphoma: a distinct diffuse large B-cell lymphoma subtype showing characteristic morphologic and immunophenotypic features." *Histopathology* 40: 31-45.

[34] Tousseyn, T., De Wolf-Peeters, C. 2011. "T cell/histiocyte-rich large B-cell lymphoma: an update on its biology and classification." *Virchows Arch* 459: 557-563.

[35] Oyama, T., Yamamoto, K., Asano, N., Oshiro, A., Suzuki, R., Kagami, Y., Morishima, Y., et al. 2007. "Age-related EBV-associated B-cell lymphoproliferative disorders constitute a distinct clinicopathologic group: a study of 96 patients." *Clin. Cancer Res.* 13: 5124-5132.

[36] Beltran, B. E., Morales, D., Quinones, P., Medeiros, L. J., Miranda, R. N., Castillo, J. J. 2011. "EBV-positive diffuse large b-cell lymphoma in young immunocompetent individuals." *Clin. Lymphoma Myeloma Leuk.* 11: 512-516.

[37] Tun, H. W., Personett, D., Baskerville, K. A., Menke, D. M., Jaeckle, K. A., Kreinest, P., Edenfield, B., et al. 2008. "Pathway analysis of primary central nervous system lymphoma." *Blood* 111: 3200-3210.

[38] Sung, C. O., Kim, S. C., Karnan, S., Karube, K., Shin, H. J., Nam, D. H., Suh, Y. L., et al. 2011. "Genomic profiling combined with gene expression profiling in primary central nervous system lymphoma." *Blood* 117: 1291-1300.

[39] Al-Abbadi, M. A., Hattab, E. M., Tarawneh, M. S., Amr, S. S., Orazi, A., Ulbright, T. M. 2006. "Primary testicular diffuse large B-cell lymphoma belongs to the nongerminal center B-cell-like subgroup: A study of 18 cases." *Mod. Pathol.* 19: 1521-1527.

[40] Booman, M., Szuhai, K., Rosenwald, A., Hartmann, E., Kluin-Nelemans, H., de Jong, D., Schuuring, E., Kluin, P. 2008. "Genomic alterations and gene expression in primary diffuse large B-cell lymphomas of immune-privileged sites: the importance of apoptosis and immunomodulatory pathways." *J. Pathol.* 216: 209-217.

[41] Hoefnagel, J. J., Dijkman, R., Basso, K., Jansen, P. M., Hallermann, C., Willemze, R., Tensen, C. P., Vermeer, M. H. 2005. "Distinct types of primary cutaneous large B-cell lymphoma identified by gene expression profiling." *Blood* 105: 3671-3678.

[42] Ponzoni, M., Ferreri, A. J., Campo, E., Facchetti, F., Mazzucchelli, L., Yoshino, T., Murase, T., et al. 2007. "Definition, diagnosis, and management of intravascular large B-cell lymphoma: proposals and perspectives from an international consensus meeting." *J. Clin. Oncol.* 25: 3168-3173.

[43] Burg, G., Kempf, W., Cozzio, A., Feit, J., Willemze, R., E, S. Jaffe, Dummer, R., et al. 2005. "WHO/EORTC classification of cutaneous lymphomas 2005: histological and molecular aspects." *J. Cutan. Pathol.* 32: 647-674.

[44] Morgan, E. A., Nascimento, A. F. 2012. "Anaplastic lymphoma kinase-positive large B-cell lymphoma: an underrecognized aggressive lymphoma." *Adv. Hematol.* 2012: 529572.

[45] Colomo, L., Loong, F., Rives, S., Pittaluga, S., Martinez, A., Lopez-Guillermo, A., Ojanguren, J., et al. 2004. "Diffuse large B-cell lymphomas with plasmablastic differentiation represent a heterogeneous group of disease entities." *Am. J. Surg. Pathol.* 28: 736-747.

[46] Vega, F., Chang, C. C., Medeiros, L. J., Udden, M. M., Cho-Vega, J. H., Lau, C. C., Finch, C. J., et al. 2005. "Plasmablastic lymphomas and plasmablastic plasma cell myelomas have nearly identical immunophenotypic profiles." *Mod. Pathol.* 18: 806-815.

[47] Taddesse-Heath, L., Meloni-Ehrig, A., Scheerle, J., Kelly, J. C., Jaffe, E. S. 2010. "Plasmablastic lymphoma with MYC translocation: evidence for a common pathway in the generation of plasmablastic features." *Mod. Pathol.* 23: 991-999.

[48] Beaty, M. W., Kumar, S., Sorbara, L., Miller, K., Raffeld, M., Jaffe, E. S. 1999. "A biophenotypic human herpesvirus 8--associated primary bowel lymphoma." *Am. J. Surg. Pathol.* 23: 992-994.

[49] Petitjean, B., Jardin, F., Joly, B., Martin-Garcia, N., Tilly, H., Picquenot, J. M., Briere, J., et al. 2002. "Pyothorax-associated lymphoma: a peculiar clinicopathologic entity derived from B cells at late stage of differentiation and with occasional aberrant dual B- and T-cell phenotype." *Am. J. Surg. Pathol.* 26: 724-732.

[50] Aukema, S. M., Siebert, R., Schuuring, E., van Imhoff, G. W., Kluin-Nelemans, H. C., Boerma, E. J., Kluin, P. M. 2011. "Double-hit B-cell lymphomas." *Blood* 117: 2319-2331.

[51] Tomita, N., Tokunaka, M., Nakamura, N., Takeuchi, K., Koike, J., Motomura, S., Miyamoto, K., et al. 2009. "Clinicopathological features of lymphoma/leukemia patients carrying both BCL2 and MYC translocations." *Haematologica* 94: 935-943.

[52] Johnson, N. A., Savage, K. J., Ludkovski, O., Ben-Neriah, S., Woods, R., Steidl, C., Dyer, M. J., et al. 2009. "Lymphomas with concurrent BCL2 and MYC translocations: the critical factors associated with survival." *Blood* 114: 2273-2279.

[53] Hummel, M., Bentink, S., Berger, H., Klapper, W., Wessendorf, S., Barth, T. F., Bernd, H. W., *et al.* 2006. "A biologic definition of Burkitt's lymphoma from transcriptional and genomic profiling." *N. Engl. J. Med.* 354: 2419-2430.

[54] Jaffe, E. S., Pittaluga, S. 2011. "Aggressive B-cell lymphomas: a review of new and old entities in the WHO classification." *Hematology Am. Soc. Hematol. Educ. Program* 2011: 506-514.

[55] Traverse-Glehen, A., Pittaluga, S., Gaulard, P., Sorbara, L., Alonso, M. A., Raffeld, M., Jaffe, E. S. 2005. "Mediastinal gray zone lymphoma: the missing link between classic Hodgkin's lymphoma and mediastinal large B-cell lymphoma." *Am. J. Surg. Pathol.* 29: 1411-1421.

[56] Eberle, F. C., Rodriguez-Canales, J., Wei, L., Hanson, J. C., Killian, J. K., Sun, H. W., Adams, L. G., et al. 2011. "Methylation profiling of mediastinal gray zone lymphoma reveals a distinctive signature with elements shared by classical Hodgkin's lymphoma and primary mediastinal large B-cell lymphoma." *Haematologica* 96: 558-566.

[57] Fisher, R. I., Gaynor, E. R., Dahlberg, S., Oken, M. M., Grogan, T. M., Mize, E. M., Glick, J. H., Coltman, C. A., Jr., Miller, T. P. 1993. "Comparison of a standard regimen (CHOP) with three intensive chemotherapy regimens for advanced non-Hodgkin's lymphoma." *N. Engl. J. Med.* 328: 1002-1006.

[58] Bjorkholm, M., Andersson, T., Ahlbom, A., Osby, E. 2008. "CNOP (mitoxantrone) chemotherapy is inferior to CHOP (doxorubicin) in the treatment of patients with aggressive non-Hodgkin lymphoma (meta-analysis)." *Eur. J. Haematol.* 80: 477-482.

[59] Bartlett, N. L., Petroni, G. R., Parker, B. A., Wagner, N. D., Gockerman, J. P., Omura, G. A., Canellos, G. P., et al. 2001. "Dose-escalated cyclophosphamide, doxorubicin, vincristine, prednisone, and etoposide (CHOPE) chemotherapy for patients with diffuse lymphoma: Cancer and Leukemia Group B studies 8852 and 8854." *Cancer* 92: 207-217.

[60] Sparano, J. A., Weller, E., Nazeer, T., Habermann, T., Traynor, A. E., Manalo, J., Cassileth, P. 2002. "Phase 2 trial of infusional cyclophosphamide, doxorubicin, and etoposide in patients with poor-prognosis, intermediate-grade non-Hodgkin lymphoma: an Eastern Cooperative Oncology Group trial (E3493)." *Blood* 100: 1634-1640.

[61] Coiffier, B., Lepage, E., Briere, J., Herbrecht, R., Tilly, H., Bouabdallah, R., Morel, P., et al. 2002. "CHOP chemotherapy plus rituximab compared with CHOP alone in elderly patients with diffuse large-B-cell lymphoma." *N. Engl. J. Med.* 346: 235-242.

[62] Coiffier, B., Thieblemont, C., Van Den Neste, E., Lepeu, G., Plantier, I., Castaigne, S., Lefort, S., et al. 2010. "Long-term outcome of patients in the LNH-98.5 trial, the first randomized study comparing rituximab-CHOP to standard CHOP chemotherapy in DLBCL patients: a study by the Groupe d'Etudes des Lymphomes de l'Adulte." *Blood* 116: 2040-2045.

[63] Habermann, T. M., Weller, E. A., Morrison, V. A., Gascoyne, R. D., Cassileth, P. A., Cohn, J. B., Dakhil, S. R., et al. 2006. "Rituximab-CHOP versus CHOP alone or with maintenance rituximab in older patients with diffuse large B-cell lymphoma." *J. Clin. Oncol.* 24: 3121-3127.

[64] Pfreundschuh, M., Trumper, L., Osterborg, A., Pettengell, R., Trneny, M., Imrie, K., Ma, D., et al. 2006. "CHOP-like chemotherapy plus rituximab versus CHOP-like chemotherapy alone in young patients with good-prognosis diffuse large-B-cell lymphoma: a randomised controlled trial by the MabThera International Trial (MInT) Group." *Lancet Oncol.* 7: 379-391.

[65] Pfreundschuh, M., Trumper, L., Kloess, M., Schmits, R., Feller, A. C., Rube, C., Rudolph, C., et al. 2004. "Two-weekly or 3-weekly CHOP chemotherapy with or without etoposide for the treatment of elderly patients with aggressive lymphomas: results of the NHL-B2 trial of the DSHNHL." *Blood* 104: 634-641.

[66] Verdonck, L. F., Notenboom, A., de Jong, D. D., MacKenzie, M. A., Verhoef, G. E., Kramer, M. H., Ossenkoppele, G. J., et al. 2007. "Intensified 12-week CHOP (I-CHOP) plus G-CSF compared with standard 24-week CHOP (CHOP-21) for patients with intermediate-risk aggressive non-Hodgkin lymphoma: a phase 3 trial of the Dutch-Belgian Hemato-Oncology Cooperative Group (HOVON)." *Blood* 109: 2759-2766.

[67] Ohmachi, K., Tobinai, K., Kobayashi, Y., Itoh, K., Nakata, M., Shibata, T., Morishima, Y., et al. 2011. "Phase III trial of CHOP-21 versus CHOP-14 for aggressive non-Hodgkin's lymphoma: final results of the Japan Clinical Oncology Group Study, JCOG 9809." *Ann. Oncol.* 22: 1382-1391.

[68] Cunningham, D., Hawkes, E. A., Jack, A., Qian, W., Smith, P., Mouncey, P., Pocock, C., et al. 2013. "Rituximab plus cyclophosphamide, doxorubicin, vincristine, and prednisolone in patients with newly diagnosed diffuse large B-cell non-Hodgkin lymphoma: a phase 3 comparison of dose intensification with 14-day versus 21-day cycles." *Lancet* 381: 1817-1826.

[69] Delarue, R., Tilly, H., Mounier, N., Petrella, T., Salles, G., Thieblemont, C., Bologna, S., et al. 2013. "Dose-dense rituximab-CHOP compared with standard rituximab-CHOP in elderly patients with diffuse large B-cell lymphoma (the LNH03-6B study): a randomised phase 3 trial." *Lancet Oncol.* 14: 525-533.

[70] Pfreundschuh, M., Schubert, J., Ziepert, M., Schmits, R., Mohren, M., Lengfelder, E., Reiser, M., et al. 2008. "Six versus eight cycles of bi-weekly CHOP-14 with or without rituximab in elderly patients with aggressive CD20+ B-cell lymphomas: a randomised controlled trial (RICOVER-60)." *Lancet Oncol.* 9: 105-116.

[71] Recher, C., Coiffier, B., Haioun, C., Molina, T. J., Ferme, C., Casasnovas, O., Thieblemont, C., et al. 2011. "Intensified chemotherapy with ACVBP plus rituximab versus standard CHOP plus rituximab for the treatment of diffuse large B-cell lymphoma (LNH03-2B): an open-label randomised phase 3 trial." *Lancet* 378: 1858-1867.

[72] Molina, T. J., Canioni, D., Copie-Bergman, C., Recher, C., Briere, J., Haioun, C., Berger, F., et al. 2014. "Young patients with non-germinal center B-cell-like diffuse large B-cell lymphoma benefit from intensified chemotherapy with ACVBP plus rituximab compared with CHOP plus rituximab: analysis of data from the Groupe d'Etudes des Lymphomes de l'Adulte/lymphoma study association phase III trial LNH 03-2B." *J. Clin. Oncol.* 32: 3996-4003.

[73] Dunleavy, K., Little, R. F., Pittaluga, S., Grant, N., Wayne, A. S., Carrasquillo, J. A., Steinberg, S. M., et al. 2010. "The role of tumor histogenesis, FDG-PET, and short-course EPOCH with dose-dense rituximab (SC-EPOCH-RR) in HIV-associated diffuse large B-cell lymphoma." *Blood* 115: 3017-3024.

[74] Garcia-Suarez, J., Banas, H., Arribas, I., De Miguel, D., Pascual, T., Burgaleta, C. 2007. "Dose-adjusted EPOCH plus rituximab is an effective regimen in patients with poor-prognostic untreated diffuse large B-cell lymphoma: results from a prospective observational study." *Br. J. Haematol.* 136: 276-285.

[75] Dunleavy, K., Pittaluga, S., Maeda, L. S., Advani, R., Chen, C. C., Hessler, J., Steinberg, S. M., et al. 2013. "Dose-adjusted EPOCH-rituximab therapy in primary mediastinal B-cell lymphoma." *N. Engl. J. Med.* 368: 1408-1416.

[76] Fitoussi, O., Belhadj, K., Mounier, N., Parrens, M., Tilly, H., Salles, G., Feugier, P., et al. 2011. "Survival impact of rituximab combined with ACVBP and upfront

consolidation autotransplantation in high-risk diffuse large B-cell lymphoma for GELA." *Haematologica* 96: 1136-1143.

[77] Stiff, P. J., Unger, J. M., Cook, J. R., Constine, L. S., Couban, S., Stewart, D. A., Shea, T. C., et al. 2013. "Autologous transplantation as consolidation for aggressive non-Hodgkin's lymphoma." *N. Engl. J. Med.* 369: 1681-1690.

[78] Vitolo, U., Chiappella, A., Brusamolino, E. 2011. "A randomized multicentre phase III study for first line treatment of young patients with high risk (aaIPI 2-3) diffuse large B-cell lymphoma (DLBCL): rituximab (R) plus dose-dense chemotherapy CHOP14/megaCHOP14 with or without intensified high-dose chemotherapy (HDC) and autologous stem cell transplantation (ASCT). results of DLCL04 trial of Italian Lymphoma Foundation Annals of Oncology." 22 (4).

[79] Schmitz, N., Nickelsen, M., Ziepert, M., Haenel, M., Borchmann, P., Schmidt, C., Viardot, A., et al. 2012. "Conventional chemotherapy (CHOEP-14) with rituximab or high-dose chemotherapy (MegaCHOEP) with rituximab for young, high-risk patients with aggressive B-cell lymphoma: an open-label, randomised, phase 3 trial (DSHNHL 2002-1)." *Lancet Oncol.* 13: 1250-1259.

[80] Milipied, N, Legouill, S, Lamy, T. 2010. "'No Benefit of First-Line Rituximab (R) - High-Dose Therapy (R-HDT) Over R-CHOP14 for Young Adults with Diffuse Large B-Cell Lymphoma. Preliminary Results of the GOELAMS 075 Prospective Multicentre Randomized Trial' paper presented at 53rd ASH Annual Meeting and Exposition." *Blood*.

[81] Kwak, L. W., Halpern, J., Olshen, R. A., Horning, S. J. 1990. "Prognostic significance of actual dose intensity in diffuse large-cell lymphoma: results of a tree-structured survival analysis." *J. Clin. Oncol.* 8: 963-977.

[82] Peyrade, F., Jardin, F., Thieblemont, C., Thyss, A., Emile, J. F., Castaigne, S., Coiffier, B., et al. 2011. "Attenuated immunochemotherapy regimen (R-miniCHOP) in elderly patients older than 80 years with diffuse large B-cell lymphoma: a multicentre, single-arm, phase 2 trial." *Lancet Oncol.* 12: 460-468.

[83] Fields, P. A., Townsend, W., Webb, A., Counsell, N., Pocock, C., Smith, P., Jack, A., et al. 2014. "De novo treatment of diffuse large B-cell lymphoma with rituximab, cyclophosphamide, vincristine, gemcitabine, and prednisolone in patients with cardiac comorbidity: a United Kingdom National Cancer Research Institute trial." *J. Clin. Oncol.* 32:2 82-287.

[84] Chao, N. J., Rosenberg, S. A., Horning, S. J. 1990. "CEPP(B): an effective and well-tolerated regimen in poor-risk, aggressive non-Hodgkin's lymphoma." *Blood* 76: 1293-1298.

[85] Moccia, A. , Schaff, K. , Hoskins, P. , Klasa, R. 2009. "R-CHOP with Etoposide Substituted for Doxorubicin (R-CEOP): Excellent Outcome in Diffuse Large B Cell Lymphoma for Patients with a Contraindication to Anthracyclines." *Blood* 408.

[86] Barta, S. K., Xue, X., Wang, D., Tamari, R., Lee, J. Y., Mounier, N., Kaplan, L. D., et al. 2013. "Treatment factors affecting outcomes in HIV-associated non-Hodgkin lymphomas: a pooled analysis of 1546 patients." *Blood* 122: 3251-3262.

[87] Zinzani, P. L., Martelli, M., Bertini, M., Gianni, A. M., Devizzi, L., Federico, M., Pangalis, G., et al. 2002. "Induction chemotherapy strategies for primary mediastinal large B-cell lymphoma with sclerosis: a retrospective multinational study on 426 previously untreated patients." *Haematologica* 87: 1258-1264.

[88] Wilson, W., Gerecitano, J., Goy, A., de Vos, S., Kenkre, V., Barr, P. 2012. "The Bruton's Tyrosine Kinase (BTK) Inhibitor, Ibrutinib (PCI-32765), Has Preferential Activity in the ABC Subtype of Relapsed/Refractory De Novo Diffuse Large B-Cell Lymphoma (DLBCL): Interim Results of a Multi- center, Open-Label, Phase 2 Study." *Blood* 120.

[89] Cortelazzo, S., Rambaldi, A., Rossi, A., Oldani, E., Ghielmini, M., Benedetti, F., Tarella, C., et al. 2001. "Intensification of salvage treatment with high-dose sequential chemotherapy improves the outcome of patients with refractory or relapsed aggressive non-Hodgkin's lymphoma." *Br. J. Haematol.* 114: 333-341.

[90] Thieblemont, C., Briere, J., Mounier, N., Voelker, H. U., Cuccuini, W., Hirchaud, E., Rosenwald, A., et al. 2011. "The germinal center/activated B-cell subclassification has a prognostic impact for response to salvage therapy in relapsed/refractory diffuse large B-cell lymphoma: a bio-CORAL study." *J. Clin. Oncol.* 29: 4079-4087.

[91] Escalon, M. P., Champlin, R. E., Saliba, R. M., Acholonu, S. A., Hosing, C., Fayad, L., Giralt, S., et al. 2004. "Nonmyeloablative allogeneic hematopoietic transplantation: a promising salvage therapy for patients with non-Hodgkin's lymphoma whose disease has failed a prior autologous transplantation." *J. Clin. Oncol.* 22: 2419-2423.

[92] Goede, V., Fischer, K., Busch, R., Engelke, A., Eichhorst, B., Wendtner, C. M., Chagorova, T., et al. 2014. "Obinutuzumab plus chlorambucil in patients with CLL and coexisting conditions." *N. Engl. J. Med.* 370: 1101-1110.

[93] Palanca-Wessels, M., Salles, G., Czuczman, M. 2013. "Final results of a phase I study of the anti-CD79b antibody-drug conjugate DCDS4501A in relapsed or refractory (R/R) B-cell non-Hodgkin lymphoma (NHL)." *Blood* 122: 4400.

[94] Fayad, L., Offner, F., Smith, M. R., Verhoef, G., Johnson, P., Kaufman, J. L., Rohatiner, A., et al. 2013. "Safety and clinical activity of a combination therapy comprising two antibody-based targeting agents for the treatment of non-Hodgkin lymphoma: results of a phase I/II study evaluating the immunoconjugate inotuzumab ozogamicin with rituximab." *J. Clin. Oncol.* 31: 573-583.

[95] Jiang, Y., Melnick, A. 2015. "The epigenetic basis of diffuse large B-cell lymphoma." *Semin. Hematol.* 52: 86-96.

[96] Knutson, S. K., Wigle, T. J., Warholic, N. M., Sneeringer, C. J., Allain, C. J., Klaus, C. R., Sacks, J. D., et al. 2012. "A selective inhibitor of EZH2 blocks H3K27 methylation and kills mutant lymphoma cells." *Nat. Chem. Biol.* 8: 890-896.

[97] Cerchietti, L. C., Yang, S. N., Shaknovich, R., Hatzi, K., Polo, J. M., Chadburn, A., Dowdy, S. F., Melnick, A. 2009. "A peptomimetic inhibitor of BCL6 with potent antilymphoma effects in vitro and in vivo." *Blood* 113: 3397-3405.

[98] Furman, R. R., Martin, P., Ruan, J., Cheung, Y. K., Vose, J. M., LaCasce, A. S., Elstrom, R., Coleman, M., Leonard, J. P. 2010. "Phase 1 trial of bortezomib plus R-CHOP in previously untreated patients with aggressive non-Hodgkin lymphoma." *Cancer* 116: 5432-5439.

[99] Goy, A., Younes, A., McLaughlin, P., Pro, B., Romaguera, J. E., Hagemeister, F., Fayad, L., et al. 2005. "Phase II study of proteasome inhibitor bortezomib in relapsed or refractory B-cell non-Hodgkin's lymphoma." *J. Clin. Oncol.* 23: 667-675.

[100] Ruan, J., Martin, P., Furman, R. R., Lee, S. M., Cheung, K., Vose, J. M., Lacasce, A., et al. 2011. "Bortezomib plus CHOP-rituximab for previously untreated diffuse large B-cell lymphoma and mantle cell lymphoma." *J. Clin. Oncol.* 29: 690-697.

[101] B., Foran, J. M., Nelson, G. D., Thompson, C. A., et al. 2015. "Lenalidomide combined with R-CHOP overcomes negative prognostic impact of non-germinal center B-cell phenotype in newly diagnosed diffuse large B-Cell lymphoma: a phase II study." *J. Clin. Oncol.* 33: 251-257.

[102] Younes, A., Thieblemont, C., Morschhauser, F., Flinn, I., Friedberg, J. W., Amorim, S., Hivert, B., et al. 2014. "Combination of ibrutinib with rituximab, cyclophosphamide, doxorubicin, vincristine, and prednisone (R-CHOP) for treatment-naive patients with CD20-positive B-cell non-Hodgkin lymphoma: a non-randomised, phase 1b study." *Lancet Oncol.* 15: 1019-1026.

[103] Kochenderfer, J. N., Yu, Z., Frasheri, D., Restifo, N. P., Rosenberg, S. A. 2010. "Adoptive transfer of syngeneic T cells transduced with a chimeric antigen receptor that recognizes murine CD19 can eradicate lymphoma and normal B cells." *Blood* 116: 3875-3886.

[104] Kochenderfer, J. N., Dudley, M. E., Kassim, S. H., Somerville, R. P., Carpenter, R. O., Stetler-Stevenson, M., Yang, J. C., et al. 2015. "Chemotherapy-refractory diffuse large B-cell lymphoma and indolent B-cell malignancies can be effectively treated with autologous T cells expressing an anti-CD19 chimeric antigen receptor." *J. Clin. Oncol.* 33: 540-549.

In: Diffuse Large B-Cell Lymphoma (DLBCL)
Editor: Haipeng Shao
ISBN: 978-1-63484-402-4

Chapter 3

The Evolving Role of Radiation Therapy in the Management of Diffuse Large B-Cell Lymphoma

Kamran A. Ahmed and Sungjune Kim*
Department of Radiation Oncology, H. Lee Moffitt
Cancer Center and Research Institute, Tampa, FL, US

Abstract

Historically, radiation therapy (RT) was the primary curative treatment for limited stage diffuse large B-cell lymphoma (DLBCL). Today, with the advancement of combined chemotherapy regimens including CHOP (cyclophosphamide, doxorubicin, vincristine, and prednisone) with the addition of the anti-CD20 antibody rituximab (R-CHOP), radiation treatment has evolved to a consolidative role following primary chemotherapy. Radiation therapy continues to play a significant role in the management of DLBCL both in the limited and advanced stages. However, due to a scarcity of data in the era of R-CHOP, radiation practices differ widely amongst individual practitioners and institutions. Critics of consolidative RT are often influenced by the risk of late toxicities from historical RT techniques. In this chapter, we will outline the role of RT in the management of DLBCL. In addition, we will describe the evolution of RT techniques in the management of DLBCL. Finally, we will outline research questions, which currently exist and future directions for prospective randomized studies to address controversial areas in the management of DLBCL.

Introduction

Diffuse large B-cell lymphoma (DLBCL) is the most common subtype of Non-Hodgkin lymphoma (NHL). The majority of patients present with advanced disease (≥ stage 3); however, a third of patients present with limited stage disease (stages I-II) [1, 2]. Although

* Corresponding author: Sungjune Kim. E-mail: Sungjune.Kim@moffitt.org, phone: 813-745-7898.

chemotherapy now plays a significant role in the management of DLBCL, historically radiation treatment alone played the central management role in DLBCL [1, 3].

Long-term results from the British National Lymphoma Investigation led to CR rates of 98% in low-grade disease and 84% in high grade disease with radiation therapy [3]. However, systemic control remained an issue with progression free survival (PFS) of 47% and 45% in low and high grade disease, respectively at 10 years [3]. Similar findings were noted in studies of patients treated in the 1970s and 1980s [4]. Although, local control was preserved in patients treated with radiotherapy alone, the high rate of systemic pathogenesis of DLBCL and the high rate of relapse in sites outside of the radiation treatment field led to investigation of chemotherapy treatment options. The use of adjuvant chemotherapy in the management of DLBCL took place in a series of studies in the 1970s and 1980s. The studies showed significant benefit of combined modality management with increasing relapse free survival (RFS) and overall survival (OS) rates.

The Era of CHOP

Prospective Trials

Studies over the past several decades have revealed the benefits of combined modality treatment in the management of DLBCL. A summary of these prospective studies is located in Table 1. One of the first trials to assess combined modality management and reveal the benefits of the addition of chemotherapy was the Southwest Oncology Group (SWOG) study 8736 [5]. The study was designed to test eight cycles of CHOP (cyclophosphamide, adriamycin, oncovin, and prednisone) or a reduction of chemotherapy to three cycles of CHOP alongside involved field radiation therapy (IFRT) of 40 to 55 Gy. Radiation doses were determined by the radiation oncologist with higher doses generally delivered to patients with residual disease. Five-year results revealed a significant benefit in OS (82% vs.72%, respectively, $p = 0.02$) [5]. Similarly, 5 year PFS was noted to be superior in those patients treated with CHOP + IFRT (77% vs. 64%, respectively, $p = 0.03$). In addition, there were a larger proportion of patients unable to tolerate the arm with extended chemotherapy due to increased toxicity. Reported rates were 2% vs. 13% $p < 0.01$. A subsequent report of this study was published only in abstract form [6]. In this follow-up study, the authors reported convergence of survival curves between the arms. However, without further details on the patterns of failure and causes of death, this result with longer follow-up is difficult to interpret.

The Eastern Cooperative Oncology Group (ECOG) 1484 study attempted to answer whether RT could be eliminated in patients with a complete response (CR) following the delivery of 8 cycles of CHOP [7]. A total of 352 stage I and II patients were enrolled. All patients received 8 cycles of CHOP. Patients who were noted to have a partial response (PR) received IFRT to 40 Gy. The patients with a CR following chemotherapy were randomized to IFRT to 30 Gy or observation. Notably there was a high dropout rate of patients with CR. Twenty percent of complete responding patients did not receive their assigned treatment. This high dropout rate has been attributed in part to CHOP related toxicity noted during extended regimens.

Table 1. Summary of CHOP +/- RT Prospective Trials

Trial	Patient Characteristics	No. of Patients	Arms	Results	P-value
SWOG 8736	Median age: 59 Normal LDH: 80% PS 0-1: 97% Stage II: 33% Excluded bulky Stage II	401	CHOP X 3 + RT or CHOP X 8	CHOP X 3 +RT: 5-year PFS 77%; 5-year OS 92% CHOP X 8: 5-year PFS 64%; 5-year OS 72%	PFS: P = 0.03 OS: P = 0.02
ECOG 1484	Median age: 59 PS 0-1: 92% Stage II: 68% Bulky: 31%	399	CHOP X 8 if CR randomized to +/- RT. If PR received RT	CR with RT: 6-year DFS 69%; 5-year OS 87% CR without RT: 6-year DFS 53%; 6-year OS 73%	DFS: P = 0.05 OS: P = 0.23
LNH 93-1	Median age: 47 Normal LDH, PS 0-1 Stage II: 32% Bulky: 11%	647	CHOP X 3 + RT or ACVBP	CHOP X 3 RT: 5-year EFS 74%; 5-year OS 81% ACVBP: 5-year EFS 82%; 5-year OS 90%	EFS: P < 0.001 OS: P = 0.001
LNH 93-4	Median age: 68 Normal LDH, PS 0-1 Stage II: 32% Bulky: 8%	574	CHOP X 4 + RT or CHOP X 4	CHOP X 4 + RT: 5-year EFS 64%; 5-year OS 68% CHOP X 4: 5-year EFS 61%; 5-year OS 72%	EFS: P = 0.56 OS: P = 0.54

LDH, lactate dehydrogenase; PS, performance status; CHOP, cyclophosphamide, adriamycin, oncovin, and prednisone; ACVBP, doxorubicin, cyclophosphamide, vindesine, bleomycin, and prednisone; EFS, event free survival; OS, overall survival; PFS, progression free survival; DFS, disease free survival; and RT, radiation therapy.

In addition, 26% of patients in the consolidation RT group versus 17% in the chemotherapy alone arm had bulky disease, p = 0.13. At 6 years, a benefit in disease free survival (DFS) was observed in patients who received consolidation IFRT compared with observation alone (69% vs. 53%, respectively, p = 0.05), based on the intent to treat analysis. Similarly, failure free survival (FFS) was favored in the IFRT arm (70% vs. 53%, respectively, p = 0.06). OS at 5, 10 and 15 years was higher in patients who received IFRT compared with observation alone (87%, 68% and 60% vs. 73%, 65% and 44%, respectively; based on the as treated analysis). However, these large OS differences were not statistically significant. Toxicity was an issue in this study with grade 4 neutropenia reported in 32% of patients with four treatment related deaths (attributed to infection and congestive heart failure) from prolonged doxorubicin based regimens. DFS was the primary end point of this trial. This study was not powered to detect an OS difference between arms given the high dropout rate. Despite the limits of this study a DFS benefit was noted with the addition of RT.

Critics of consolidation RT most often point to two trials performed by the Groupe d'Etude des Lymphomes de l'Adulte (GELA) in patients with early stage DLBCL. It is important to note that both studies were performed in the pre-PET and pre-rituximab eras. The GELA LNH 931 trial tested whether consolidation IFRT could be replaced by an aggressive, dose intense chemotherapy regimen [8]. A total of 647 patients with stage III NHL were enrolled in this trial with patients randomized to either intensive chemotherapy alone with three cycles of induction with dose intense doxorubicin, cyclophosphamide, vindesine, bleomycin, and prednisone (ACVBP) followed by sequential consolidation with two cycles of methotrexate, four cycles of etoposide and ifosfamide, and then two cycles of cytarabine (IVAM) (n = 318), or three cycles of CHOP followed by IFRT (n = 329). All patients were under 61 years of age and did not have any adverse prognostic factors, as defined by the age-adjusted IPI.

At 5 years, event free survival (EFS) and OS were both superior in the intensive chemotherapy alone group compared with chemoradiotherapy, which was statistically significant (82% vs. 74%, and 90% vs. 81%, respectively). It is important to note that this study was not designed to test the value of consolidation RT, but rather was testing a more potent alternative to abbreviated CHOP plus consolidation RT, which constituted the standard of care at the time.

The patterns of failure differed between the two cohorts. In the group receiving consolidation RT, 23% of relapses occurred in local sites only, compared to 41% of relapses in the intensive chemotherapy group [8]. However, there was a strong benefit in the ACVBP arm in terms of distant control with a rate of 38% compared to 72% in the arm receiving CHOP plus consolidation RT. However, there was more toxicity noted in the ACVBP arm. Acutely, ACVBP was noted to have a 12% risk of grade 3 or 4 infections in the intensive chemotherapy arm, compared to only 1% in the arm of abbreviated CHOP chemotherapy and consolidation RT. ACVBP has also been found to have significant late toxicities with a pooled analysis from the GELA studies noting neoplastic rates of 3% and late toxicity rates of 5% [9]. There was a particularly high rate of secondary MDS/AML with a 6-fold increase in men and a 20-fold increase noted in females in comparison to the general population. Due to these risks, ACVBP has not been widely accepted into common clinical practice.

A second trial from the GELA group, the GELA LNH 934 trial, assessed the efficacy of adding consolidation RT to four cycles of CHOP in patients over 60 years with NHL [10]. A total of 576 patients were randomized to four cycles of CHOP alone followed by either observation (n = 277) or 39.6 Gy of IFRT (n = 299). At 5 years, no significant differences were observed between the chemotherapy alone and chemoradiotherapy arms in EFS and OS (61% vs. 64% and 72% vs. 68%, respectively). On multivariate analysis (MVA), stage II disease and male sex affected OS. In the chemotherapy alone group, 47% of patients had local relapses while, 16% of relapses were both local and distant at the time of relapse, and the remaining cases were exclusively distant (37%). By contrast, only 21% of the relapses in the chemoradiotherapy group were exclusively local, 13% were both local and distant, and 66% of cases were exclusively distant. Toxicity did not significantly differ between the two arms.

There were several issues regarding the quality of RT delivery in the GELA LNH 934 trial. First, only 77% of patients received the actual recommended dose of 40 Gy, and 5% of patients began radiation approximately 3 months after chemotherapy. In addition, 12% of patients in the consolidation RT arm never received the prescribed radiation therapy. As EFS and OS were calculated based on an intent-to-treat analysis, these unirradiated patients were included in the consolidation RT arm for analysis. Re-evaluation of the trial outcome with the as treated analysis revealed a 5 year EFS of 71% in the chemoradiotherapy arm and 64% in the chemotherapy alone arm, which was not statistically significant. However, the trial may have been underpowered to detect the difference between the arms. Although oncologists often quote this trial as a rationale to omit RT, the flaws in this trial both in the dose and delivery of radiation therapy renders it difficult to draw firm conclusions on the use of RT.

Retrospective Studies

Several key retrospective series have also evaluated the role of RT in patients treated with DLBCL. The British Columbia Cancer Agency (BCCA) reported the long-term results of 308 patients with nonbulky stage IA or IIA disease treated with three cycles of doxorubicin based chemotherapy followed by IFRT [11]. Patients were treated to a dose equivalent of 30 Gy in 10 fractions. At 5 and 10 years the PFS rates were 81% and 74%, and OS rates were 80% and 63%, respectively. The OS and PFS rates for all patients, as well as PFS and OS rates according to stage modified IPI risk factors were similar to results from SWOG 8736 providing further evidence that combined chemoradiotherapy is a good treatment option for early stage DLBCL.

A Surveillance, Epidemiology and End Results (SEER) study also examined consolidation RT in patients with limited stage DLBCL [12]. The study assessed approximately 13,000 patients with stage I, IE, II, or IIE DLBCL treated between 1988 and 2004. Approximately 40% of patients received RT while 60% did not. The receipt of RT was associated with a significant disease specific survival improvement and OS benefit that lasted 15 years [hazard ratio (HR), 0.82, $p < 0.0001$], which remained significant on MVA. Although the study is large and shows a clear survival benefit to the receipt of RT, one of the main limitations of analyses from the SEER database is the lack of chemotherapy details. In a separate publication, the authors assessed cardiac specific mortality (CSM) in NHL patients who were treated with or without RT in the SEER database [13]. The exclusion of RT from the treatment regimen was associated with a significant increase in CSM. It can be assumed that patients that did not receive RT likely received more intensive chemotherapy regimens involving adriamycin suggesting side effects of extended chemotherapy regimens leading to increased cardiac events.

R-CHOP Studies

Rituximab is a CD20 antibody that has offered a targeted management approach to patients with DLBCL. The first clinical trial to assess the effect of the addition of rituximab to CHOP chemotherapy was the SWOG 0014 study [14]. In this phase II study, a total of 60 patients with limited stage DLBCL with at least one risk factor as defined by the stage-modified International Prognostic Index (IPI) were included. Risk factors included patients with nonbulky stage II disease, age >60 years, WHO performance status of 2, and/or elevated serum lactate dehydrogenase. All patients in this study received three cycles of CHOP and four doses of rituximab, which was followed by IFRT with radiation doses ranging between 40 and 46 Gy. The study found that at 4 years, PFS and OS rates were 88% and 92%, respectively. These results have been compared in a retrospective fashion to patients treated on the SWOG 8736 trial with 3 cycles of CHOP with IFRT. In this analysis, both PFS and OS were improved with the addition of rituximab with rates of 88% compared to 78% and 92% vs. 88%, respectively.

A retrospective series from MD Anderson Cancer Center assessed the efficacy of consolidation RT, following R-CHOP chemotherapy, an area where prospective data is lacking and questions regarding best clinical practice remains. The study assessed a total of 469 patients, 40% with stage I or II disease and the remaining with advanced stage III or IV disease [15]. At least 6 cycles of R-CHOP were received by most patients (70%) with 30% of patients treated with IFRT to doses between 30-39.6 Gy. With a median follow-up of 36 months (range: 8-85 months) MVA revealed that RT ($p < .0001$) influenced OS and PFS. The 5 year PFS and OS rates for all patients who received chemoradiotherapy were 82% and 91%, respectively. PFS and OS rates in patients treated with chemotherapy alone were 59% and 68%, respectively. A matched pair analysis based on three factors: bulky disease, response to therapy, and IPI score was conducted on patients with stage I or II disease who received six to eight cycles of R-CHOP chemotherapy. A significant benefit to the addition of consolidation RT was observed with a similar trend in patients with stage III or IV disease. In addition, the study noted no infield relapses in patients receiving consolidation RT. This study is important due to its use of modern radiation therapy techniques as well as the analysis in patients treated with R-CHOP, which is now the standard chemotherapy regimen of choice in DLBCL.

Further study into the use of consolidation RT in the era of R-CHOP has been provided by the recent study from Dabaja et al. [16]. The study utilized the NCCN outcomes database to assess 841 patients with stage I-IV DLBCL. The majority of patients (84%) received R-CHOP and 35% received consolidative radiation therapy. At 5 years, both OS and FFS rates were better for patients who received RT versus those who did not (OS, 91% vs. 83%, $p = 0.01$; FFS, 83% vs. 76%, $p = 0.05$). A matched pair analysis was conducted with 217 pairs matched by age, stage, IPI, B symptoms, disease bulk, and response to chemotherapy. This analysis revealed there to be a trend with receipt of RT improving OS (HR 0.53, $p = 0.07$) and FFS (HR 0.77, $p = 0.34$) for patients with stage III/IV disease, but too few events took place among those with stage I/II disease for meaningful comparisons.

A recent analysis of outcomes from the National Cancer Data Base of over 59,000 patients treated for stage I and II DLBCL with multiagent chemotherapy alone or chemotherapy plus consolidative RT between 1998 and 2012 has provided more evidence on the benefits of consolidation RT following R-CHOP [17]. A significant decline in the use of RT was noted in the study with 47% of patients receiving RT in 2000 and 32% in 2012. With a median follow-up of 60 months, the estimated 5 and 10 year OS rates were, respectively, 79% and 59% for all patients, 75% and 55% for patients receiving chemotherapy alone, and 82% and 64% for patients receiving combined modality therapy ($p < .001$). After adjusting for immortal times and indication bias, combined modality therapy was associated with better OS (HR 0.66; 95% CI, 0.61 to 0.71, $p < .001$) than chemotherapy alone. This study gives further evidence to the use of radiation combined with R-CHOP chemotherapy in the management of DLBCL. A retrospective review of 257 DLBCL patients treated from the International Oncology Network between 2005 and 2012 similarly found low rates of utilization of RT following R-CHOP chemotherapy with 78% of patients undergoing active surveillance, 13% receiving maintenance rituximab-based treatment, and 6% receiving radiation therapy [18]. Relapse rates among patients receiving maintenance rituximab, active surveillance, and radiation therapy were 28% (6/21), 19% (24/124), and 0%, (0/10), respectively ($p = 0.08$). This study indicates the low rate of utilization of consolidative RT.

Retrospective evidence of the benefit of consolidative IFRT to R-CHOP has also been provided by an analysis of 216 stage I-IV DLBCL patients who were enrolled in two clinical trials at Italian Lymphoma Study Group sites [19]. IFRT treatment yielded significant EFS benefit, with a 66% reduction in the risk of death and/or disease progression. Cox analysis, when adjusted for age, gender, stage, performance status, lactate dehydrogenase (LDH), and disease bulk, confirmed the significant EFS benefit of IFRT.

Advanced Stage

Although consolidative RT is an established treatment option for patients with early stage DLBCL, limited data exists to suggest whether consolidative RT should be a mainstay in the management of advanced stage DLBCL. As such the current National Comprehensive Cancer Network (NCCN) guidelines fail to mention RT as a preferred treatment option. Patients presenting with stage III or IV DLBCL are at higher risk of treatment failure than those presenting with limited stage disease. Several studies have assessed the management of DLBCL with RT.

A study from Milan from Ferreri et al. of 94 patients with stage III or IV DLBCL assessed outcomes in 40 patients that received consolidation radiotherapy to bulky (≥10 cm) ($n = 20$) or semibulky lesions (6-9 cm) ($n = 20$) while 54 (18 with bulky disease) did not [20]. Twenty-eight patients were irradiated to the involved field and 12 to the extended field with a dose of 30-46 Gy. In patients with bulky disease, a prolonged time to relapse (TTR) ($p = 0.05$) and improved 5 year OS (73 vs. 57%, $p = 0.05$) was noted in patients that received radiation. Consolidation radiotherapy reduced relapses in semibulky lesions as well with a prolonged TTR ($p = 0.01$) and improved 5 year OS (59 vs. 41%, $p = 0.09$). These analyses were confirmed on MVA and the treatment with radiation was noted to be well tolerated.

Prospective evidence has been published from Aviles et al. on the role of adjuvant RT in patients with bulky ≥10 cm diameter stage IV DLBCL [21]. In the study, 218 patients were initially treated with combined chemotherapy CEOP-bleo (cyclophosphamide, epirubicin, vincristine, prednisone, bleomycin) alternating with DAC (dexamethasone, cytosine arabinoside, and cisplatin). Of the 155 patients who achieved CR, 88 patients with initial bulky disease were randomly assigned to either receive (43 patients) or not receive radiotherapy (45 patients). Doses ranged from 40-50 Gy. Results revealed that at 5 years 72% of the patients treated with the combined therapy remained disease free compared to 35% in the control group. OS was also improved (81% vs. 55%, $p < 0.01$) in patients with bulky stage IV disease who achieved a CR to chemotherapy. Another trial addressed the role of adjuvant RT for patients with advanced stage disease achieving a PR to chemotherapy [22]. A total of 166 patients with stage III-IV disease with residual disease <5 cm after six cycles of anthracycline based chemotherapy with CHOP or CEOP were randomly assigned to receive 30 Gy in 20 fractions or observation. With a median follow-up of 135 months, 5-year PFS was 86% vs. 32%, ($p < 0.001$) and OS 89% vs. 58%, ($p < 0.001$) with both favoring the group receiving RT. However, results from this group should be interpreted with caution [21, 22]. An additional trial conducted by Aviles et al. was subsequently retracted calling the results of these other prospective trials into question [23, 24].

A prospective study from MD Anderson of 32 patients with stage III and 27 patients with stage IV disease analyzed the impact of IFRT on patients that responded to CHOP chemotherapy [25]. At least six cycles of chemotherapy were delivered to 92% of the patients. IFRT (39.6-40.0 Gy in 20-22 fractions in 74% of cases) was administered to 28/59 (47%) patients beginning 3-4 weeks after chemotherapy. With a median follow-up of 53 months, RT improved 5 year local control 89% vs. 52%, $p = 0.001$ for stages III and IV combined. RT also improved 5 year rates of FFP 85% vs. 51%, $p = 0.003$ for stages III and IV combined. On MVA, radiotherapy was the most significant factor affecting local control and FFP. However, these improvements in local control and FFP did not significantly improve OS.

The role of consolidative radiation in the management of advanced stage DLBCL is further complicated by the availability of data in the era of rituximab. In the study from MD Anderson, 60% of patients presented with stage III – IV disease [15]. RT was given to only 39 (14%) of 279 patients with stage III – IV disease of whom 59% had bulky disease. With a median follow-up of 36 months, RT significantly improved outcomes across all stages. For stage III – IV patients, the 5 year PFS (76% vs. 55%, $p = 0.003$) and OS (89% vs. 66%, $p = 0.008$) were also in favor of the RT group. On MVA, administration of RT and response to chemotherapy were the strongest prognostic factors affecting PFS and OS. The study concluded that in the era of R-CHOP chemotherapy, consolidative RT was associated with significant improvements in PFS and OS for all patients with DLBCL, regardless of disease stage or disease bulk. However, it should be noted that only a small percentage of patients in this study with advanced stage disease received RT and it is not clear what criteria were used to select those patients who would receive RT.

Duke University reported a retrospective review of their experience treating patients with stage III-IV DLBCL to evaluate the impact of consolidative RT in patients who achieved CR post-chemotherapy [26]. Sixty-five percent of patients received R-CHOP, and rituximab was incorporated in 72% of the chemotherapy regimens. Approximately half of patients received consolidative RT to involved sites of disease with a median dose of 25 Gy. Receipt of consolidation RT was associated with improvement in field control (92% vs. 69%, respectively, p = 0.028) and EFS (85% vs. 65%, respectively, p = 0.014) but no difference in OS (85% vs. 78%, respectively, p = 0.15) when compared to patients who did not receive consolidation RT. On MVA, no RT was predictive of increased risk of local failure (HR 8.01, p = 0.014) and worse EFS (HR 4.3, p = 0.014). Both the Duke and MDACC studies further strengthen the rationale for RT in current practice for the management of advanced stage disease.

Prospective Evaluation in the Era of R-CHOP

Debate continues on the optimal management of DLBCL in the era of rituximab. To date, there are few prospective data regarding the role of consolidation radiation therapy in the context of improved outcome with rituximab-based systemic therapy. The main prospective study evaluating the role of radiation therapy is an amended protocol for the RICOVER-60 trial, which tested the role of RT following R-CHOP [27]. In the RICOVER-60 trial, elderly patients (ages 61-80 years) were randomly assigned to six or eight cycles of CHOP-14 (CHOP administered once every 2 weeks) with or without eight administrations of rituximab [28]. Additive RT was administered to sites of initial bulky disease (≥7.5 cm) and extralymphatic involvement. Six cycles of R-CHOP with two additional cycles of rituximab was the best of the four treatment arms and significantly improved EFS, PFS, and OS over six cycles of CHOP-14. In this recent prospective amendment to the RICOVER-60 trial, the best arm of the RICOVER-60 trial (6 cycles of R-CHOP with two additional cycles of rituximab) plus IFRT (36 Gy) was compared with a cohort receiving the same immunochemotherapy but without RT. After a median observation time of 39 months, MVA of the intention to treat population, adjusting for IPI risk factors and age (>70 years), revealed EFS of patients with bulky disease was inferior without additive RT (HR 2.1; 95% CI, 1.3 to 3.5, p = .005), with trends for inferior PFS (HR 1.8; 95% CI, 1.0 to 3.3, p = .058) and OS (HR 1.6; 95% CI, 0.9 to 3.1, p = .127). In a per-protocol analysis with 11 patients excluded for receiving unplanned RT, MVA revealed HRs of 2.7 (95% CI, 1.3 to 5.9, p = .011) for EFS, 4.4 (95% CI, 1.8 to 10.6, p = .001) for PFS, and 4.3 (95% CI, 1.7 to 11.1, p = .002) for OS for patients not receiving RT to bulky disease. This study provides evidence for the addition of radiation to sites of bulky disease in elderly patients with aggressive B-cell lymphoma.

There is an ongoing phase III prospective randomized trial, UNFOLDER, by the German High Grade Non-Hodgkin's Lymphoma Study Group (DHSNHL) (ClinicalTrials.gov identifier, NCT00278408). This trial compares two different schedules of R-CHOP (R-CHOP 21 or R-CHOP 14) for 6 cycles with or without consolidative RT in patients with aggressive B cell lymphoma. Young patients (aged 18-60 years) with bulky disease ≥7.5 cm or extranodal involvement who achieved a CR to chemotherapy were further randomized to consolidative RT. Interim analysis revealed that the R-CHOP alone resulted in excess relapse with inferior OS compared to those that received consolidation RT. Therefore, R-CHOP without radiotherapy arm for bulky limited-stage DLBCL was closed early. Of note, patients in the UNFOLDER trial include not only those patients with DLBCL but also patients with grade 3 follicular lymphoma, Burkitt lymphoma, primary mediastinal B cell lymphoma, marginal zone lymphoma, and mantle cell lymphoma. Further details will be available once the full manuscript is published to more clearly delineate the histology and stages with significant benefit from RT; however, at this point the study does indicate that RT still play a significant role in disease management in the era of R-CHOP.

Another phase III trial from the Lysa/Goelams Group evaluated the role of consolidation radiation therapy in non-bulky limited stage DLBCL [29]. 301 patients were randomized to R-CHOP alone vs. R-CHOP with RT. With a median follow-up of 51 months, EFS and OS were not statistically different between the two arms. This study concluded limited role for consolidation radiation therapy in early stage non-bulky DLBCL.

Radiation Techniques

Radiation techniques and treatment design have evolved significantly over the years. One of the biggest concerns of older radiation techniques in this patient population of long-term survivors was the risk of secondary malignancy and other long-term toxicities to organs including the heart and lungs. Previous radiation techniques involved a larger radiation field for more significant coverage of uninvolved lymphoid tissue. Multiple lymph node chains were covered with as few radiation fields as possible to avoid gaps or overlaps within the field junctions. The "mantle field" was used to treat the lymph nodes in the upper part of the body and the "inverted Y" was used to treat lymph nodes in the abdomen, pelvis, and groins. The combination of the "inverted Y" and "mantle fields" was termed "total lymphoid irradiation" and if the pelvis was excluded "subtotal lymphoid irradiation." The primary concern with these larger fields was the risk of secondary malignancy in a cohort of patients with long-term survival.

Modern RT techniques are designed to achieve comparable DFS while minimizing unnecessary radiation and toxicity. Until recently the standard of care has been IFRT. By focusing on the regions involved by the disease prior to chemotherapy, an excellent disease control has been achieved [5, 7, 8, 30]. IFRT was adapted from similar treatment concepts used in Hodgkin lymphoma to limit radiation treatment fields used in DLBCL [31].

It was believed that further field reductions to exclude adjacent, uninvolved nodal areas would further improve toxicity profiles while not sacrificing DFS. This has provided the rationale for involved site radiation therapy (ISRT) [32]. ISRT has now become the standard radiation treatment planning method and requires modern CT based simulation and planning capabilities. An example of an ISRT treatment plan with corresponding pre-chemotherapy PET imaging is seen in Figure 1. Prechemotherapy imaging studies including PET, MRI, and CT scans assist in treatment volume determination. This treatment field focuses on irradiation of the initial lymph node volume prior to chemotherapy or surgery respecting anatomic boundaries with some modifications to avoid unnecessary radiation to critical uninvolved organs or muscles. Possible movement of the target by respiratory motion is also taken into account with 4D-CT treatment planning. ISRT requires a careful assessment of pre and post chemotherapy imaging. This technique has not compromised local control or overall outcomes of PFS or OS over IFRT [31]. Further field reductions may be possible if pre-treatment imaging is obtained in the radiation treatment position, further reducing the size of the treatment fields [33]. This concept of involved nodal radiation therapy (INRT) defines radiation fields based on a planned pre-chemotherapy imaging study obtained in the same radiation treatment position and immobilization. This requires a careful multidisciplinary planning prior to chemotherapy, which is not always feasible in clinical practice. Therefore, ISRT remains the most common. A comparison of the evolution of radiation treatment fields is seen in Figure 2. The majority of radiation treatment is delivered with photons and electrons. Proton therapy is another treatment option for radiation oncologists. There are unique physical properties of protons distinct from photons and electrons that allow for reduced radiation exit dose. As the beam of protons travels through tissue maintaining velocity and energy, it begins to slow near the end of its path. An abrupt deposition of its dose at the end of its path, known as the Bragg peak, allows decreased dose to normal structures in certain clinical scenarios. As long term cure is often possible with DLBCL patients following combined chemotherapy and radiotherapy, they are at increased risk of developing late adverse effects from radiation therapy including secondary malignancies, cardiac toxicities, and pulmonary toxicities. For this reason, proton therapy may have a potential role in younger patient cohorts with DLBCL [34, 35]. Further study is needed to determine the long-term reduction in late toxicity utilizing proton therapy in DLBCL.

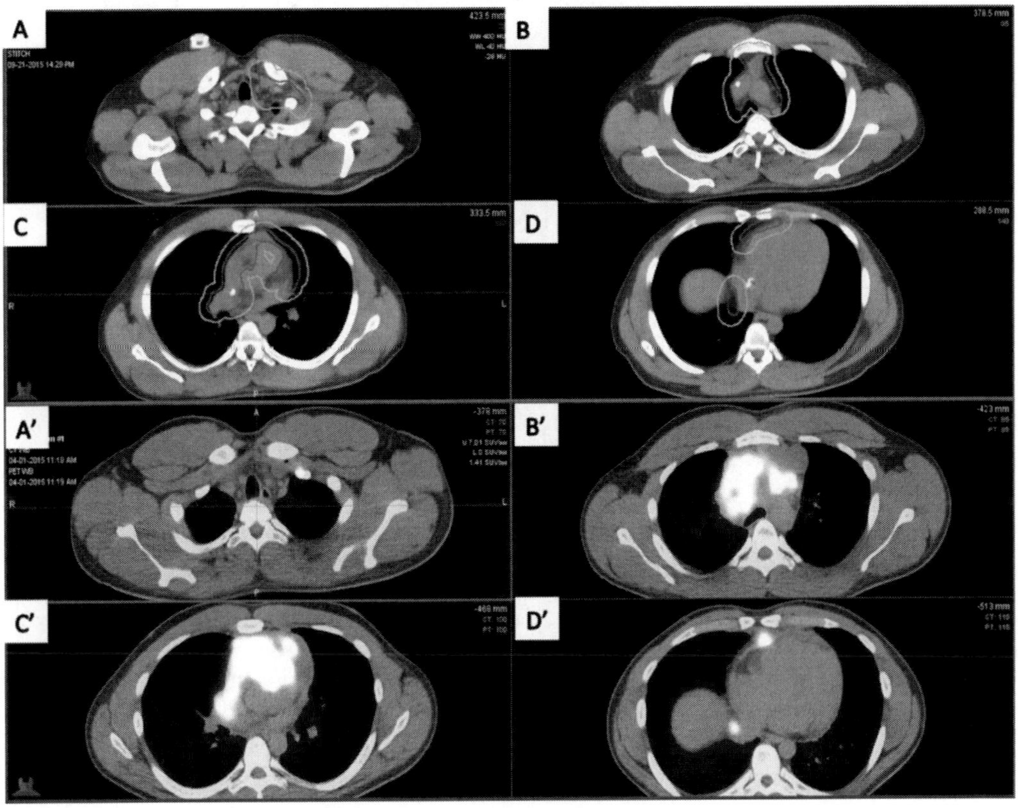

Figure 1. Radiation treatment volumes for an involved site radiation therapy (ISRT) plan. Patient treated for Stage 2B bulky mediastinal DLBCL post 6 cycles of R-CHOP. Clinical target volume (CTV) is in red with an 8 mm expansion to the planning target volume (PTV) in orange. A-D represent contours on CT imaging and A'-D' represent corresponding pre-chemotherapy PET images.

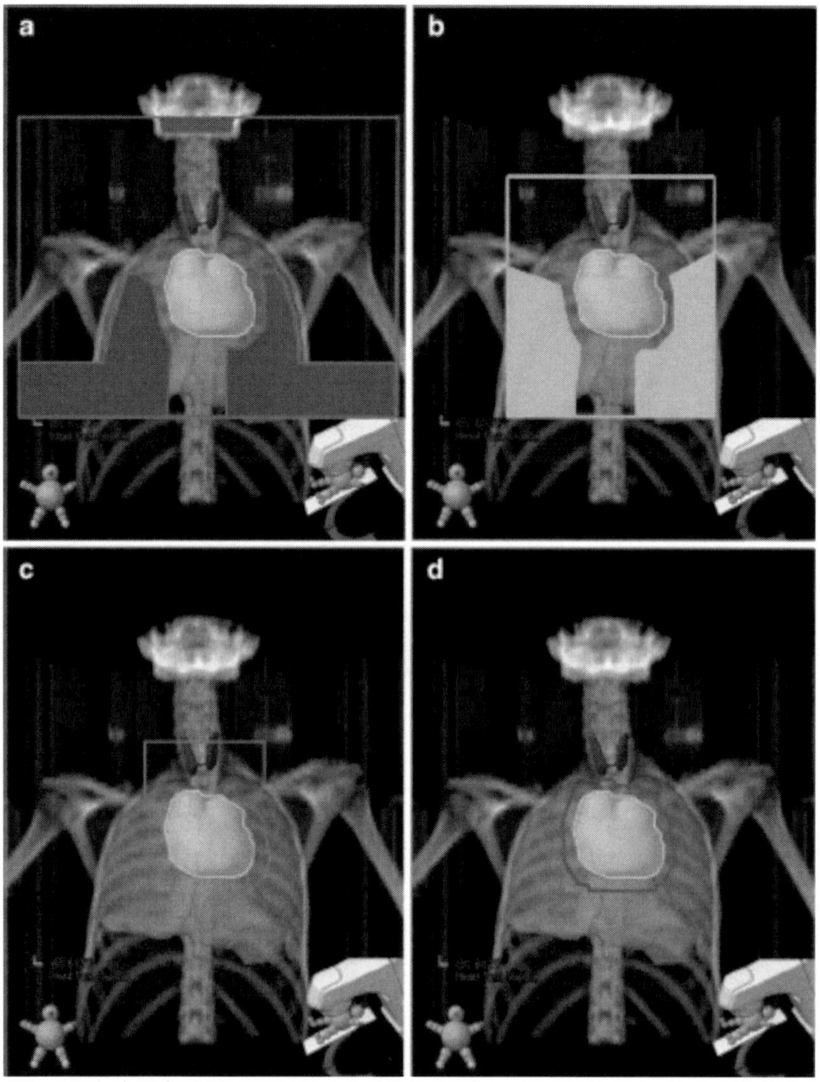

Reprinted with permission from Campbell BA. The role of radiation therapy in the treatment of stage I-II diffuse large B-cell lymphoma. *Curr. Hematol. Malig. Rep*. 2013; 8:236-242.

Figure 2. Prechemotherapy nodal volume: light blue; organs at risk: thyroid (dark blue), lungs (brown), heart (light green). (a) Mantle field radiation therapy is outlined in green; solid areas represent shielding of normal tissues. (b) Involved field radiation therapy (IFRT) is outlined in orange; solid areas represent shielding of normal tissues. (c) Involved site radiation therapy (ISRT) is outlined in purple. (d) Involved node radiation therapy (INRT) is outlined in red.

Risk-Adapted Treatment Selection

As we move closer to tailoring patient specific approaches to management of malignancies, prognostic factors may help us stratify patients into different management approaches. This may help facilitate sparing patients with low risk disease from the excess toxicity of unnecessary treatment while intensifying treatment for those patients more prone to disease relapse.

A number of studies have assessed the role of PET imaging in identifying patients who may benefit from intensification of treatment. A systematic review was published in 2009, which assessed results of interim PET analysis in 311 DLBCL patients [36]. Due to heterogeneity in the studies available, no conclusions could be drawn on the utility of interim PET for prognostic purposes. In order for PET imaging to help determine prognosis and help facilitate treatment decisions the definition of PET positivity must be more clearly delineated [37-39] as well as the optimal timing of PET imaging [39]. However, PET imaging does offer promise in identifying patients who may particularly benefit from radiation. For instance, a retrospective study from Emory University revealed that in patients with stage III or IV DLBCL, who underwent a CR to chemotherapy and did not receive RT with tumors <5 cm with an SUV max ≥ 15 may be particularly prone to recurrence [40]. However, future prospective trials are required to establish the role of PET/CT in the management of patients with DLBCL, and the use of interim PET/CT to help guide treatment decisions and offer prognostic information is considered investigational at the present time.

Conclusion

Great strides have been made in improving outcomes for DLBCL patients while limiting toxicity. There is increasing evidence that in the era of rituximab, RT should strongly be considered as a standard management approach in early and advanced stage patients. Recent advances in radiation treatment delivery and field design have dramatically reduced normal tissue radiation and resultant acute and long-term sequelae while maintaining high rates of local disease control. In the current era of risk adapted and personalized therapy, further investigation is needed to determine the role PET imaging and genetic profiling in determining prognosis and in guiding treatment decisions.

References

[1] Ng, A. K. 2007. "Diffuse large B-cell lymphoma." *Semin. Radiat. Oncol.* 17:169-175.

[2] Persky, D. O., Miller, T. P. 2009. "Localized large cell lymphoma: is there any need for radiation therapy?" *Curr. Opin. Oncol.* 21:401-406.

[3] Vaughan Hudson, B., Vaughan Hudson, G., MacLennan, K. A., Anderson, L., Linch, D. C. 1994. "Clinical stage 1 non-Hodgkin's lymphoma: long-term follow-up of patients treated by the British National Lymphoma Investigation with radiotherapy alone as initial therapy." *Br. J. Cancer* 69:1088-1093.

[4] Kaminski, M. S., Coleman, C. N., Colby, T. V., Cox, R. S., Rosenberg, S. A. 1986. "Factors predicting survival in adults with stage I and II large-cell lymphoma treated with primary radiation therapy." *Ann. Intern. Med.* 104:747-756.

[5] Miller, T. P., Dahlberg, S., Cassady, J. R., Adelstein, D. J., Spier, C. M., Grogan, T. M., LeBlanc, M. et al. 1998. "Chemotherapy alone compared with chemotherapy plus radiotherapy for localized intermediate- and high-grade non-Hodgkin's lymphoma." *N. Engl. J. Med.* 339:21-26.

[6] Miller, T. P., Leblanc, M., Spier, C. 2001. "CHOP alone compared to CHOP plus radiotherapy for early stage aggressive non-Hodgkin's lymphomas: update of the Southwest Oncology Group (SWOG) randomized trial." *Blood* 98:742a-743.

[7] Horning, S. J., Weller, E., Kim, K., Earle, J. D., O'Connell, M. J., Habermann, T. M., Glick, J. H. 2004. "Chemotherapy with or without radiotherapy in limited-stage diffuse aggressive non-Hodgkin's lymphoma: Eastern Cooperative Oncology Group study 1484." *J. Clin. Oncol.* 22:3032-3038.

[8] Reyes, F., Lepage, E., Ganem, G., Molina, T. J., Brice, P., Coiffier, B., Morel, P. et al. 2005. "ACVBP versus CHOP plus radiotherapy for localized aggressive lymphoma." *N. Engl. J. Med.* 352:1197-1205.

[9] Andre, M., Mounier, N., Leleu, X., Sonet, A., Brice, P., Henry-Amar, M., Tilly, H. et al. 2004. "Second cancers and late toxicities after treatment of aggressive non-Hodgkin lymphoma with the ACVBP regimen: a GELA cohort study on 2837 patients." *Blood* 103:1222-1228.

[10] Bonnet, C., Fillet, G., Mounier, N., Ganem, G., Molina, T. J., Thieblemont, C., Ferme, C. et al. 2007. "CHOP alone compared with CHOP plus radiotherapy for localized aggressive lymphoma in elderly patients: a study by the Groupe d'Etude des Lymphomes de l'Adulte." *J. Clin. Oncol.* 25:787-792.

[11] Shenkier, T. N., Voss, N., Fairey, R., Gascoyne, R. D., Hoskins, P., Klasa, R., Klimo, P. et al. 2002. "Brief chemotherapy and involved-region irradiation for limited-stage diffuse large-cell lymphoma: an 18-year experience from the British Columbia Cancer Agency." *J. Clin. Oncol.* 20:197-204.

[12] Ballonoff, A., Rusthoven, K. E., Schwer, A., McCammon, R., Kavanagh, B., Bassetti, M., Newman, F., Rabinovitch, R. 2008. "Outcomes and effect of radiotherapy in patients with stage I or II diffuse large B-cell lymphoma: a surveillance, epidemiology, and end results analysis." *Int. J. Radiat. Oncol. Biol. Phys.* 72:1465-1471.

[13] Pugh, T. J., Ballonoff, A., Rusthoven, K. E., McCammon, R., Kavanagh, B., Newman, F., Rabinovitch, R. 2010. "Cardiac mortality in patients with stage I and II diffuse large B-cell lymphoma treated with and without radiation: a surveillance, epidemiology, and end-results analysis." *Int. J. Radiat. Oncol. Biol. Phys.* 76:845-849.

[14] Persky, D. O., Unger, J. M., Spier, C. M., Stea, B., LeBlanc, M., McCarty, M. J., Rimsza, L. M. et al. 2008. "Phase II study of rituximab plus three cycles of CHOP and involved-field radiotherapy for patients with limited-stage aggressive B-cell lymphoma: Southwest Oncology Group study 0014." *J. Clin. Oncol.* 26:2258-2263.

[15] Phan, J., Mazloom, A., Medeiros, L. J., Zreik, T. G., Wogan, C., Shihadeh, F., Rodriguez, M. A. et al. 2010. "Benefit of consolidative radiation therapy in patients with diffuse large B-cell lymphoma treated with R-CHOP chemotherapy." *J. Clin. Oncol.* 28:4170-4176.

[16] Dabaja, B. S., Vanderplas, A. M., Crosby-Thompson, A. L., Abel, G. A., Czuczman, M. S., Friedberg, J. W., Gordon, L. I. et al. 2015. "Radiation for diffuse large B-cell lymphoma in the rituximab era: analysis of the National Comprehensive Cancer Network lymphoma outcomes project." *Cancer* 121:1032-1039.

[17] Vargo, J. A., Gill, B. S., Balasubramani, G. K., Beriwal, S. 2015. "Treatment Selection and Survival Outcomes in Early-Stage Diffuse Large B-Cell Lymphoma: Do We Still Need Consolidative Radiotherapy?" *J. Clin. Oncol.*

[18] Mytelka, D. S., Li, L., Stafkey-Mailey, D., Liepa, A. M., Hess, L. M., Farrelly, E., Eaddy, M. 2014. "Treatment patterns and outcomes among patients with high-intermediate/high-risk diffuse large B-cell lymphoma in the US." *Hematology.*

[19] Marcheselli, L., Marcheselli, R., Bari, A., Liardo, E. V., Morabito, F., Baldini, L., Brugiatelli, M. et al. 2011. "Radiation therapy improves treatment outcome in patients with diffuse large B-cell lymphoma." *Leuk. Lymphoma* 52:1867-1872.

[20] Ferreri, A. J., Dell'Oro, S., Reni, M., Ceresoli, G. L., Cozzarini, C., Ponzoni, M., Villa, E. 2000. "Consolidation radiotherapy to bulky or semibulky lesions in the management of stage III-IV diffuse large B cell lymphomas." *Oncology* 58:219-226.

[21] Aviles, A., Delgado, S., Nambo, M. J., Alatriste, S., Diaz-Maqueo, J. C. 1994. "Adjuvant radiotherapy to sites of previous bulky disease in patients stage IV diffuse large cell lymphoma." *Int. J. Radiat. Oncol. Biol. Phys.* 30:799-803.

[22] Aviles, A., Neri, N., Delgado, S., Perez, F., Nambo, M. J., Cleto, S., Talavera, A., Huerta-Guzman, J. 2005. "Residual disease after chemotherapy in aggressive malignant lymphoma: the role of radiotherapy." *Med. Oncol.* 22:383-387.

[23] Aviles, A., Fernandezb, R., Perez, F., Nambo, M. J., Neri, N., Talavera, A., Castaneda, C., Gonzalez, M., Cleto, S. 2004. "Adjuvant radiotherapy in stage IV diffuse large cell lymphoma improves outcome." *Leuk. Lymphoma* 45:1385-1389.

[24] Polliack, A., Van Besien, K., Seymour, J., Treadway, A. 2013. "Statement of retraction. Aviles, A., Fernandezb, R., Perez, F., Nambo, M. J., Neri, N., Talavera, A., Castaneda, C., Gonzalez, M., Cleto. Adjuvant radiotherapy in stage IV diffuse large cell lymphoma improves outcome." *Leuk. Lymphoma* 54:1571.

[25] Schlembach, P. J., Wilder, R. B., Tucker, S. L., Ha, C. S., Rodriguez, M. A., Hess, M. A., Cabanillas, F. F., Cox, J. D. 2000. "Impact of involved field radiotherapy after CHOP-based chemotherapy on stage III-IV, intermediate grade and large-cell immunoblastic lymphomas." *Int. J. Radiat. Oncol. Biol. Phys.* 48:1107-1110.

[26] Dorth, J. A., Prosnitz, L. R., Broadwater, G., Diehl, L. F., Beaven, A. W., Coleman, R. E., Kelsey, C. R. 2012. "Impact of consolidation radiation therapy in stage III-IV diffuse large B-cell lymphoma with negative post-chemotherapy radiologic imaging." *Int. J. Radiat. Oncol. Biol. Phys.* 84:762-767.

[27] Held, G., Murawski, N., Ziepert, M., Fleckenstein, J., Poschel, V., Zwick, C., Bittenbring, J. et al. 2014. "Role of radiotherapy to bulky disease in elderly patients with aggressive B-cell lymphoma." *J. Clin. Oncol.* 32:1112-1118.

[28] Pfreundschuh, M., Schubert, J., Ziepert, M., Schmits, R., Mohren, M., Lengfelder, E., Reiser, M. et al. 2008. "Six versus eight cycles of bi-weekly CHOP-14 with or without rituximab in elderly patients with aggressive CD20 + B-cell lymphomas: a randomised controlled trial (RICOVER-60)." *Lancet Oncol.* 9:105-116.

[29] Lamy, T., Damaj, G., Gyan, E., Soubeyran, P., Bouabdallah, K., Cartron, G., Gressin, R., Cornillon, J., Banos, A., Moles, M., Katell Le Dû, K., Benchalal, M., Costes, V., Bene, M., Delwail, V. "R-CHOP with or without radiotherapy in non-bulky limited-stage diffuse large B cell lymphoma (DLBCL): Preliminary results of the prospective randomized phase III 02-03 trial from the Lysa/Goelams Group." *2014 ASH Annual Meeting.*

[30] Kamath, S. S., Marcus, R. B., Jr., Lynch, J. W., Mendenhall, N. P. 1999. "The impact of radiotherapy dose and other treatment-related and clinical factors on in-field control

in stage I and II non-Hodgkin's lymphoma." *Int. J. Radiat. Oncol. Biol. Phys.* 44:563-568.

[31] Campbell, B. A., Connors, J. M., Gascoyne, R. D., Morris, W. J., Pickles, T., Sehn, L. H. 2012. "Limited-stage diffuse large B-cell lymphoma treated with abbreviated systemic therapy and consolidation radiotherapy: involved-field versus involved-node radiotherapy." *Cancer* 118:4156-4165.

[32] Illidge, T., Specht, L., Yahalom, J., Aleman, B., Berthelsen, A. K., Constine, L., Dabaja, B. et al. 2014. "Modern radiation therapy for nodal non-Hodgkin lymphoma-target definition and dose guidelines from the International Lymphoma Radiation Oncology Group." *Int. J. Radiat. Oncol. Biol. Phys.* 89:49-58.

[33] Girinsky, T., van der Maazen, R., Specht, L., Aleman, B., Poortmans, P., Lievens, Y., Meijnders, P. et al. 2006. "Involved-node radiotherapy (INRT) in patients with early Hodgkin lymphoma: concepts and guidelines." *Radiother. Oncol.* 79:270-277.

[34] Ho, C. K., Flampouri, S., Hoppe, B. S. 2014. "Proton therapy in the management of lymphoma." *Cancer J.* 20:387-392.

[35] Sachsman, S., Flampouri, S., Li, Z., Lynch, J., Mendenhall, N. P., Hoppe, B. S. 2015. "Proton therapy in the management of non-Hodgkin lymphoma." *Leuk. Lymphoma* 1-5.

[36] Terasawa, T., Lau, J., Bardet, S., Couturier, O., Hotta, T., Hutchings, M., Nihashi, T., Nagai, H. 2009. "Fluorine-18-fluorodeoxyglucose positron emission tomography for interim response assessment of advanced-stage Hodgkin's lymphoma and diffuse large B-cell lymphoma: a systematic review." *J. Clin. Oncol.* 27:1906-1914.

[37] Moskowitz, C. H. 2012. "Interim PET-CT in the management of diffuse large B-cell lymphoma." *Hematology Am. Soc. Hematol. Educ. Program* 2012:397-401.

[38] Cashen, A. F., Dehdashti, F., Luo, J., Homb, A., Siegel, B. A., Bartlett, N. L. 2011. "18F-FDG PET/CT for early response assessment in diffuse large B-cell lymphoma: poor predictive value of international harmonization project interpretation." *J. Nucl. Med.* 52:386-392.

[39] Michallet, A. S., Trotman, J., Tychyj-Pinel, C. 2010. "Role of early PET in the management of diffuse large B-cell lymphoma." *Curr. Opin. Oncol.* 22:414-418.

[40] Jegadeesh, N., Rajpara, R., Esiashvili, N., Shi, Z., Liu, Y., Okwan-Duodu, D., Flowers, C. R., Khan, M. K. 2015. "Predictors of local recurrence after rituximab-based chemotherapy alone in stage III and IV diffuse large B-cell lymphoma: guiding decisions for consolidative radiation." *Int. J. Radiat. Oncol. Biol. Phys.* 92:107-112.

In: Diffuse Large B-Cell Lymphoma (DLBCL)
Editor: Haipeng Shao
ISBN: 978-1-63484-402-4

Chapter 4

AUTOLOGOUS AND ALLOGENEIC HEMATOPOIETIC STEM CELL TRANSPLANTATION FOR DIFFUSE LARGE B-CELL LYMPHOMA

Vijaya Raj Bhatt[1,*], Smith Giri[2], Guru Subramanian Guru Murthy[3] and R. Gregory Bociek[1]

[1]Division of Hematology-Oncology, Department of Internal Medicine, University of Nebraska Medical Center, Omaha, NE, US
[2]Department of Medicine, University of Tennessee Health Science Center, Memphis, TN, US
[3]Division of Hematology-Oncology, Department of Internal Medicine, Medical college of Wisconsin, Milwaukee, WI, US

ABSTRACT

Diffuse large B-cell lymphoma (DLBCL) accounts for approximately one-third of all non-Hodgkin lymphomas (NHL) and is the most common aggressive NHL. It can arise *de novo* or as a transformation of an indolent lymphoma. Although rituximab-based immunochemotherapy has improved overall survival (OS) in DLBCL, high-intermediate or high-risk disease is associated with a 4-year OS of approximately 50-60%. Stem cell transplant (SCT) has been extensively investigated in DLBCL in both upfront and salvage settings. Several trials have failed to show an OS benefit with upfront autologous SCT in DLBCL or other aggressive NHL. Therefore, upfront SCT is not currently indicated in an unselected population of patients with aggressive NHL. Approximately 10-15% of patients with DLBCL are refractory to primary rituximab-based therapy or progress soon afterwards. An additional one-third of patients relapse within 2-3 years after initial therapy. Outcomes are generally poor in these patients with chemotherapy

* Corresponding author: Vijaya Raj Bhatt. Division of Hematology-Oncology, Department of Internal Medicine, University of Nebraska Medical Center, Omaha, NE, US. E-mail: vijaya. bhatt@unmc.edu, phone: (402) 559-5600, fax: (402) 559-6520.

alone. Patients, who have chemosensitive relapse are generally taken to autologous SCT if they are transplant candidates. Several strategies including the use of radioimmunotherapy and rituximab have been investigated to improve the outcomes of autologous SCT; however, there is no conclusive evidence of their benefits. Conversely, radiotherapy may have a role and should be utilized before or after SCT in patients with bulky or residual disease in non-irradiated areas. Patients with DLBCL who fail multiple chemotherapies or autologous SCT have poor outcomes with a median OS of approximately 10 months in the rituximab era; such patients should be considered for allogeneic SCT or novel clinical trials. Outcomes with allogeneic SCT are better in patients with good performance status, young age, chemosensitive disease and those who relapse >12 months after autologous SCT. Reduced intensity conditioning or nonmyeloablative conditioning may reduce non-relapse mortality associated with allogeneic SCT, possibly expanding its utilization to older patients. Haploidentical transplant and cord blood transplant are emerging techniques that allow alternative donor options. Advances in the field of autologous and allogeneic SCT continue to change the landscape of hematologic malignancies such as DLBCL.

INTRODUCTION

Diffuse large B-cell lymphoma (DLBCL), which can arise *de novo* or as a transformation of indolent lymphoma [1], is the most common aggressive non-Hodgkin lymphoma (NHL) throughout the world, consisting of approximately one-third of all NHL [1, 2]. DLBCL is a heterogeneous group of lymphomas with various morphologic appearances, protein-expression patterns, and gene-expression profiles [1]. Based on gene-expression profiling, it can be divided into 3 subtypes with varying outcomes; these subtypes include germinal-center type, the activated B-cell type, and mediastinal large B-cell lymphoma type [1, 3]. The introduction of rituximab in upfront immunochemotherapy has improved the overall survival (OS) of patients with DLBCL in recent years [4, 5]. While the OS of patients with DLBCL with low or intermediate-risk disease is more than 80-90% at 4 years, only about half of patients with high-intermediate or high-risk disease are alive at 4 years [6]. Similarly, the outcomes of double-HIT DLBCL [7], activated B-cell type, DLBCL transformed from indolent lymphoma [1] and leukemic DLBCL [8] remain generally poor. Therefore, hematopoietic stem cell transplant (SCT) has been extensively investigated in DLBCL in both upfront and salvage setting with hope to improve outcomes [9]. The current management strategy of patients with DLBCL is summarized in Figure 1.

UPFRONT CONSOLIDATION WITH AUTOLOGOUS STEM CELL TRANSPLANTATION

The use of upfront consolidation with high-dose chemotherapy (HDT) and autologous stem cell transplantation (autoSCT) has not been shown to improve OS in DLBCL, hence not indicated in an unselected population of DLBCL. This is highlighted by a meta-analysis of 15 randomized controlled trials of 3079 patients with aggressive NHL that demonstrated a higher complete remission rate ($p = .004$) and similar event-free survival (EFS) ($p = .31$) or OS ($p = .58$) with HDT/auto-SCT versus chemotherapy alone [10].

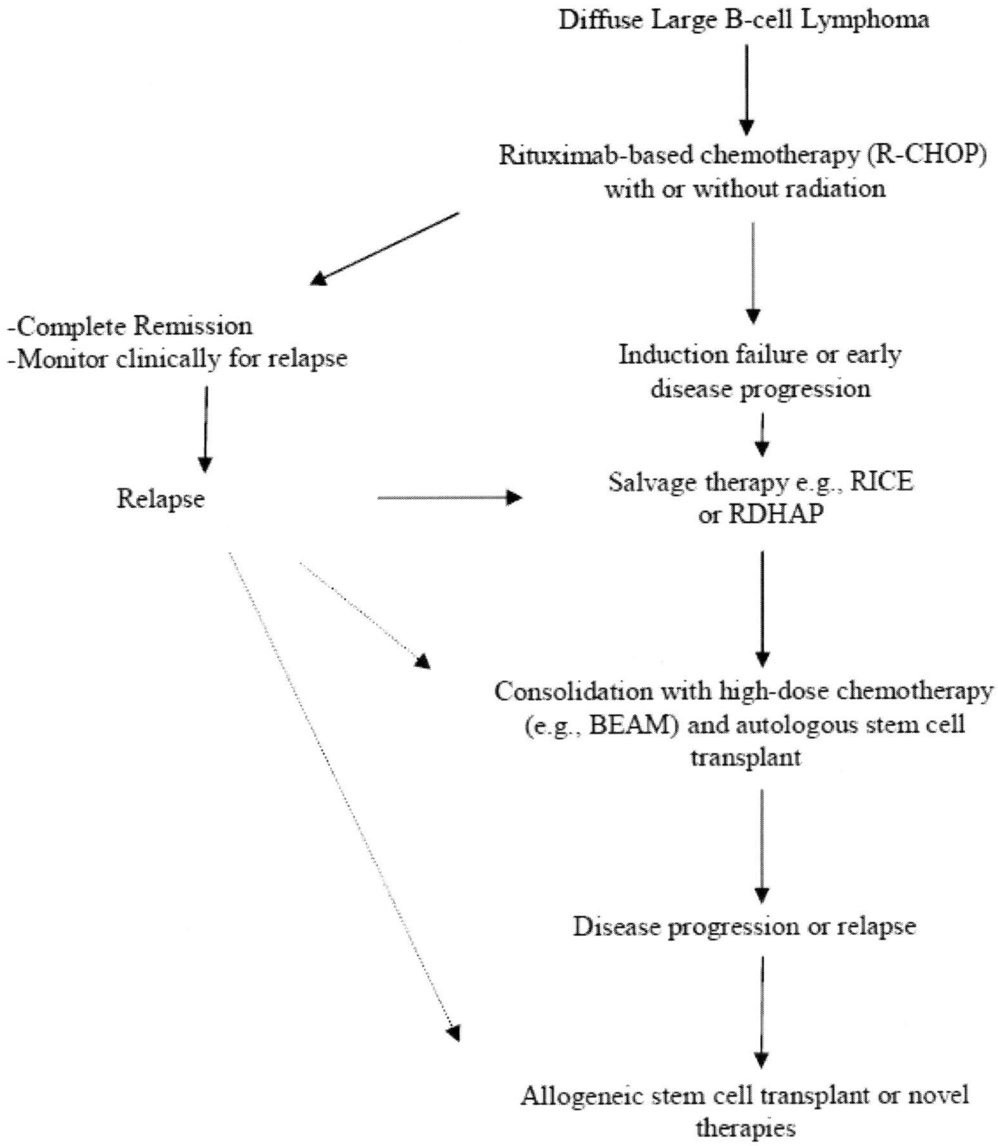

BEAM, carmustine, etoposide, cytarabine and melphalan; RCHOP, rituximab, cyclophosphamide, doxorubicin, vincristine and prednisone; RDHAP, rituximab, dexamethasone, high-dose cytarabine, and cisplatin; RICE, rituximab, ifosfamide, etoposide, and carboplatin.

Figure 1. Management of patients with diffuse large B-cell lymphoma outside of a trial.

Then, the next question is whether upfront autoSCT is of any value in patients with high-intermediate or high-risk DLBCL, who have significant risk of relapse [6, 11]. A retrospective subgroup analysis of LNH-87, one of the early trials of upfront auto-SCT in aggressive lymphomas, indicated an improved progression-free survival (PFS) and OS in high-intermediate and high-risk patients [12]. A recent Southwest Oncology Group (SWOG) trial 9704 of high-intermediate risk or high-risk aggressive NHL, however, demonstrated a higher PFS (69% vs. 55%, $p = 0.005$) but similar OS at 2 years (74% vs. 71%, $p = 0.30$) with auto-SCT, compared to chemotherapy with cyclophosphamide, doxorubicin, vincristine and prednisone (CHOP) or CHOP-rituximab (CHOP-R). The lack of OS advantage was the result of successful use of salvage therapy in relapsed patients. In a subset analysis, patients with high-risk disease (by age adjusted International Prognostic Index score) had an improvement in OS with autoSCT (82% vs. 64%, p = 0.01). The use of HDT/autoSCT was associated with greater risk of grade 3-4 toxicities [13].

Even in patients with high-risk disease, prior trials with important differences in their designs, have failed to demonstrate an OS advantage with autoSCT [14-16].

It should also be understood that no randomized trial in this patient population has used positron emission tomography (PET) imaging in its design, and as such there may still be subgroups of patients that could benefit from upfront autoSCT based on PET response. Hence, the upfront HDT/autoSCT in this patient population would not be considered a standard of care at present. It may however be a reasonable consideration for a high-risk patient who can fully understand the nuances and risks and uncertainties associated with existing data. Certain subtypes of DLBCL such as activated B-cell subtype, double-hit or gray-zone lymphomas have poor prognosis. Whether upfront HDT/autoSCT has a role in such situation remain unclear and is an area for future research.

Salvage Consolidation with Autologous Stem Cell Transplantation

Although the incorporation of rituximab to upfront chemotherapy has reduced the risk of relapsed/refractory disease, up to 15% of patients with DLBCL are primary refractory to rituximab-based immunochemotherapy or develop disease progression soon after initial therapy [9]. The majority of DLBCL relapses occur within 2-3 years after initial therapy; such relapses consist of one-third of responding patients [17, 18]. A few late relapses, as far out as 15-20 years after the initial therapy, may be noted [1]. Such patients are initially treated with salvage chemotherapy such as rituximab, ifosfamide, etoposide, and carboplatin (RICE), or rituximab, dexamethasone, high-dose cytarabine, and cisplatin (RDHAP). However, long-term survival of patients with relapsed/refractory DLBCL is dismal with salvage chemotherapy alone. Hence, transplant-eligible patients responding to salvage therapy should undergo HDT/autoSCT. In such setting, the use of HDT/autoSCT has been shown to improve OS [19-22] (Table 1).

There are two major trials that have shaped our current therapeutic approach to patients with relapsed/refractory DLBCL. The PARMA trial demonstrated the survival advantage of HDT/autoSCT in relapsed NHL. In this trial of 215 patients, the use of HDT/autoSCT as compared with conventional chemotherapy showed improved response rate (84% vs. 44%), event-free survival (EFS) (46% vs. 12%) and OS at 5 years (53% vs. 32%) [20].

The Collaborative Trial in Relapsed Aggressive Lymphoma (CORAL) trial aimed to compare the outcomes of relapsed/refractory DLBCL with the use of two salvage regimens, RICE and RDHAP, frequently utilized prior to HDT/autoSCT. The response rate after 3 cycles of chemotherapy (63% vs. 62%) as well as PFS (31% vs. 42%, p = 0.4) and OS at 3 years (47% vs. 51%, p = 0.4) were similar for RICE and RDHAP arms. An important finding of this study was the demonstration of poor outcomes among patients with an early relapse after initial rituximab-based therapy.

Table 1. Autologous Hematopoietic Stem Cell Transplantation for Patients with Relapsed or Refractory Diffuse large B-cell lymphoma

Year	Number of patients	Salvage strategy	EFS/PFS	OS	Reference
Comparative studies					
1995	215	DHAP vs. HDT/autoSCT	12% vs. 46% at 5 years	53% vs. 32% at 5 years	[20]
2004	429	HDT/autoSCT in first relapse vs. second remission	28% vs. 38% at 3 years	38% vs. 55% at 3 years	[29]
2010	396	RICE vs. RDHAP prior to HDT/autoSCT	26% vs. 35% at 3 years	47% vs. 51% at 3 years	[23]
Non-comparative studies					
2000	85	ICE prior to HDT/autoSCT	44% at 3 years	52% at 3 years	[22]
2001	184	Various prior to HDT/autoSCT	31% at 5 years	37% at 5 years	[21]
2004	36	RICE prior to HDT/autoSCT	54% at 2 years	67% at 2 years	[57]
2005	67	High-dose R plus chemotherapy prior to HDT/autoSCT	67% at 2 years	80% at 2 years	[41]

EFS, event-free survival; HDT, indicates high-dose chemotherapy; N, number; OS, overall survival; PFS, progression-free survival; R, rituximab; DHAP, rituximab, dexamethasone, high-dose cytarabine, and cisplatin; ICE, rituximab, ifosfamide, etoposide, and carboplatin; SCT, stem cell transplantation.

Conversely, prior rituximab use failed to influence EFS in patients who relapsed >12 months after diagnosis [23]. A subsequent analysis of this trial indicated a higher 3-year PFS (52% vs. 32%, p = 0.01) and OS (61% vs. 45%) with the use of RDHAP for germinal center B-cell (GCB) versus non-GCB type of DLBCL although this was based on a relatively small subset analysis of cases for which such data was available and it did not appear that the OS difference remained after adjustment for other variables in a multivariate analysis. The use of RICE therapy, however, resulted in similar 3-year PFS (31% vs. 27%, p = 0.81) and OS (50% vs. 49%) for GCB and non-GCB DLBCL. These results indicate that the use of RDHAP may improve outcomes for relapsed/refractory GCB DLBCL patients, who are healthy enough to tolerate the therapy [24]. This study also demonstrated the prognostic role of the cell of origin [24], which was, however, not confirmed in other studies [25, 26]. The PARMA and CORAL trials demonstrated that HDT/autoSCT should be considered for eligible patients with relapsed/refractory DLBCL, and that RDHAP may be a preferred salvage therapy for young and fit patients with GCB DLBCL.

The outcome for patients with primary refractory DLBCL is significantly worse than those with relapsed DLBCL; the outcomes may even be better with longer time to relapse [19, 23]. Nonetheless, the use of salvage therapy followed by HDT/autoSCT with or without radiation may achieve prolonged disease control and possible cure in a subset of patients with primary refractory disease [21, 22]. In an Autologous Blood and Marrow Transplant Registry study, 184 patients with primary refractory diffuse aggressive NHL achieved a complete remission rate of 44% and 5-year PFS and OS of 31% and 37% respectively, with the use of HDT/auto-SCT [21]. The outcomes were worse for older patients, patients with Karnofsky performance score <80 and those with chemoresistance disease [21]. The use of involved-field radiation therapy before or after autoSCT may improve outcomes [21].

ROLE OF PROGNOSTIC FACTORS IN THERAPY SELECTION

Patients with high-risk disease based on age-adjusted international prognostic index [22, 23, 27, 28], multiple extranodal site of disease [22] or increased lactate dehydrogenase [29] have poor outcomes. Older patients [21, 29] and those with poor performance status [21] are at risk of greater toxicities and worse survival. Chemorefractory disease [21, 29], disease relapse within 12 months of diagnosis [23, 28, 29] and a history of ≥3 prior chemotherapy regimens [21] also portend poor prognosis. While useful for patient education and informed decision, these prognostic indicators may also guide therapy selection. For example, older unfit patients with high-risk or chemorefractory disease are likely to have significant toxicities yet lower benefit from HDT/autoSCT. Hence, subjecting such patients to the excess risk may not always be appropriate. Conversely, young fit patients with late relapses should undergo salvage therapy followed by autoSCT in first relapse to improve chances of cure. Young fit patients with chemorefractory disease, heavily pretreated disease or high-risk disease may be considered for an allogeneic SCT (alloSCT) over autoSCT.

ADVANCING THE BENEFITS OF TRANSPLANT STRATEGY

Involved field radiation therapy (IFRT), if not previously utilized, may be used before or after autoSCT in patients with bulky (>5 cm) or residual disease [22]. In a retrospective study of 164 relapsed or refractory DLBCL, the use of 30 Gy IFRT was associated with a low risk of local relapse and minimal transplant-related mortality (TRM) [30]. The use of radioimmunotherapy (^{131}I-tositumomab or ^{90}Y-ibritumomab tiuxetan) with HDT prior to autoSCT, although demonstrated initial promising results [31-36], failed to improve PFS or OS in a subsequent phase III Blood and Marrow Transplant Clinical Trials Network (BMT CTN) 0401 trial [37]. Incorporation of rituximab during HDT improves outcomes in patients not previously exposed to rituximab [38-40]. However, in rituximab era, all patients are treated with upfront rituximab-based therapy, hence the benefit of incorporation of rituximab during HDT remain unclear. Similarly, the role of rituximab maintenance after HDT/autoSCT is controversial [28, 41]. In indolent lymphoma, obinutuzumab [42] is active even in rituximab-refractory cases but the role of obinutuzumab in rituximab-refractory DLBCL is still not established.

ROLE OF ALLOGENEIC STEM CELL TRANSPLANTATION

AlloSCT has a higher potential to control disease as a result of tumor kill by conditioning therapy and the graft-versus-lymphoma effect. This advantage of lower disease relapse, however, is offset by higher TRM. Hence, the timing and role of alloSCT, as compared to autoSCT, is not clear and depends on the specific context, institutional guidelines, patient's and physician's preferences. Nonetheless, the OS of heavily pretreated DLBCL patients, particularly those with disease progression after autoSCT, is dismal [43]. Such patients with multiple relapses should be evaluated for alloSCT. A large Center for International Blood and Marrow Transplant Research (CIBMTR) study compared the outcomes of first autoSCT (n = 837) or matched sibling myeloablative alloSCT (n = 79) in DLBCL. Compared to autoSCT recipients, alloSCT recipients had higher-risk features such as higher stage disease, marrow involvement at diagnosis, more prior chemotherapy regimens and resistant disease. The use of alloSCT was associated with a higher TRM (41% vs. 12% at one year post transplant) and lower progression/relapse (33% vs. 40%) and OS (22% vs. 49%) at 5 years [44]. In the European Bone Marrow Transplantation Registry (EBMTR) study, the use of alloSCT among patients with disease relapse after autoSCT was associated with TRM, relapse rate, PFS and OS of 28%, 30%, 41% and 53% respectively. TRM associated with alloSCT was higher for older patients (≥45 years) and patients who relapsed <12 months after autoSCT. Relapse rate was lower with chemosensitive disease [45]. This study demonstrated a therapeutic role of alloSCT even after failure of autoSCT; the results are better among patients <45 years and those with >12 months of remission with the use of autoSCT.

Reduced-Intensity Conditioning Allogeneic Transplant

Graft-versus-lymphoma effect allows the use of reduced-intensity conditioning (RIC) alloSCT, where the graft-versus-lymphoma effect is exploited in the management of DLBCL. Such option may be reasonable in patients with well controlled disease before alloSCT and permits the use of alloSCT in older and less-fit patients. The lower TRM associated with RIC alloSCT is offset by a higher risk of relapse, thus resulting in similar OS, compared to myeloablative alloSCT. For example, in a CIBMTR study of refractory or relapsed DLBCL, the use of myeloablative compared to RIC and nonmyeloablative conditioning alloSCT was associated with a higher TRM, lower relapse/progression and similar PFS and OS at 5 years. The presence of lower Karnofsky performance status (<90), prior relapse resistant disease, and the use of unrelated donor were also associated with a higher TRM [46].

Alternative Donor Strategy

Haploidentical donor transplant and umbilical cord blood transplant are emerging strategies aimed to provide alternative donor options. Although the details are outside of the scope of this chapter, the use of haploidentical SCT using post-transplant high-dose cyclophosphamide [47] and umbilical cord blood alloSCT [48] have shown promising results in many hematologic malignancies including non-Hodgkin lymphoma. Such donor options may allow timely and easy access to stem cells, hence may be considered for the management of select patients with relapsed/refractory DLBCL in the absence of related donors.

Survivorship Issues and Follow-Up Plan

Transplant recipients are at risk of disease relapse and other long-term complications such as therapy-related myeloid neoplasms (with autoSCT) [49], solid malignancies, infections, organ failure, and graft-versus-host disease (with alloSCT patients) [50, 51]. Despite an improvement in the OS of lymphoma patients in recent years, disease relapse remains to the most important cause of deaths within the first 5 years of autoSCT [52]. Hence, strategies to reduce relapse after SCT should be investigated. Such strategy may include monitoring of minimal residual disease and utilization of newer therapies such as ibrutinib [53] obinutuzumab [42], immune checkpoint inhibitors [54] and anti-CD19 chimeric antigen receptor (CAR) T cells [55] for trials on post-transplant maintenance and pre-emptive therapy. In the context of prevention and appropriate management of long-term complications, a comprehensive survivorship plan should be formulated and communicated to the SCT recipients and primary care providers [56]. Supportive care, management of late effects, survivorship issues and socioeconomic counseling are equally important aspect of transplant care and can improve long-term outcomes and quality of life of transplant recipients.

Acknowledgments

This work was supported in part by the University of Nebraska Medical Center, College of Medicine, Physician-Scientist Training Program Grant 2015-2016 to Vijaya Bhatt.

References

[1] Armitage, J. O. 2007. "How I treat patients with diffuse large B-cell lymphoma." *Blood* 110:29-36.

[2] Morton, Lindsay M., Wang, Sophia S., Devesa, Susan S., Hartge, Patricia, Weisenburger, Dennis D., Linet, Martha S. 2006. "Lymphoma incidence patterns by WHO subtype in the United States, 1992-2001." *Blood* 107:265-276.

[3] Bhatt, V. R., Mourya, R., Shrestha, R., Armitage, J. O. 2015. "Primary mediastinal large B-cell lymphoma." *Cancer Treat. Rev*.

[4] Shah, B. K., Bista, A., Shafii, B. 2014. "Survival in advanced diffuse large B-cell lymphoma in pre- and post-rituximab Eras in the United States." *Anticancer Res.* 34: 5117-5120.

[5] Shenoy, P. J., Malik, N., Nooka, A., Sinha, R., Ward, K. C., Brawley, O. W., Lipscomb, J., Flowers, C. R. 2011. "Racial differences in the presentation and outcomes of diffuse large B-cell lymphoma in the United States." *Cancer* 117:2530-2540.

[6] Sehn, L. H., Berry, B., Chhanabhai, M., Fitzgerald, C., Gill, K., Hoskins, P., Klasa, R. et al. 2007. "The revised International Prognostic Index (R-IPI) is a better predictor of outcome than the standard IPI for patients with diffuse large B-cell lymphoma treated with R-CHOP." *Blood* 109:1857-1861.

[7] Armitage, J. O., Bociek, R. G. 2014. "Increasing complexity of high-grade B-cell lymphomas." *Cancer* 120:1611-1613.
[8] Bhatt, V. R., Bociek, R. G., Yuan, J., Fu, K., Greiner, T. C., Dave, B. J., Rajan, S. K., Armitage, J. O. 2015. "Leukemic diffuse large B-cell lymphoma in a patient with myeloproliferative disorder." *J. Natl. Compr. Canc. Netw.* 13:281-287.
[9] Bhatt, V. R., Vose, J. M. 2014. "Hematopoietic stem cell transplantation for non-Hodgkin lymphoma." *Hematol. Oncol. Clin. North Am.* 28:1073-1095.
[10] Greb, A., Bohlius, J., Schiefer, D., Schwarzer, G., Schulz, H., Engert, A. 2008. "High-dose chemotherapy with autologous stem cell transplantation in the first line treatment of aggressive non-Hodgkin lymphoma (NHL) in adults." *Cochrane Database Syst. Rev.* CD004024.
[11] Ziepert, M., Hasenclever, D., Kuhnt, E., Glass, B., Schmitz, N., Pfreundschuh, M., Loeffler, M. 2010. "Standard International prognostic index remains a valid predictor of outcome for patients with aggressive CD20 + B-cell lymphoma in the rituximab era." *J. Clin. Oncol.* 28:2373-2380.
[12] Haioun, C., Lepage, E., Gisselbrecht, C., Salles, G., Coiffier, B., Brice, P., Bosly, A. et al. 2000. "Survival benefit of high-dose therapy in poor-risk aggressive non-Hodgkin's lymphoma: final analysis of the prospective LNH87-2 protocol--a groupe d'Etude des lymphomes de l'Adulte study." *J. Clin. Oncol.* 18:3025-3030.
[13] Stiff, P. J., Unger, J. M., Cook, J. R., Constine, L. S., Couban, S., Stewart, D. A., Shea, T. C. et al. 2013. "Autologous transplantation as consolidation for aggressive non-Hodgkin's lymphoma." *N. Engl. J. Med.* 369:1681-1690.
[14] U. Vitolo, A. Chiappella, E. Brusamolino, E. Angelucci, M. Balzarotti, A. M. Carella, G. Ciccone et al. 2011. "A randomized multicentre phase III study for first line treatment of young patients with high risk (aaIPI 2-3) diffuse large B-cell lymphoma (DLBCL): rituximab plus dose-dense chemotherapy CHOP-14/MEGACHOP 14 with or without intensified high-dose chemotherapy (HDC) and autologous stem cell transplantation (ASCT): results of DLCL04 trial of Italian lymphoma foundation (FIL)." *Annals of Oncology* 22:106.
[15] Milpied, Noel-Jean, Legouill, Steven, Lamy, Thierry, Delwail, Vincent, Gressin, Remy, Guyotat, Denis, Damaj, Gandhi et al. 2010. "No Benefit of First-Line Rituximab (R) -High-Dose Therapy (R-HDT) Over R-CHOP14 for Young Adults with Diffuse Large B-Cell Lymphoma. Preliminary Results of the GOELAMS 075 Prospective Multicentre Randomized Trial." *ASH Annual Meeting Abstracts* 116:685-.
[16] Schmitz, N., Nickelsen, M., Ziepert, M., Haenel, M., Borchmann, P., Schmidt, C., Viardot, A. et al. 2012. "Conventional chemotherapy (CHOEP-14) with rituximab or high-dose chemotherapy (MegaCHOEP) with rituximab for young, high-risk patients with aggressive B-cell lymphoma: an open-label, randomised, phase 3 trial (DSHNHL 2002-1)." *Lancet Oncol.* 13:1250-1259.
[17] Coiffier, Bertrand, Lepage, Eric, Brière, Josette, Herbrecht, Raoul, Tilly, Hervé, Bouabdallah, Reda, Morel, Pierre et al. 2002. "CHOP Chemotherapy plus Rituximab Compared with CHOP Alone in Elderly Patients with Diffuse Large-B-Cell Lymphoma." *New England Journal of Medicine* 346:235-242.
[18] Pfreundschuh, M., Schubert, J., Ziepert, M., Schmits, R., Mohren, M., Lengfelder, E., Reiser, M. et al. 2008. "Six versus eight cycles of bi-weekly CHOP-14 with or without

rituximab in elderly patients with aggressive CD20 + B-cell lymphomas: a randomised controlled trial (RICOVER-60)." *Lancet Oncol.* 9:105-116.

[19] Philip, T., Armitage, J. O., Spitzer, G., Chauvin, F., Jagannath, S., Cahn, J. Y., Colombat, P. et al. 1987. "High-dose therapy and autologous bone marrow transplantation after failure of conventional chemotherapy in adults with intermediate-grade or high-grade non-Hodgkin's lymphoma." *N. Engl. J. Med.* 316:1493-1498.

[20] Philip, T., Guglielmi, C., Hagenbeek, A., Somers, R., Van der Lelie, H., Bron, D., Sonneveld, P. et al. 1995. "Autologous bone marrow transplantation as compared with salvage chemotherapy in relapses of chemotherapy-sensitive non-Hodgkin's lymphoma." *N. Engl. J. Med.* 333:1540-1545.

[21] Vose, J. M., Zhang, M. J., Rowlings, P. A., Lazarus, H. M., Bolwell, B. J., Freytes, C. O., Pavlovsky, S. et al. 2001. "Autologous transplantation for diffuse aggressive non-Hodgkin's lymphoma in patients never achieving remission: a report from the Autologous Blood and Marrow Transplant Registry." *J. Clin. Oncol.* 19:406-413.

[22] Kewalramani, T., Zelenetz, A. D., Hedrick, E. E., Donnelly, G. B., Hunte, S., Priovolos, A. C., Qin, J. et al. 2000. "High-dose chemoradiotherapy and autologous stem cell transplantation for patients with primary refractory aggressive non-Hodgkin lymphoma: an intention-to-treat analysis." *Blood* 96:2399-2404.

[23] Gisselbrecht, C., Glass, B., Mounier, N., Singh Gill, D., Linch, D. C., Trneny, M., Bosly, A. et al. 2010. "Salvage regimens with autologous transplantation for relapsed large B-cell lymphoma in the rituximab era." *J. Clin. Oncol.* 28:4184-4190.

[24] Thieblemont, C., Briere, J., Mounier, N., Voelker, H. U., Cuccuini, W., Hirchaud, E., Rosenwald, A. et al. 2011. "The germinal center/activated B-cell subclassification has a prognostic impact for response to salvage therapy in relapsed/refractory diffuse large B-cell lymphoma: a bio-CORAL study." *J. Clin. Oncol.* 29:4079-4087.

[25] Moskowitz, C. H., Zelenetz, A. D., Kewalramani, T., Hamlin, P., Lessac-Chenen, S., Houldsworth, J., Olshen, A. et al. 2005. "Cell of origin, germinal center versus nongerminal center, determined by immunohistochemistry on tissue microarray, does not correlate with outcome in patients with relapsed and refractory DLBCL." *Blood* 106:3383-3385.

[26] Gu, K., Weisenburger, D. D., Fu, K., Chan, W. C., Greiner, T. C., Aoun, P., Smith, L. M. et al. 2012. "Cell of origin fails to predict survival in patients with diffuse large B-cell lymphoma treated with autologous hematopoietic stem cell transplantation." *Hematol. Oncol.* 30:143-149.

[27] Hamlin, P. A., Zelenetz, A. D., Kewalramani, T., Qin, J., Satagopan, J. M., Verbel, D., Noy, A. et al. 2003. "Age-adjusted International Prognostic Index predicts autologous stem cell transplantation outcome for patients with relapsed or primary refractory diffuse large B-cell lymphoma." *Blood* 102:1989-1996.

[28] Gisselbrecht, C., Schmitz, N., Mounier, N., Singh Gill, D., Linch, D. C., Trneny, M., Bosly, A. et al. 2012. "Rituximab maintenance therapy after autologous stem-cell transplantation in patients with relapsed CD20(+) diffuse large B-cell lymphoma: final analysis of the collaborative trial in relapsed aggressive lymphoma." *J. Clin. Oncol.* 30: 4462-4469.

[29] Vose, J. M., Rizzo, D. J., Tao-Wu, J., Armitage, J. O., Bashey, A., Burns, L. J., Christiansen, N. P. et al. 2004. "Autologous transplantation for diffuse aggressive non-

Hodgkin lymphoma in first relapse or second remission." *Biol. Blood Marrow Transplant.* 10:116-127.

[30] Hoppe, B. S., Moskowitz, C. H., Filippa, D. A., Moskowitz, C. S., Kewalramani, T., Zelenetz, A. D., Yahalom, J. 2008. "Involved-field radiotherapy before high-dose therapy and autologous stem-cell rescue in diffuse large-cell lymphoma: long-term disease control and toxicity." *J. Clin. Oncol.* 26:1858-1864.

[31] Winter, J. N., Inwards, D. J., Spies, S., Wiseman, G., Patton, D., Erwin, W., Rademaker, A. W. et al. 2009. "Yttrium-90 ibritumomab tiuxetan doses calculated to deliver up to 15 Gy to critical organs may be safely combined with high-dose BEAM and autologous transplantation in relapsed or refractory B-cell non-Hodgkin's lymphoma." *J. Clin. Oncol.* 27:1653-1659.

[32] Nademanee, A., Forman, S., Molina, A., Fung, H., Smith, D., Dagis, A., Kwok, C. et al. 2005. "A phase 1/2 trial of high-dose yttrium-90-ibritumomab tiuxetan in combination with high-dose etoposide and cyclophosphamide followed by autologous stem cell transplantation in patients with poor-risk or relapsed non-Hodgkin lymphoma." *Blood* 106:2896-2902.

[33] Press, O. W., Eary, J. F., Gooley, T., Gopal, A. K., Liu, S., Rajendran, J. G., Maloney, D. G. et al. 2000. "A phase I/II trial of iodine-131-tositumomab (anti-CD20), etoposide, cyclophosphamide, and autologous stem cell transplantation for relapsed B-cell lymphomas." *Blood* 96:2934-2942.

[34] Decaudin, D., Mounier, N., Tilly, H., Ribrag, V., Ghesquieres, H., Bouabdallah, K., Morschhauser, F. et al. 2011. "(90)Y ibritumomab tiuxetan (Zevalin) combined with BEAM (Z-BEAM) conditioning regimen plus autologous stem cell transplantation in relapsed or refractory low-grade CD20-positive B-cell lymphoma. A GELA phase II prospective study." *Clin. Lymphoma Myeloma Leuk.* 11:212-218.

[35] Vose, J. M., Bierman, P. J., Loberiza, F. R., Enke, C., Hankins, J., Bociek, R. G., Chan, W. C., Weisenburger, D. D., Armitage, J. O. 2013. "Phase II trial of 131-Iodine tositumomab with high-dose chemotherapy and autologous stem cell transplantation for relapsed diffuse large B cell lymphoma." *Biol. Blood Marrow Transplant.* 19:123-128.

[36] Briones, J., Novelli, S., Garcia-Marco, J. A., Tomas, J. F., Bernal, T., Grande, C., Canales, M. A. et al. 2013. "Autologous stem cell transplantation after conditioning with Yttrium-90 ibritumomab tiuxetan plus beam in refractory non-Hodgkin diffuse large B-cell lymphoma: results of a prospective, multicenter, phase II clinical trial." *Haematologica.*

[37] Vose, J. M., Carter, S., Burns, L. J., Ayala, E., Press, O. W., Moskowitz, C. H., Stadtmauer, E. A. et al. 2013. "Phase III randomized study of rituximab/carmustine, etoposide, cytarabine, and melphalan (BEAM) compared with iodine-131 tositumomab/ BEAM with autologous hematopoietic cell transplantation for relapsed diffuse large B-cell lymphoma: results from the BMT CTN 0401 trial." *J. Clin. Oncol.* 31:1662-1668.

[38] Glass, B., Ziepert, M., Reiser, M., Freund, M., Trumper, L., Metzner, B., Feller, A. et al. 2010. "High-dose therapy followed by autologous stem-cell transplantation with and without rituximab for primary treatment of high-risk diffuse large B-cell lymphoma." *Ann. Oncol.* 21:2255-2261.

[39] Coso, D., Sebban, C., Boulat, O., Biron, P., Rey, J., Aurran, T., Chabannon, C. et al. 2006. "A phase II trial of rituximab as adjuvant to intensive sequential chemotherapy in

patients under 60 years with untreated poor-prognosis diffuse large B-cell lymphoma." *Bone Marrow Transplant.* 38:217-222.

[40] Sieniawski, M., Staak, O., Glossmann, J. P., Reineke, T., Scheuss, H., Diehl, V., Engert, A., Josting, A. 2007. "Rituximab added to an intensified salvage chemotherapy program followed by autologous stem cell transplantation improved the outcome in relapsed and refractory aggressive non-Hodgkin lymphoma." *Ann. Hematol.* 86:107-115.

[41] Khouri, I. F., Saliba, R. M., Hosing, C., Okoroji, G. J., Acholonu, S., Anderlini, P., Couriel, D. et al. 2005. "Concurrent administration of high-dose rituximab before and after autologous stem-cell transplantation for relapsed aggressive B-cell non-Hodgkin's lymphomas." *J. Clin. Oncol.* 23:2240-2247.

[42] Sehn, Laurie Helen, Chua, Neil Sun, Mayer, Jiri, Dueck, Gregory Scott, Trn, #x011B, ny, Marek et al. 2015. "GADOLIN: Primary results from a phase III study of obinutuzumab plus bendamustine compared with bendamustine alone in patients with rituximab-refractory indolent non-Hodgkin lymphoma." *ASCO Meeting Abstracts* 33: LBA8502.

[43] Nagle, S. J., Woo, K., Schuster, S. J., Nasta, S. D., Stadtmauer, E., Mick, R., Svoboda, J. 2013. "Outcomes of patients with relapsed/refractory diffuse large B-cell lymphoma with progression of lymphoma after autologous stem cell transplantation in the rituximab era." *Am. J. Hematol.* 88:890-894.

[44] Lazarus, H. M., Zhang, M. J., Carreras, J., Hayes-Lattin, B. M., Ataergin, A. S., Bitran, J. D., Bolwell, B. J. et al. 2010. "A comparison of HLA-identical sibling allogeneic versus autologous transplantation for diffuse large B cell lymphoma: a report from the CIBMTR." *Biol. Blood Marrow Transplant.* 16:35-45.

[45] van Kampen, R. J., Canals, C., Schouten, H. C., Nagler, A., Thomson, K. J., Vernant, J. P., Buzyn, A. et al. 2011. "Allogeneic stem-cell transplantation as salvage therapy for patients with diffuse large B-cell non-Hodgkin's lymphoma relapsing after an autologous stem-cell transplantation: an analysis of the European Group for Blood and Marrow Transplantation Registry." *J. Clin. Oncol.* 29:1342-1348.

[46] Bacher, U., Klyuchnikov, E., Le-Rademacher, J., Carreras, J., Armand, P., Bishop, M. R., Bredeson, C. N. et al. 2012. "Conditioning regimens for allotransplants for diffuse large B-cell lymphoma: myeloablative or reduced intensity?" *Blood* 120:4256-4262.

[47] McCurdy, S. R., Kanakry, J. A., Showel, M. M., Tsai, H. L., Bolanos-Meade, J., Rosner, G. L., Kanakry, C. G. et al. 2015. "Risk-stratified outcomes of nonmyeloablative HLA-haploidentical BMT with high-dose posttransplantation cyclophosphamide." *Blood* 125:3024-3031.

[48] Rodrigues, C. A., Sanz, G., Brunstein, C. G., Sanz, J., Wagner, J. E., Renaud, M., de Lima, M. et al. 2009. "Analysis of risk factors for outcomes after unrelated cord blood transplantation in adults with lymphoid malignancies: a study by the Eurocord-Netcord and lymphoma working party of the European group for blood and marrow transplantation." *J. Clin. Oncol.* 27:256-263.

[49] Akhtari, M., Bhatt, V. R., Tandra, P. K., Krishnamurthy, J., Horstman, H., Dreessen, A., Chen, P. X., Armitage, J. O. 2013. "Therapy-related myeloid neoplasms after autologous hematopoietic stem cell transplantation in lymphoma patients." *Cancer Biol. Ther.* 14:1077-1088.

[50] Savani, B. N., Griffith, M. L., Jagasia, S., Lee, S. J. 2011. "How I treat late effects in adults after allogeneic stem cell transplantation." *Blood* 117:3002-3009.

[51] Burns, L. J. 2009. "Late effects after autologous hematopoietic cell transplantation." *Biol. Blood Marrow Transplant.* 15:21-24.

[52] Bhatt, V. R., Loberiza, F. R., Jr., Jing, H., Bociek, R. G., Bierman, P. J., Maness, L. J., Vose, J. M., Armitage, J. O., Akhtari, M. 2015 "Mortality Patterns Among Recipients of Autologous Hematopoietic Stem Cell Transplantation for Lymphoma and Myeloma in the Past Three Decades." *Clin. Lymphoma Myeloma Leuk.*

[53] Wilson, W. H., Young, R. M., Schmitz, R., Yang, Y., Pittaluga, S., Wright, G., Lih, C. J. et al. 2015 [Epub. ahead of print]. "Targeting B cell receptor signaling with ibrutinib in diffuse large B cell lymphoma." *Nat. Med.*

[54] Lesokhin, Alexander M., Ansell, Stephen M., Armand, Philippe, Scott, Emma C., Halwani, Ahmad, Gutierrez, Martin, Millenson, Michael M. et al. 2014. "Preliminary Results of a Phase I Study of Nivolumab (BMS-936558) in Patients with Relapsed or Refractory Lymphoid Malignancies." *Blood* 124:291.

[55] Kochenderfer, James N., Dudley, Mark E., Kassim, Sadik H., Somerville, Robert P. T., Carpenter, Robert O., Stetler-Stevenson, Maryalice, Yang, James C. et al. 2015. "Chemotherapy-Refractory Diffuse Large B-Cell Lymphoma and Indolent B-Cell Malignancies Can Be Effectively Treated With Autologous T Cells Expressing an Anti-CD19 Chimeric Antigen Receptor." *Journal of Clinical Oncology* 33:540-549.

[56] Majhail, N. S., Rizzo, J. D., Lee, S. J., Aljurf, M., Atsuta, Y., Bonfim, C., Burns, L. J. et al. 2012. "Recommended screening and preventive practices for long-term survivors after hematopoietic cell transplantation." *Biol. Blood Marrow Transplant.* 18:348-371.

[57] Kewalramani, T., Zelenetz, A. D., Nimer, S. D., Portlock, C., Straus, D., Noy, A., O'Connor, O. et al. 2004. "Rituximab and ICE as second-line therapy before autologous stem cell transplantation for relapsed or primary refractory diffuse large B-cell lymphoma." *Blood* 103:3684-3688.

In: Diffuse Large B-Cell Lymphoma (DLBCL)
Editor: Haipeng Shao
ISBN: 978-1-63484-402-4

Chapter 5

PRIMARY MEDIASTINAL LARGE B-CELL LYMPHOMA

Andreas Saltos and Lubomir Sokol [*]
Department of Malignant Hematology, H. Lee Moffitt Cancer Center and Research Institute, Tampa, FL, US

ABSTRACT

Primary mediastinal large B-cell lymphoma is a distinct subtype of diffuse large B-cell lymphoma which occurs predominantly in young patients and is characterized by a large mediastinal mass but without frequent sites of distant disease. Histologic and genetic features overlap with classical Hodgkin lymphoma, although tumor cells express pan-B cell markers and exhibit a response to anti-CD20 therapy. Treatment with immuno-chemotherapy regimens containing rituximab, in many cases followed by consolidative mediastinal radiation therapy, has led to good response rates and overall survival. Early post-treatment remission evaluated by positron emission tomography has been demonstrated to have a high negative predictive value for durable response, and may be used to avoid the need for radiation therapy in many cases. However, refractory cases and relapses still occur and existing second-line therapies are limited. Molecular profiling has demonstrated a high proportion of tumors with activation of JAK-STAT and NF-κB pathways, as well as overexpression of PDL-1 and PDL-2. Novel targeted and immunotherapeutic approaches tailored to these findings hold promise to further enhance survival and limit toxicities associated with current therapies.

INTRODUCTION

Primary mediastinal large B-cell lymphoma (PMBCL) is a distinct clinical entity, generally regarded as a subtype of diffuse large B-cell lymphoma (DLBCL), which is thought to arise from thymic medullary B-cells. It is a clinically aggressive lymphoma, characterized

[*] Corresponding author: Lubomir Sokol. Department of Malignant Hematology, H. Lee Moffitt Cancer Center and Research Institute, Tampa, FL, US. E-mail: Lubomir.Sokol@moffitt.org, phone: 813-745-8212.

by a biological and molecular profile as well as clinical features common to both DLBCL and nodular sclerosis classical Hodgkin lymphoma (cHL) [1-3]. PMBCL was first reported in the 1980s [4-6], and in 2001 was incorporated into the WHO classification of tumors of hematopoietic and lymphoid tissues as a distinct entity under mature B-cell lymphomas. Because it is relatively uncommon and also only relatively recently recognized, optimal therapeutic regimens remain somewhat controversial.

EPIDEMIOLOGY

PMBCL is relatively uncommon, accounting for 2-4% of all non-Hodgkin Lymphomas (NHLs), and 6-12% of all DLBCLs. It predominantly occurs in adolescents and young adults (median age of 35), a notably younger population than other subtypes of DLBCL. There is also a female preponderance, with approximately two-thirds of cases reported in females [7-9]. There are no known environmental risk factors, although a familial inheritance was demonstrated in a single Finnish family in which three siblings were diagnosed with PMBCL and shared a single missense mutation in the MLL gene (5533C > A (His1845Asn) variant) [10].

CELL OF ORIGIN

PMBCL cells are generally regarded to be of thymic B-cell origin. The thymus is primarily involved in maturation of T-cells during childhood and early adolescence, although B-cell populations are also present in the thymic medulla and corticomedullary junction [11]. These cells have been shown to express CD19, CD20, and CD22, with the absence of CD21 [12, 13], an immunophenotypic profile similar to that seen in PMBCL [5, 6]. The thymus, or its remnants, is generally also involved within the primary tumor mass in PMBCL, supporting thymic origin. Biopsy specimens may be found to contain thymic structures including Hassall's corpuscles, thymic lobules, or epithelial lined cysts [14].

HISTOLOGY AND IMMUNOPHENOTYPE

The pathologic appearance of PMBCL can be variable, and frequently shares features in common with DLBCL or nodular sclerosis classical Hodgkin lymphoma. Morphologically, PMBCL is often characterized by sheets of medium to large cells, with abundant pale cytoplasm and round or lobulated nuclei (or possibly multinucleated, in some cases resembling Reed-Sternberg/Hodgkin cells). Strands of background sclerosis are often present, which may compartmentalize tumor cells, and focal nodularity and/or necrosis may also be seen [4-7].

Tumor cells are positive for pan-B cell antigens (CD19, CD20, CD22, CD79a), CD45 and also in most cases CD23, and MAL and to a lesser degree, CD30. PMBCL cells typically lack CD10, CD15 and CD21 [9, 15, 16]. They may also stain positive for TRAF-1 and nuclear c-REL, a pattern also seen in the Reed-Sternberg cells of classical Hodgkin lymphoma [17]. Another hallmark of PMBCL is the typically lack of expression of surface immunoglobulin (CD79a is generally the only component of the B-cell receptor which is present), and thus it is not possible to establish clonality by κ and λ staining [16]. BCL-6 is generally positive by immunohistochemistry, and nuclear transcription factors OCT-2, BOB.1 and PU.1 are typically expressed [16, 18].

The particular pathologic features and immunophenotype in PMBCL are not generally regarded as having prognostic significance. However, at least one Japanese study proposed a positive prognostic association of expression of BCL-6 or MUM1, the presence of pale cytoplasm, and BCL-2 negativity [19].

Molecular Biology

Although no single cytogenetic change is diagnostic of or defines PMBCL, there are signature gene expression patterns in PMBCL. These molecular transcriptional changes were described in two major independent studies of gene expression profiling, demonstrating a pattern in PMBCL which was distinct from DLBCL but with similarities to cHL [2, 20]. These findings have led to better definition of PMBCL as a distinct biological entity and better understanding of therapeutic targets for novel therapies.

Among features shared between PMBCL and cHL are frequent gains in chromosome 9p and 2p. Gains in chromosome 2p are found in about 20% of cases of PMBCL, and are associated with increased expression of the REL proto-oncogene, leading to increased NF-κB activity and tumor resistance to apoptosis. The REL gene is also implicated in tumorigenesis in other hematologic malignancies [2, 20, 21]. Gains in chromosome 9p occur in 50-75% of PMBCL cases, and are associated with overexpression of the Janus Kinase 2 (JAK2) gene, leading to activation of JAK-STAT pathway. Also contained within chromosome 9p are the genes encoding the ligands for the programmed cell death receptor, PDL-1 and PDL-2. These ligands play a critical role in suppressing T-cell antitumor function. Activation of the JAK-STAT pathway also leads to increased expression of PDL-1 [20, 22, 23].

BCL-6 gene somatic hypermutation is frequently detected, supporting the germinal center origin of PMBCL. Of note, the nature of BCL-6 mutations observed in PMBCL differs from those seen in DLBCL and follicular lymphoma [16, 24].

Clinical Manifestations

PMBCL generally presents with a large anterior mediastinal mass, often impinging (or involving by direct extension) surrounding structures including the pleura, lungs and airways, heart and superior vena cava (SVC). Approximately 50% of cases present with pleural and/or pericardial effusions [25]. At initial diagnosis, involvement is typically limited to the mediastinum with possible cervical involvement, while distant disease is less common (the majority of patients present with stage I or II disease). Conversely, patients presenting with recurrent disease often have lymphoma spread to distant extranodal sites such as the liver, kidneys, adrenal glands, and central nervous system [9, 26, 27].

Typical radiographic features characterized in one series of 21 patients included an anterior mediastinal mass with median size of 9.7 cm, with regular contour (67%) and the absence of cervical and abdominal lymphadenopathy (0%). The presence of vascular encasement (62%) was associated with an increased likelihood of PMBCL compared to classical Hodgkin lymphoma or T-cell lymphoblastic lymphoma. Roughly half of cases presented with pericardial effusions. Local invasion into lung, chest wall, or skin were each seen in roughly 10-20% of cases [28]. See Figure 1 below for an example of representative radiographic findings in PMBCL.

The most common clinical symptoms associated with PMBCL include chest pain, cough (with possible hemoptysis), dyspnea, and B-symptoms (including fever, night sweats, and/or weight loss). Dysphagia, hoarseness and venous thrombosis may also occur as a result of compression of local structures [29].

Oncologic Emergencies

Patients may also present with oncologic emergencies because of the tumor location near critical cardiovascular structures. SVC syndrome occurs frequently, with one series demonstrating its presence in 10 out of 30 cases [29]. SVC syndrome may manifest as dyspnea (most common symptom), facial, upper extremity, or chest swelling and plethora, or even headaches or altered mental status as a result of cerebral edema. Symptoms may be exacerbated while bending forward or lying supine. Traditionally, emergent radiation therapy was instituted in cases of SVC syndrome although this is no longer felt to be necessary in most cases. Radiation prior to obtaining a biopsy could potentially obscure the pathologic diagnosis which can be critical in selecting appropriate treatment [30]. In addition, deferring therapy until after appropriate diagnostic studies can be completed has not been shown to adversely influence outcomes [31].

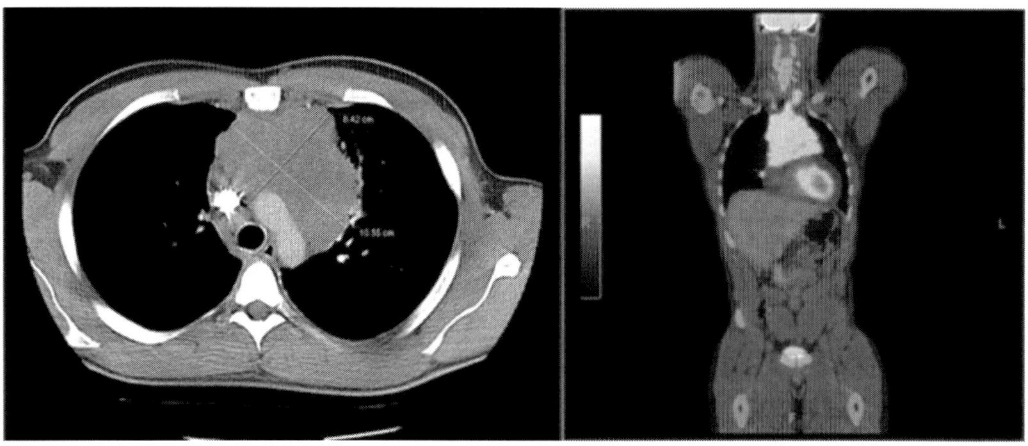

Figure 1. Representative radiographic presentation of PMBCL. On the left, axial contrast-enhanced CT reveals a large anterior mediastinal mass (>10 cm) with regular contour and mass-effect on adjacent structures. On the right, coronal PET/CT fusion images demonstrate high metabolic activity of the mediastinal mass, as well as significant pericardial effusion. There is associated supraclavicular and mediastinal activity but no evidence for involvement in the abdomen or pelvis.

Patients may also present with respiratory distress either due to compression of the trachea or due to phrenic nerve involvement resulting in diaphragmatic paralysis. Particular attention should be paid to patients undergoing general anesthesia for a biopsy procedure due to the possible mass effect of the tumor on the airway requiring high pressures to maintain patency.

Pericardial tamponade can also occur, manifesting with dyspnea, chest discomfort, and/or hypotension. Large tumor bulk is often present and can be associated with tumor lysis syndrome, resulting in electrolyte disturbances and renal injury or failure due to deposition of uric acid and/or calcium phosphate crystals into renal tubules [29, 32].

DIAGNOSIS

The diagnosis of PMBCL is primarily pathological, made on the basis of histologic appearance and immunohistochemical staining. Because of the typical anatomic localization with mediastinal involvement without frequent involvement of peripheral lymph nodes, a more invasive diagnostic biopsy is often required. Usually biopsy can be performed through mediastinoscopy, anterior mediastinotomy, or percutaneous computed tomography (CT)-guided core needle biopsy. Sufficient tissue samples should be taken whenever possible, as extensive fibrosis, crush artifact, or necrosis may limit the diagnostic quality of the specimen in small biopsies.

Hoeller et al. have described a strategy for distinguishing PMBCL from cHL using primarily three immunohistochemical markers which were determined to be among the most predictive: BOB.1, CD79a, and cyclin E. Applying these three markers enabled correct classification of 97-98% of patients to either PMBCL or cHL [33]. Recommended examinations and procedures to determine clinical stage include history and physical examination (with attention to performance status, B-symptoms, adenopathy, hepatosplenomegaly, and evaluation for the presence of urgent or emergent complications discussed above), F-fluorodeoxyglucose positron emission tomography (PET) CT or whole body CT, bone marrow aspiration and biopsy, complete blood count with differential, and blood chemistry studies. Serum LDH and uric acid measurements can evaluate for tumor lysis. An elevation in serum LDH is present in 70-80% of cases. β2-microglobulin is not typically elevated. Hepatitis B virus serology should be obtained due to possible reactivation with rituximab therapy, and other viral serology including HIV and Hepatitis C virus should be considered. Pregnancy testing is recommended for women of child-bearing age [34].

An assessment of left ventricular function is necessary before chemotherapy which typically includes an anthracycline; an echocardiogram may also evaluate for pericardial effusion and rule out tamponade physiology. Fertility counseling and preservation should be discussed with patients when appropriate. PET is preferred over CT for the purposes of identifying and selecting site for biopsy, as well as for staging [35]. Clinical stage is classified using the Ann Arbor staging system. Stage IV at presentation is uncommon, and the majority of patients present with clinical stage I or II disease.

The role of lumbar puncture for staging and/or delivery of central nervous system (CNS) prophylaxis is somewhat unclear. CNS involvement is uncommon, with observed rates of CNS relapse of around 2% in modern series, although rates as high as 7-9% have been reported. Risk of CNS involvement appears increased with increased extranodal disease burden (or nasopharyngeal, sinus, or testicular involvement) and may be more common at disease relapse [26, 36]. In at least one recent prospective study, CNS prophylaxis with intrathecal methotrexate was given to patients with elevated LDH and 2 or more extranodal sites of involvement (similar to current guidelines for DLBCL) [37].

Differential Diagnosis

The differential diagnosis of PMBCL includes other tumors which commonly present with mediastinal involvement, including thymoma, germ cell tumors, or metastatic carcinomas.

Differential diagnoses also include other lymphomas- classical Hodgkin Lymphoma often presents in the same demographic and with similar clinical features to PMBCL. In addition, histologic appearance may be similar even with the presence of Reed-Sternberg cells in PMBCL. Other non-Hodgkin Lymphomas may also present similarly to PMBCL. T-cell lymphoblastic lymphoma may also present with bulky mediastinal involvement. DLBCL with anterior mediastinal involvement should be suspected in cases with involvement of bone marrow or distant lymph nodes. Immunohistochemistry can aid in distinguishing these cases [9, 15].

A distinct subtype of NHL named mediastinal "gray zone" lymphoma, also known as B-cell lymphoma, unclassifiable, with features intermediate between DLBCL and cHL, is less common than PMBL and has only been recently recognized. In contrast to PMBCL, tumors generally stain positive for CD15. These mediastinal gray zone lymphomas predominantly affect males, and although they have been treated with a similar approach, they are associated with a worse prognosis than that of PMBCL [15, 38, 39].

Prognosis

Risk assessment in NHL is generally performed using the standard international prognostic index (IPI) although its applicability to PMBCL has been called into question. Two of the five factors included in the IPI (age greater than 60 and clinical stage III or IV) are generally not present in patients with PMBCL. Additionally, retrospective analyses have failed to show prognostic significance of the IPI [40, 41]. Aoki et al. described the PMBL prognostic index (PMBIPI) which stratifies patients into low, intermediate, or high-risk categories according to two factors: the presence of pleural or pericardial effusion, and standard IPI high/intermediate or high risk [42].

As suggested by the PMBIPI, the presence of pleural or pericardial effusions has been proposed as a negative prognostic indicator, as has high total-lesion glycolysis on baseline PET scan [43, 44]. Response to initial therapy is a strong predictive marker for progression-free survival, with those patients with a complete response and no residual hypermetabolic activity in the mediastinum having a low risk of relapse [45]. The role of FDG-PET as a marker has emerged as a potential strategy to identify patients who may require additional therapy - most often for decisions regarding consolidation radiation therapy [46]. However, it is important to note that while the negative predictive value for PET is good, a positive PET after initial treatment is not necessarily predictive of outcome and a repeat biopsy is recommended before changing or considering additional therapy [47].

Relapses generally occur within the first few months after treatment, and late relapses (after 2 years) are uncommon [20, 40, 48]. Although initial experience suggested a poorer response to treatment and prognosis than that of DLBCL, response rates and overall survival are generally good (over 85-90% in many series as highlighted in recent reviews) [49-51]. However, as discussed below, there is a lack of effective second-line therapies for those patients who experience a relapse or refractory disease.

TREATMENT

Because PMBCL is a relatively uncommon subtype of NHL, and also because it has been recognized only over the past few decades, prospective data to guide treatment is limited and there are no randomized controlled trials. Therefore, some uncertainty and controversy exists in the optimal up-front treatment approach, although modern rituximab-containing regimens have resulted in generally favorable outcomes.

It is important to note that because outcomes in second and further lines of therapy in PMBCL are poor [52, 53], accurate diagnosis and selection of appropriate treatment in the up-front setting is considered imperative.

Early Chemotherapy Experience

During the early experience of treatment for PMBCL in the pre-rituximab era, treatment initially consisted of chemotherapeutic regimens used for DLBCL, primarily with cyclophosphamide, doxorubicin, vincristine, and prednisone (CHOP). Early studies using this approach suggested an aggressive clinical course with high rates of primary refractory disease and early progression. Results from multiple published series of treatment with CHOP-like chemotherapy alone demonstrate response rates between 60-80% but with frequent early relapses and long-term overall survival of around 40-55% [41, 52, 54, 55].

These limited results prompted investigation into more intensive chemotherapy regimens. Among the most notable positive results were from studies utilizing third-generation regimens of combinations of doxorubicin, cyclophosphamide, vincristine, prednisone, and bleomycin with either methotrexate (MACOP-B) or etoposide (VACOP-B). It was also noted that the addition of consolidative involved-field radiation therapy (IFRT) after chemotherapy significantly improved both complete response rates and progression-free survival [25, 52, 54]. Thus, the institution of intensive chemotherapy regimens including MACOP-B or VACOP-B with consolidation radiation therapy was proposed as a standard of care for PMBCL in the pre-rituximab era. Complete response rates approaching 90% were reported using this approach, with long-term overall survival of approximately 80% [52, 54, 56].

Immunochemotherapy and Modern Treatment Regimens

The addition of the anti-CD20 monoclonal antibody rituximab to CHOP-like chemotherapy was demonstrated to significantly improve response rates as well as survival in patients with DLBCL, ushering in a new era of immunochemotherapy for this disease [57-59]. One of the seminal studies demonstrating this benefit was the MabThera International Trial (MInT), which included 87 patients with PMBCL (11% of all DLBCL patients included in the trial). The study population was restricted to patients under age 60 with clinical stage II-IV (or I bulky) and an age-adjusted IPI of 0 or 1. A subgroup analysis of these PMBCL patients demonstrated that the addition of rituximab produced a significant improvement in complete response (84% vs 54%, p = 0.015), less early disease progression (2.5% vs 24%, p = 0.006), and an improvement in 3-year event free survival (78% vs 52%, p = 0.012). Although the overall survival benefit (89% vs 78%, p = 0.158) did not reach statistical significance, this was felt to be related to a lack of power for the smaller subgroup of patients. Of note, without the addition of rituximab the risk of progressive disease was much higher for PMBCL than for DLBCL (24% vs 10%), and this difference was largely eliminated with the addition of rituximab [60].

The benefit of adding rituximab to CHOP chemotherapy (R-CHOP) has also been confirmed in multiple retrospective cohorts, with long-term overall survival improvements from 65-70% without rituximab to approximately 90% [40, 42]. Based upon these data, first-line therapy with R-CHOP for 6 cycles followed by consolidative radiation therapy is one recommended approach as outlined in the National Comprehensive Cancer Network (NCCN) guidelines as of 2015 [34].

However, some concerns remain over a significant remaining proportion of patients who do not achieve a durable response with R-CHOP therapy. One study which included a broader population of PMBCL patients (including those with higher risk based on IPI who were excluded in the MInT trial discussed above) demonstrated 21% of patients with primary refractory after primary treatment with R-CHOP with or without radiation, with 5-year progression-free and overall survival rates of 68% and 79%, respectively [48]. It is interesting to note that the addition of rituximab to third-generation regimens MACOP-B or VACOP-B did not appear to show an improvement in response or relapse-free survival rates [61].

Alternative immuno-chemotherapeutic regimens have also been explored in the interest of improved response rates as well as to possibly spare the need for radiation therapy. One alternative regimen which has been explored prospectively at Memorial Sloan-Kettering Cancer Center involved dose-dense R-CHOP (every 14 days) for 4 cycles followed by consolidation with ifosfamide, carboplatin and etoposide (ICE) for 3 cycles, with reported long-term progression-free and overall survival of 79% and 90%, respectively [47]. Another alternative intensified rituximab and methotrexate-based regimen (GMALL B-ALL/NHL 2002 protocol) was examined in a small (n = 15) European series, with response rates and long-term overall survival of 100% [62]. A phase II study conducted by the NCI investigated the use of 6-8 cycles of infusional dose-adjusted etoposide, doxorubicin, cyclophosphamide, vincristine, and prednisone in combination with rituximab (da-EPOCH-R) as initial therapy in PMBCL. Consolidative radiation therapy was omitted for patients who responded to therapy. The results using this approach were quite promising, with reported 5-year event-free and overall survival rates of 93% and 97%, respectively [37]. Of these approaches, both the da-EPOCH-R and the dose-dense R-CHOP followed by consolidative ICE approaches are also recommended as alternatives to R-CHOP per NCCN guidelines as of 2015 [34]. Although these intensified regimens appear to have improved survival results, their direct comparison to R-CHOP has not been evaluated in a prospective, randomized setting, and their possible benefits should be weighed against greater potential for toxicities.

Role for Radiation Therapy

As mentioned above, the addition of consolidative radiation therapy after chemotherapy has been shown to significantly improve both response rates and progression-free survival, most notably with earlier chemotherapeutic regimens without rituximab. This remains the standard of care for many patients in the modern era, including those patients with evidence of residual disease after initial therapy. Typical treatment protocols for radiation therapy involve targeting the originally involved area of disease (IFRT), delivering a dose of 30-40 Gy over 4-5 weeks [25, 54, 56].

However, radiation therapy is associated with toxicities which can be significant in young patients with curable disease. Thus there is interest in sparing the need for consolidative radiation therapy when possible. Data from multiple series suggest that patients who achieve a complete response to initial therapy have equally good outcomes without the need for radiotherapy [36, 40, 42]. An emerging strategy that has been proposed is the use of FDG-PET as a marker to identify patients who may require consolidation radiation therapy. This is based on evidence that a complete metabolic response on PET is prognostic for good progression-free survival [36, 45, 46].

There are no prospective randomized data comparing results with versus without radiation therapy after immunochemotherapy, but this is currently being evaluated in one randomized trial [www.clinicaltrials.gov; NCT01599559]. The use of more intensive immunochemotherapy induction regimens such as da-EPOCH-R, as discussed above, have demonstrated high response rates which may obviate the need for radiation therapy in many cases. However, consolidation IFRT remains standard for patients with residual disease after therapy and also remains a consideration for patients with bulky disease at presentation and those treated with R-CHOP.

Relapsed/Refractory Disease and Role for Hematopoietic Stem Cell Transplantation

For patients with relapsed or refractory disease, treatment strategies are generally similar to those for DLBCL, although outcomes are generally unfavorable. Salvage chemotherapy has not resulted in significant benefit, with 2-year survival of only 15% demonstrated in one series [53].

High dose therapy followed by autologous stem cell transplantation has been evaluated and shown to improve survival in some patients. Published series have demonstrated long-term survival rates of 58-67% for autologous transplant in the setting of primary refractory disease, although significantly worse (27% in one series) for relapsed disease. Transplant outcomes have been correlated with disease status at transplantation as well as degree of response to recent prior chemotherapy [53, 63]. The use of front-line therapy with autologous stem cell transplantation was explored as well, but results have generally not been superior to more standard regimens discussed above, with 5-year progression-free survival rates of around 83-90% [64, 65].

Targeted/Emerging Therapies

Although modern immuno-chemotherapeutic regimens have improved survival for PMBCL, many patients still may not experience a durable response. This combined with the lack of effective second-line therapies has spurred ongoing interest in targeted therapy based on recent advances in understanding of the molecular biology of PMBCL. Currently, three targeted agents have been studied in clinical trials.

As stated above, the disease specific amplification of the 9p24.1 chromosome region includes the JAK2 locus. JAK2 amplification and induced PD-1 ligand transcription result in increased sensitivity to JAK2 inhibition [22]. Preclinical data with JAK2 inhibitors in PMBCL has shown antitumor activity [66]. This data has provided rationale for clinical trials testing monotherapy with JAK 1/2 kinase inhibitor ruxolitinib [NCT01965119] and anti-PD-1 monoclonal antibody pembrolizumab [NCT02576990] in patients with relapsed or refractory PMBCL [67].

Brentuximab-vedotin is a monoclonal antibody against CD30 which is conjugated to the antitubulin agent monomethyl auristatin E. There is interest in its use as targeted therapy in PMBCL since there is often expression of CD30 (albeit more weakly than seen in Hodgkin lymphoma). Early clinical evidence has been encouraging [68, 69], and clinical trials further investigating its use are ongoing [NCT01994850; NCT02423291].

Conclusion

PMBCL is a clinically and biologically distinct subtype of DLBCL, and particular attention should be paid to the appropriate identification of cases given its clinical and pathologic overlap with other lymphoma subtypes. Establishment of the correct diagnosis is also imperative because of the importance of selecting appropriate up-front treatment in this predominantly young population with potentially curable disease.

Early clinical experience in the pre-rituxumab era suggested a poorer response to therapy than conventional DLBCL, but recent advances in understanding of the biology of and treatment of PMBCL as a distinct entity have resulted in immunochemotherapy regimens with significant improvements in cure rates and a prognosis which is in fact better than that of conventional DLBCL. Consolidative radiation therapy has traditionally been considered standard for most cases; however there is interest in identifying patients for whom radiation therapy can be spared without an adverse effect on outcomes.

Despite these advances in therapy, relapses still occur and neither current second-line therapies nor bone marrow transplantation have demonstrated significant efficacy, highlighting the importance of further research in this disease. Recent advances in the understanding of the biology of PMBCL have driven interest in novel targeted therapies, and enrollment in a clinical trial remains a highly encouraged treatment option particularly for those patients with relapsed or refractory disease.

REFERENCES

[1] Yonetani, N., Kurata, M., Nishikori, M., Haga, H., Ohmori, K., Yamabe, H., Uchiyama, T., Ohno, H. 2001. "Primary mediastinal large B-cell lymphoma: a comparative study with nodular sclerosis-type Hodgkin's disease." *Int. J. Hematol.* 74:178-185.

[2] Savage, K. J., Monti, S., Kutok, J. L., Cattoretti, G., Neuberg, D., De Leval, L., Kurtin, P. et al. 2003. "The molecular signature of mediastinal large B-cell lymphoma differs from that of other diffuse large B-cell lymphomas and shares features with classical Hodgkin lymphoma." *Blood* 102:3871-3879.

[3] Steidl, C., Gascoyne, R. D. 2011. "The molecular pathogenesis of primary mediastinal large B-cell lymphoma." *Blood* 118:2659-2669.

[4] Yousem, S. A., Weiss, L. M., Warnke, R. A. 1985. "Primary mediastinal non-Hodgkin's lymphomas: a morphologic and immunologic study of 19 cases." *Am. J. Clin. Pathol.* 83:676-680.

[5] Menestrina, F., Chilosi, M., Bonetti, F., Lestani, M., Scarpa, A., Novelli, P., Doglioni, C. et al. 1986. "Mediastinal large-cell lymphoma of B-type, with sclerosis: histopathological and immunohistochemical study of eight cases." *Histopathology* 10: 589-600.

[6] Lamarre, L., Jacobson, J. O., Aisenberg, A. C., Harris, N. L. 1989. "Primary large cell lymphoma of the mediastinum. A histologic and immunophenotypic study of 29 cases." *Am. J. Surg. Pathol.* 13:730-739.

[7] Lazzarino, M., Orlandi, E., Paulli, M., Boveri, E., Morra, E., Brusamolino, E., Kindl, S. et al. 1993. "Primary mediastinal B-cell lymphoma with sclerosis: an aggressive tumor with distinctive clinical and pathologic features." *J. Clin. Oncol.* 11:2306-2313.

[8] Armitage, J. O., Weisenburger, D. D. 1998. "New approach to classifying non-Hodgkin's lymphomas: clinical features of the major histologic subtypes. Non-Hodgkin's Lymphoma Classification Project." *J. Clin. Oncol.* 16:2780-2795.

[9] Swerdllow, S. H., Campo, Elias, Harris, N. Lee. 2008; *WHO classification of tumours of haematopoietic and lymphoid tissues*. France: IARC Press, 2008.

[10] Saarinen, S., Kaasinen, E., Karjalainen-Lindsberg, M. L., Vesanen, K., Aavikko, M., Katainen, R., Taskinen, M. et al. 2013. "Primary mediastinal large B-cell lymphoma segregating in a family: exome sequencing identifies MLL as a candidate predisposition gene." *Blood* 121:3428-3430.

[11] Pearse, G. 2006. "Normal structure, function and histology of the thymus." *Toxicol. Pathol.* 34:504-514.

[12] Isaacson, P. G., Norton, A. J., Addis, B. J. 1987. "The human thymus contains a novel population of B lymphocytes." *Lancet* 2:1488-1491.

[13] Hofmann, W. J., Momburg, F., Moller, P. 1988. "Thymic medullary cells expressing B lymphocyte antigens." *Hum. Pathol.* 19:1280-1287.

[14] Addis, B. J., Isaacson, P. G. 1986. "Large cell lymphoma of the mediastinum: a B-cell tumour of probable thymic origin." *Histopathology* 10:379-390.

[15] Harris, N. L. 2013. "Shades of gray between large B-cell lymphomas and Hodgkin lymphomas: differential diagnosis and biological implications." *Mod. Pathol.* 26 Suppl. 1:S57-70.

[16] Pileri, S. A., Gaidano, G., Zinzani, P. L., Falini, B., Gaulard, P., Zucca, E., Pieri, F. et al. 2003. "Primary mediastinal B-cell lymphoma: high frequency of BCL-6 mutations and consistent expression of the transcription factors OCT-2, BOB.1, and PU.1 in the absence of immunoglobulins." *Am. J. Pathol.* 162:243-253.

[17] Rodig, S. J., Savage, K. J., LaCasce, A. S., Weng, A. P., Harris, N. L., Shipp, M. A., Hsi, E. D., Gascoyne, R. D., Kutok, J. L. 2007. "Expression of TRAF1 and nuclear c-Rel distinguishes primary mediastinal large cell lymphoma from other types of diffuse large B-cell lymphoma." *Am. J. Surg. Pathol.* 31:106-112.

[18] de Leval, L., Ferry, J. A., Falini, B., Shipp, M., Harris, N. L. 2001. "Expression of bcl-6 and CD10 in primary mediastinal large B-cell lymphoma: evidence for derivation from germinal center B cells?" *Am. J. Surg. Pathol.* 25:1277-1282.

[19] Maeshima, A. M., Taniguchi, H., Miyamoto, K., Fukuhara, S., Munakata, W., Maruyama, D., Kim, S. W. et al. 2014. "Prognostic significance of immunophenotypes and a nodular pattern in primary mediastinal large B-cell lymphoma." *Pathol. Int.* 64: 382-387.

[20] Rosenwald, A., Wright, G., Leroy, K., Yu, X., Gaulard, P., Gascoyne, R. D., Chan, W. C. et al. 2003. "Molecular diagnosis of primary mediastinal B cell lymphoma identifies a clinically favorable subgroup of diffuse large B cell lymphoma related to Hodgkin lymphoma." *J. Exp. Med.* 198:851-862.

[21] Joos, S., Otano-Joos, M. I., Ziegler, S., Bruderlein, S., du Manoir, S., Bentz, M., Moller, P., Lichter, P. 1996. "Primary mediastinal (thymic) B-cell lymphoma is characterized by gains of chromosomal material including 9p and amplification of the REL gene." *Blood* 87:1571-1578.

[22] Green, M. R., Monti, S., Rodig, S. J., Juszczynski, P., Currie, T., O'Donnell, E., Chapuy, B. et al. 2010. "Integrative analysis reveals selective 9p24.1 amplification, increased PD-1 ligand expression, and further induction via JAK2 in nodular sclerosing Hodgkin lymphoma and primary mediastinal large B-cell lymphoma." *Blood* 116:3268-3277.

[23] Chen, B. J., Chapuy, B., Ouyang, J., Sun, H. H., Roemer, M. G., Xu, M. L., Yu, H. et al. 2013. "PD-L1 expression is characteristic of a subset of aggressive B-cell lymphomas and virus-associated malignancies." *Clin. Cancer Res.* 19:3462-3473.

[24] Malpeli, G., Barbi, S., Moore, P. S., Scardoni, M., Chilosi, M., Scarpa, A., Menestrina, F. 2004. "Primary mediastinal B-cell lymphoma: hypermutation of the BCL6 gene targets motifs different from those in diffuse large B-cell and follicular lymphomas." *Haematologica* 89:1091-1099.

[25] Savage, K. J., Al-Rajhi, N., Voss, N., Paltiel, C., Klasa, R., Gascoyne, R. D., Connors, J. M. 2006. "Favorable outcome of primary mediastinal large B-cell lymphoma in a single institution: the British Columbia experience." *Ann. Oncol.* 17:123-130.

[26] Bishop, P. C., Wilson, W. H., Pearson, D., Janik, J., Jaffe, E. S., Elwood, P. C. 1999. "CNS involvement in primary mediastinal large B-cell lymphoma." *J. Clin. Oncol.* 17: 2479-2485.

[27] Papageorgiou, S. G., Diamantopoulos, P., Levidou, G., Angelopoulou, M. K., Economopoulou, P., Efthimiou, A., Constantinou, N. et al. 2013. "Isolated central

nervous system relapses in primary mediastinal large B-cell lymphoma after CHOP-like chemotherapy with or without Rituximab." *Hematol. Oncol.* 31:10-17.

[28] Tateishi, U., Muller, N. L., Johkoh, T., Onishi, Y., Arai, Y., Satake, M., Matsuno, Y., Tobinai, K. 2004. "Primary mediastinal lymphoma: characteristic features of the various histological subtypes on CT." *J. Comput. Assist. Tomogr.* 28:782-789.

[29] Jacobson, J. O., Aisenberg, A. C., Lamarre, L., Willett, C. G., Linggood, R. M., Miketic, L. M., Harris, N. L. 1988. "Mediastinal large cell lymphoma. An uncommon subset of adult lymphoma curable with combined modality therapy." *Cancer* 62:1893-1898.

[30] Loeffler, J. S., Leopold, K. A., Recht, A., Weinstein, H. J., Tarbell, N. J. 1986. "Emergency prebiopsy radiation for mediastinal masses: impact on subsequent pathologic diagnosis and outcome." *J. Clin. Oncol.* 4:716-721.

[31] Schraufnagel, D. E., Hill, R., Leech, J. A., Pare, J. A. 1981. "Superior vena caval obstruction. Is it a medical emergency?" *Am. J. Med.* 70:1169-1174.

[32] van Besien, K., Kelta, M., Bahaguna, P. 2001. "Primary mediastinal B-cell lymphoma: a review of pathology and management." *J. Clin. Oncol.* 19:1855-1864.

[33] Hoeller, S., Zihler, D., Zlobec, I., Obermann, E. C., Pileri, S. A., Dirnhofer, S., Tzankov, A. 2010. "BOB.1, CD79a and cyclin E are the most appropriate markers to discriminate classical Hodgkin's lymphoma from primary mediastinal large B-cell lymphoma." *Histopathology* 56:217-228.

[34] Zelenetz, A. D., Gordon, L. I., Wierda, W. G., Abramson, J. S., Advani, R. H., Andreadis, C. B., Bartlett, N. et al. 2014. "Non-Hodgkin's lymphomas, version 4.2014." *J. Natl. Compr. Canc. Netw.* 12:1282-1303.

[35] Cheson, B. D., Fisher, R. I., Barrington, S. F., Cavalli, F., Schwartz, L. H., Zucca, E., Lister, T. A. 2014. "Recommendations for initial evaluation, staging, and response assessment of Hodgkin and non-Hodgkin lymphoma: the Lugano classification." *J. Clin. Oncol.* 32:3059-3068.

[36] Savage, Kerry J., Yenson, Paul R., Shenkier, Tamara, Klasa, Richard, Villa, Diego, Goktepe, Ozge, Steidl, Christian et al. In: *The outcome of primary mediastinal large B-cell lymphoma (PMBCL) in the R-CHOP treatment era*, ASH Annual Meeting Abstracts, 2012; p 303.

[37] Dunleavy, K., Pittaluga, S., Maeda, L. S., Advani, R., Chen, C. C., Hessler, J., Steinberg, S. M. et al. 2013. "Dose-adjusted EPOCH-rituximab therapy in primary mediastinal B-cell lymphoma." *N. Engl. J. Med.* 368:1408-1416.

[38] Wilson, W. H., Pittaluga, S., Nicolae, A., Camphausen, K., Shovlin, M., Steinberg, S. M., Roschewski, M. et al. 2014. "A prospective study of mediastinal gray-zone lymphoma." *Blood* 124:1563-1569.

[39] Evens, A. M., Kanakry, J. A., Sehn, L. H., Kritharis, A., Feldman, T., Kroll, A., Gascoyne, R. D. et al. 2015. "Gray zone lymphoma with features intermediate between classical Hodgkin lymphoma and diffuse large B-cell lymphoma: Characteristics, outcomes, and prognostication among a large multicenter cohort." *Am. J. Hematol.* 90: 778-783.

[40] Vassilakopoulos, T. P., Pangalis, G. A., Katsigiannis, A., Papageorgiou, S. G., Constantinou, N., Terpos, E., Zorbala, A. et al. 2012. "Rituximab, cyclophosphamide, doxorubicin, vincristine, and prednisone with or without radiotherapy in primary

mediastinal large B-cell lymphoma: the emerging standard of care." *Oncologist* 17:239-249.

[41] Hamlin, P. A., Portlock, C. S., Straus, D. J., Noy, A., Singer, A., Horwitz, S. M., Oconnor, O. A. et al. 2005. "Primary mediastinal large B-cell lymphoma: optimal therapy and prognostic factor analysis in 141 consecutive patients treated at Memorial Sloan Kettering from 1980 to 1999." *Br. J. Haematol.* 130:691-699.

[42] Aoki, Tomohiro, Izutsu, Koji, Suzuki, Ritsuro, Nakaseko, Chiaki, Arima, Hiroshi, Shimada, Kazuyuki, Sasaki, Makoto et al. 2013. "Novel Prognostic Model Of Primary Mediastinal Large B-Cell Lymphoma (PMBL): A Multicenter Cooperative Retrospective Study In Japan." *Blood* 122:638-638.

[43] Aoki, T., Izutsu, K., Suzuki, R., Nakaseko, C., Arima, H., Shimada, K., Tomita, A. et al. 2014. "Prognostic significance of pleural or pericardial effusion and the implication of optimal treatment in primary mediastinal large B-cell lymphoma: a multicenter retrospective study in Japan." *Haematologica* 99:1817-1825.

[44] Ceriani, L., Martelli, M., Zinzani, P. L., Ferreri, A. J., Botto, B., Stelitano, C., Gotti, M. et al. 2015. "Utility of baseline 18FDG-PET/CT functional parameters in defining prognosis of primary mediastinal (thymic) large B-cell lymphoma." *Blood* 126:950-956.

[45] Nagle, S. J., Chong, E. A., Chekol, S., Shah, N. N., Nasta, S. D., Glatstein, E., Plastaras, J. P. et al. 2015. "The role of FDG-PET imaging as a prognostic marker of outcome in primary mediastinal B-cell lymphoma." *Cancer Med.* 4:7-15.

[46] Martelli, M., Ceriani, L., Zucca, E., Zinzani, P. L., Ferreri, A. J., Vitolo, U., Stelitano, C. et al. 2014. "[18F]fluorodeoxyglucose positron emission tomography predicts survival after chemoimmunotherapy for primary mediastinal large B-cell lymphoma: results of the International Extranodal Lymphoma Study Group IELSG-26 Study." *J. Clin. Oncol.* 32:1769-1775.

[47] Moskowitz, C. H., Schoder, H., Teruya-Feldstein, J., Sima, C., Iasonos, A., Portlock, C. S., Straus, D. et al. 2010. "Risk-adapted dose-dense immunochemotherapy determined by interim FDG-PET in Advanced-stage diffuse large B-Cell lymphoma." *J. Clin. Oncol.* 28:1896-1903.

[48] Soumerai, J. D., Hellmann, M. D., Feng, Y., Sohani, A. R., Toomey, C. E., Barnes, J. A., Takvorian, R. W. et al. 2014. "Treatment of primary mediastinal B-cell lymphoma with rituximab, cyclophosphamide, doxorubicin, vincristine and prednisone is associated with a high rate of primary refractory disease." *Leuk. Lymphoma* 55:538-543.

[49] Hamlin, P. A. 2014. "Evolving treatment paradigms for primary mediastinal diffuse large B-cell lymphoma." *J. Clin. Oncol.* 32:1751-1753.

[50] Dabrowska-Iwanicka, A., Walewski, J. A. 2014. "Primary mediastinal large B-cell lymphoma." *Curr. Hematol. Malig. Rep.* 9:273-283.

[51] Bhatt, V. R., Mourya, R., Shrestha, R., Armitage, J. O. 2015. "Primary mediastinal large B-cell lymphoma." *Cancer Treat. Rev.* 41:476-485.

[52] Todeschini, G., Secchi, S., Morra, E., Vitolo, U., Orlandi, E., Pasini, F., Gallo, E. et al. 2004. "Primary mediastinal large B-cell lymphoma (PMLBCL): long-term results from a retrospective multicentre Italian experience in 138 patients treated with CHOP or MACOP-B/VACOP-B." *Br. J. Cancer* 90:372-376.

[53] Kuruvilla, J., Pintilie, M., Tsang, R., Nagy, T., Keating, A., Crump, M. 2008. "Salvage chemotherapy and autologous stem cell transplantation are inferior for relapsed or refractory primary mediastinal large B-cell lymphoma compared with diffuse large B-cell lymphoma." *Leuk. Lymphoma* 49:1329-1336.

[54] Zinzani, P. L., Martelli, M., Bertini, M., Gianni, A. M., Devizzi, L., Federico, M., Pangalis, G. et al. 2002. "Induction chemotherapy strategies for primary mediastinal large B-cell lymphoma with sclerosis: a retrospective multinational study on 426 previously untreated patients." *Haematologica* 87:1258-1264.

[55] Lazzarino, M., Orlandi, E., Paulli, M., Strater, J., Klersy, C., Gianelli, U., Gargantini, L. et al. 1997. "Treatment outcome and prognostic factors for primary mediastinal (thymic) B-cell lymphoma: a multicenter study of 106 patients." *J. Clin. Oncol.* 15: 1646-1653.

[56] Martelli, M. P., Martelli, M., Pescarmona, E., De Sanctis, V., Donato, V., Palombi, F., Todisco, E. et al. 1998. "MACOP-B and involved field radiation therapy is an effective therapy for primary mediastinal large B-cell lymphoma with sclerosis." *Ann. Oncol.* 9: 1027-1029.

[57] Pfreundschuh, M., Kuhnt, E., Trumper, L., Osterborg, A., Trneny, M., Shepherd, L., Gill, D. S. et al. 2011. "CHOP-like chemotherapy with or without rituximab in young patients with good-prognosis diffuse large-B-cell lymphoma: 6-year results of an open-label randomised study of the MabThera International Trial (MInT) Group." *Lancet Oncol.* 12: 1013-1022.

[58] Coiffier, B., Thieblemont, C., Van Den Neste, E., Lepeu, G., Plantier, I., Castaigne, S., Lefort, S. et al. 2010. "Long-term outcome of patients in the LNH-98.5 trial, the first randomized study comparing rituximab-CHOP to standard CHOP chemotherapy in DLBCL patients: a study by the Groupe d'Etudes des Lymphomes de l'Adulte." *Blood* 116:2040-2045.

[59] Habermann, T. M., Weller, E. A., Morrison, V. A., Gascoyne, R. D., Cassileth, P. A., Cohn, J. B., Dakhil, S. R. et al. 2006. "Rituximab-CHOP versus CHOP alone or with maintenance rituximab in older patients with diffuse large B-cell lymphoma." *J. Clin. Oncol.* 24:3121-3127.

[60] Rieger, M., Osterborg, A., Pettengell, R., White, D., Gill, D., Walewski, J., Kuhnt, E. et al. 2011. "Primary mediastinal B-cell lymphoma treated with CHOP-like chemotherapy with or without rituximab: results of the Mabthera International Trial Group study." *Ann. Oncol.* 22:664-670.

[61] Zinzani, P. L., Stefoni, V., Finolezzi, E., Brusamolino, E., Cabras, M. G., Chiappella, A., Salvi, F. et al. 2009. "Rituximab combined with MACOP-B or VACOP-B and radiation therapy in primary mediastinal large B-cell lymphoma: a retrospective study." *Clin. Lymphoma Myeloma* 9:381-385.

[62] Pohlen, M., Gerth, H. U., Liersch, R., Koschmieder, S., Mesters, R. M., Kessler, T., Appelmann, I., Muller-Tidow, C., Berdel, W. E. 2011. "Efficacy and toxicity of a rituximab and methotrexate based regimen (GMALL B-ALL/NHL 2002 protocol) in Burkitt's and primary mediastinal large B-cell lymphoma." *Am. J. Hematol.* 86:E61-64.

[63] Sehn, L. H., Antin, J. H., Shulman, L. N., Mauch, P., Elias, A., Kadin, M. E., Wheeler, C. 1998. "Primary diffuse large B-cell lymphoma of the mediastinum: outcome following high-dose chemotherapy and autologous hematopoietic cell transplantation." *Blood* 91:717-723.

[64] Rodriguez, J., Conde, E., Gutierrez, A., Garcia, J. C., Lahuerta, J. J., Varela, M. R., Perez, C., Albo, C., Caballero, M. D. 2008. "Primary mediastinal large cell lymphoma (PMBL): frontline treatment with autologous stem cell transplantation (ASCT). The GEL-TAMO experience." *Hematol. Oncol.* 26:171-178.

[65] Cairoli, R., Grillo, G., Tedeschi, A., Gargantini, L., Marenco, P., Tresoldi, E., Barbarano, L., Nosari, A. M., Morra, E. 2002. "Efficacy of an early intensification treatment integrating chemotherapy, autologous stem cell transplantation and radiotherapy for poor risk primary mediastinal large B cell lymphoma with sclerosis." *Bone Marrow Transplant.* 29:473-477.

[66] Hao, Y., Chapuy, B., Monti, S., Sun, H. H., Rodig, S. J., Shipp, M. A. 2014. "Selective JAK2 inhibition specifically decreases Hodgkin lymphoma and mediastinal large B-cell lymphoma growth in vitro and in vivo." *Clin. Cancer Res.* 20:2674-2683.

[67] Dunleavy, K., Steidl, C. 2015. "Emerging biological insights and novel treatment strategies in primary mediastinal large B-cell lymphoma." *Semin. Hematol.* 52:119-125.

[68] Jacobsen, E. D., Sharman, J. P., Oki, Y., Advani, R. H., Winter, J. N., Bello, C. M., Spitzer, G. et al. 2015. "Brentuximab-vedotin demonstrates objective responses in a phase 2 study of relapsed/refractory DLBCL with variable CD30 expression." *Blood* 125:1394-1402.

[69] Sotomayor, E. M., Young, K. H., Younes, A. 2014. "Clinical roundtable monograph: CD30 in lymphoma: its role in biology, diagnostic testing, and targeted therapy." *Clin. Adv. Hematol. Oncol.* 12:1-22.

In: Diffuse Large B-Cell Lymphoma (DLBCL)
Editor: Haipeng Shao
ISBN: 978-1-63484-402-4

Chapter 6

MANAGING DIFFUSE LARGE B-CELL LYMPHOMA OF THE CENTRAL NERVOUS SYSTEM

Celeste M. Bello*
Department of Malignant Hematology, H. Lee Moffitt Cancer Center and Research Institute, Tampa, FL, US

ABSTRACT

Central nervous system lymphoma is a rare but aggressive form of non-Hodgkin's lymphoma (NHL). Although grouped together as one manifestation of NHL, it is actually a heterogeneous group of lymphomas. CNS lymphoma can be defined as primary CNS lymphoma if it is restricted to the brain, eyes, leptomeninges, or spinal cord. It is referred to as secondary lymphoma when there is CNS involvement and evidence of systemic disease. The single most effective agent for the treatment of CNS lymphoma, whether it is primary or secondary, is intravenous high dose methotrexate. While the effectiveness of methotrexate in the treatment of CNS lymphoma is well established, the optimal dose and regimen remains controversial and is a matter of debate.

INTRODUCTION

The majority of central nervous system (CNS) lymphoma cases are caused by diffuse large B cell lymphoma [1]. CNS lymphoma can occur as a primary malignancy or as an extension of systemic disease (referred to as secondary involvement). Primary CNS lymphoma (PCNSL) is defined as a lymphoma that is confined to the brain, eyes, leptomeninges, or spinal cord in the absence of systemic lymphoma. Secondary involvement of the CNS can occur at the time of diagnosis during work up for systemic disease or as relapsed disease in a patient previously treated for systemic lymphoma. PCNSL is an overall rare malignancy that is estimated to make up about 1% of all lymphoma cases and about 3% of all CNS tumors [2].

* Corresponding author: E-mail: BelloCM@moffitt.org; Phone: 813-745-4294.

The biggest risk factor for developing CNS lymphoma is immunodeficiency, however, CNS lymphoma is now becoming an increasing problem in immunocompetent patients. In the United States, the overall incidence rate of PCNSL has declined since 1995 [3]. This is primarily driven by the change in incidence in young and middle-aged men. This change has been attributed to the incidence and management of HIV/AIDS over this period of time. However, the rate has continued to increase in women and in men aged 65 years and older.

The exact pathogenesis of CNS lymphoma is unknown, and the pathogenesis of PCNSL is most likely different than that of secondary CNS lymphoma. The strong association of PCNSL with immunodeficiencies suggests that the immune system most likely plays a substantial role in the development of PCNSL. Tropism for the CNS is also thought to play a role in both PCNSL and secondary CNS lymphoma. The expression of a specific gene profile related to cell-surface adhesion molecules and various chemokine receptors has been demonstrated to be more common in PCNSL when compared to non-CNS lymphoma samples [3].

CNS lymphoma has an overall poor prognosis, but it has improved over the past few decades. The blood brain barrier limits the access of many drugs to the CNS, making the treatment of this disease challenging. In addition, the rarity of the disease makes it difficult to conduct large randomized studies and most treatment recommendations are from retrospective studies or single arm phase 2 trials.

This review will go over the initial evaluation of CNS lymphoma as well as recommended treatments. The treatment recommendations are broken down into PCNSL, secondary CNS lymphoma, and CNS lymphoma prophylaxis recommendations.

Initial Evaluation

When lymphoma of the CNS is suspected, the preferred radiologic test is magnetic resonance imaging (MRI) of the brain for further evaluation and localization. If possible, the use of glucocorticoids should be avoided in these patients since these can alter the appearance of the lesions on imaging and also result in insufficient sampling on a biopsy.

The initial work up should include an HIV blood test, a lumbar puncture with flow cytometry of the cerebrospinal fluid (CSF), and an ophthalmological assessment including a slit lamp exam. Regardless of the degree of suspicion, a biopsy must be done to confirm the diagnosis. If the vitreous or CSF is positive for lymphoma, then it is reasonable to omit a brain biopsy in this circumstance.

A stereotactic biopsy is the recommended modality for obtaining tissue for histopathologic analysis. A stereotactic biopsy is usually sufficient to obtain ample tissue for analysis and has less comorbidity associated with it than surgery. In addition, there are no prospective studies showing a survival benefit in patients receiving resection versus those receiving stereotactic biopsy of the lymphoma. However, in 2012, the German PCNSL study group-1 published results of a retrospective study that showed an improvement in progression free survival (PFS) and overall survival (OS) in select patients who received a total or subtotal resection of their PCNSL [4]. This was especially true in patients with solitary lesions compared to those with multiple CNS lesions. Given these findings, patients with isolated PCNSL may benefit from a resection of the tumor if this can be done safely.

Resection in these patients does not eliminate the need for chemotherapy since radiographic and gross appearances underestimate the extent of the lymphoma.

In addition to confirming the diagnosis, a whole body positron emission tomography (PET) scan or computerized tomography (CT) scan should be done to determine if this is a PCNSL or secondary CNS lymphoma. A bone marrow biopsy should also be done to rule out marrow involvement. In the past, a testicular ultrasound was recommended in males with suspected PCNSL. However, if a PET scan was used for the initial staging, a testicular ultrasound is probably not necessary.

Treatment of Primary CNS NHL

In PCNSL the brain parenchyma is involved in more than 90% of the patients and can by multifocal in more than half of them [5]. Up to 30% can have leptomeningeal involvement, and up to 20% can have ocular disease [6, 7]. These findings demonstrate the infiltrative nature of this disease. It is considered a whole brain disease and cannot be effectively treated with local measures (i.e., surgical resection or radiation therapy) alone.

Numerous regimens have been tested for the treatment of PCNSL: regimens involving radiation therapy, intrathecal chemotherapy, and such drugs as intravenous high dose methotrexate, vincristine, procarbazine, rituximab, cytarabine, ifosfamide, temozolomide, and others. However, despite numerous reports involving these drugs, only a few have been tested in a randomized trial. Because of this, there is essentially no gold standard for the treatment of PCNSL.

One common theme throughout most of the published studies is that high dose methotrexate (MTX) appears to be the most important drug in the treatment of PCNSL. Prior to the 1980's, the main treatment for PCNSL was radiation therapy. In 1977, Skarin and colleagues published a report on the use of high dose MTX in the treatment of non-Hodgkin's lymphoma involving the CNS [8]. This prompted further studies in the 1980's evaluating the use of MTX at different doses for CNS lymphoma [9-11]. In 1990, DeAngelis published a study evaluating combination chemotherapy followed by radiation therapy in patients with PCNSL [12, 13]. This study demonstrated that a combination of high dose intravenous MTX, intra-Ommaya MTX, whole brain radiation therapy (RT), and post RT cytarabine improved progression free survival when compared to patients receiving RT alone. After the publication of this study, high dose MTX essentially became the backbone of most treatment regimens for PCNSL.

The efficacy of high dose MTX in PCNSL has been well established, but the optimal dose, frequency, and drug combination of MTX is controversial. It is thought that MTX doses of 1 g/m^2 result in tumoricidal levels in the brain parenchyma and doses of 3 g/m^2 or higher yield tumoricidal levels in the cerebrospinal fluid [14]. Studies using doses from $1g/m^2$ up to $8g/m^2$ of IV MTX have shown activity in the treatment of CNS lymphoma in humans. Skarin's study used MTX at a dose of $1g/m^2$ and showed an overall response rate of 66% [8]. Batchelor and colleagues conducted a study using single agent MTX at an increased dose of $8g/m^2$ given every 2 weeks as an induction treatment for 4-6 treatments followed by a monthly consolidation phase for 10 months [15]. This study showed an overall response rate of 74%. No head to head studies have been done to compare different doses of MTX, so the optimal dose is still a matter of debate.

In an effort to improve on the outcomes seen with single agent MTX treatment, a study was published in 2000 which attempted to improve survival by combining MTX with procarbazine, vincristine (MPV), whole brain RT, and cytarabine [16]. This study showed an improvement in disease control and overall survival when compared to previously published studies. A follow up to this study was done adding rituximab (R-MPV) to the regimen [17]. The addition of rituximab showed a further improvement in response (overall response rate of 95% and a complete response rate of 79%) and overall survival (median overall survival of 6.6 years). However, both of these multi-modality regimens were associated with neurotoxicity, especially in those patients who received RT.

Combination chemotherapy regimens and multi-modality treatments showed improved survival in patients that prior to the 1990s had an overall survival of less than a year. With these regimens, patients were living longer and the side effects such as cognitive impairment became more of a concern. A phase 3 study omitting RT was published in 2010 [18]. This study randomized newly diagnosed PCNSL patients who were treated with high dose MTX ($4g/m^2$) with or without ifosfamide to receive whole brain RT (total dose of 45Gy) or no further treatment. The study showed an improvement in median overall survival in the group that did not receive RT, but a better progression free survival in the RT group. Unfortunately, the results were not statistically significant. It also showed that the RT group had a higher percentage of patients with neurotoxicity (49% vs 26%). Other phase 2 multi-modality studies have shown durable responses using lower doses of RT, but none of these were randomized studies. There is a randomized phase 2 on-going Radiation Therapy Oncology Group study that is evaluating patients receiving methotrexate combination chemotherapy with low dose radiation consolidation to those not receiving any RT consolidation (clinicaltrials.gov identifier NCT01399372). Hopefully, this will shed light on the role of RT for PCNSL.

The ideal drug combination with MTX is also a matter for debate. While multiple studies have shown that MTX combined with multiple chemotherapeutic agents is effective in PCNSL, only one randomized study has been published comparing a combination regimen with single agent MTX. Ferreri and the International Extranodal Lymphoma Study Group conducted a randomized phase 2 study comparing cytarabine plus high dose MTX versus high dose MTX alone [19]. This study showed a superior overall response rate and complete remission rate in the cytarabine plus MTX group when compared to the MTX alone group (ORR 69% vs 40%, respectively; CR 46% vs 18%, respectively). Significant hematologic toxicities were noted in the cytarabine plus MTX group and 92% of the patients experienced a grade 3 or 4 hematologic toxicity. Temozolomide and MTX was also found to be an effective regimen without the addition of intrathecal chemotherapy or RT [20]. The combination showed an overall response rate of 55% and all of the responses were complete remissions.

The addition of intrathecal chemotherapy was initially part of the multi-drug chemotherapy regimen tested by DeAngelis and colleagues [12]. However, data by Glantz and colleagues demonstrated that high-dose intravenous administration of methotrexate produces higher cytotoxic levels of methotrexate in serum and CSF than intrathecal methotrexate at 48 and 72 hours [21]. Data has also shown that the omission of IT from induction chemotherapy did not affect the outcome in patients treated with HD-MTX IV at a dose of $3.5g/m^2$ [22]. Given these findings, the use of IT MTX in IV HD MTX containing regimens is probably best reserved for patient with leptomeningeal disease refractory to IV HD MTX treatment.

Although the combinations and doses may vary, the previously mentioned studies demonstrated that MTX is an essential component to the successful treatment of PCNSL. Recent studies have started to focus on improving the duration of response. Most experts feel that some sort of consolidation therapy is required to result in a long term disease free survival and even possibly a cure. Whether or not it's consolidation with RT or some form of high dose chemotherapy is another matter for debate. High dose chemotherapy followed by an autologous stem cell transplant (HDC-ASCT) has been evaluated as an option for newly diagnosed PCNSL. One study that showed particularly promising results evaluated conditioning with thiotepa, cyclophosphamide, and busulfan followed by an ASCT [23]. This study treated newly diagnosed PCNSL patients with the previously mentioned R-MPV regimen. Patients who received a complete remission or partial remission went on to receive the HDC-ASCT as consolidation. The 2 year progression free and overall survival was 81% in those patients who received the HDC-ASCT. At the time the study was published, no evidence of neurotoxicity was observed although 3 treatment related deaths were reported.

Treatment of Secondary CNS NHL

Secondary CNS lymphoma presents with the same challenges as PCNSL but with the additional challenge of treating systemic disease too. Systemic diffuse large B-cell lymphoma (DLBCL) is a curable form of lymphoma that has a high response rate to CHOP and Rituxan. However, this regimen does not have adequate CNS penetration and is not sufficient on its own to treat CNS disease. Secondary CNS lymphoma can occur as synchronous disease at the time of initial diagnosis or as an isolated CNS relapse after successful treatment of systemic lymphoma. The management of these should be approached differently.

In synchronous disease, intrathecal (IT) MTX and cytarabine are commonly used in addition to CHOP-R in the treatment of secondary CNS lymphoma. However, there are no prospective studies evaluating IT chemotherapy as the sole treatment of CNS lymphoma. Additionally, as mentioned previously, data has shown that intravenous administration of methotrexate produces higher cytotoxic levels of methotrexate in serum and CSF than intrathecal methotrexate [21]. Data has also shown that the omission of IT from induction chemotherapy consisting of HD IV MTX does not affect the outcome [22]. Although these results were demonstrated in PCNSL patients as part of a retrospective analysis, it is reasonable to assume that this data would also apply to patients with secondary CNS lymphoma. Given these findings, the combination of high dose IV MTX with a systemic DLBCL chemotherapy regimen such as CHOP-R is probably the optimal therapy for secondary CNS lymphoma. There is no prospective data to support this, but this is per personal observation and also the recommendation of some experts [24].

Relapsed CNS lymphoma has a worse prognosis than systemic relapse. These relapses usually occur earlier than systemic relapses and have a shorter median overall survival (2.2 months vs 9 months) [25]. In cases of isolated CNS relapse it's reasonable to manage these like PCNSL. Combination chemotherapy regimens with HD IV MTX or single agent HD IV MTX should be used in these patients. Since these patients have received prior chemotherapy treatments for their systemic disease, it is possible that they may not be in a condition to tolerate HD IV MTX, especially if they suffer from renal insufficiency. In these patients localized therapy with IT chemotherapy or whole brain radiation therapy may be appropriate options.

In both cases, consolidation is likely to improve progression free survival and possibly the rate of cure. Again, in this setting the ideal consolidation regimen has not been defined. Consolidation with etoposide and cytarabine followed by an autologous stem cell transplant showed good responses as a salvage treatment in patients with relapsed PCNSL, and may be a good option in patients who have secondary CNS lymphoma [26]. Also, a study by Korfel and colleagues showed a durable remission with autologous stem cell transplant as consolidation in patients with CNS relapse of their aggressive non-Hodgkin's lymphoma [27]. In this study 6 of the 30 patients had systemic DLBCL in addition to CNS relapse. These patients were all treated with a high dose induction chemotherapy followed by consolidation with an autologous stem cell transplant. Of these 6, four had either a CR or PR after receiving consolidation with the transplant. After a median follow up of 21 months, the time to treatment failure (TTF) for all patients who underwent consolidation with the transplant was 24.3 months. The TTF for the 6 patients with concomitant systemic DLBCL was not reported separately.

Conclusion

CNS lymphoma is an aggressive type of NHL. The blood brain barrier protects these lymphomas from most standard lymphoma chemotherapy treatments such as CHOP and Rituximab. Methotrexate is the most effective chemotherapeutic drug in the treatment of CNS lymphoma. Intravenous administration allows penetration of the brain parenchyma as well as the spinal cord and cerebrospinal fluid. The optimal dose is unknown, but it appears that doses of 3.5 g/m^2 or higher are necessary for adequate cytotoxic drug levels in the CNS. Combining MTX with other drugs that can cross the blood brain barrier such as cytarabine can make the therapy more effective but with increased toxicities. Consolidation with radiation therapy may also improve response rates marginally, but with increased neurotoxicity. Current studies are evaluating the role of combination regimens as well as consolidation treatments and will hopefully shed light on the optimal therapy for CNS lymphomas in the near future.

References

[1] Gerstner, E. R., Batchelor, T. T. 2010. "Primary central nervous system lymphoma." *Arch Neurol* 67:291-297.

[2] Villano, J. L., Koshy, M., Shaikh, H., Dolecek, T. A., McCarthy, B. J. 2011. "Age, gender, and racial differences in incidence and survival in primary CNS lymphoma." *Br J Cancer* 105:1414-1418.

[3] Tun, H. W., Personett, D., Baskerville, K. A., Menke, D. M., Jaeckle, K. A., Kreinest, P., Edenfield, B., et al. 2008. "Pathway analysis of primary central nervous system lymphoma." *Blood* 111:3200-3210.

[4] Weller, M., Martus, P., Roth, P., Thiel, E., Korfel, A., German, Pcnsl Study Group. 2012. "Surgery for primary CNS lymphoma? Challenging a paradigm." *Neuro Oncol* 14:1481-1484.

[5] Bataille, B., Delwail, V., Menet, E., Vandermarcq, P., Ingrand, P., Wager, M., Guy, G., Lapierre, F. 2000. "Primary intracerebral malignant lymphoma: report of 248 cases." *J Neurosurg* 92:261-266.

[6] Fischer, L., Martus, P., Weller, M., Klasen, H. A., Rohden, B., Roth, A., Storek, B., et al. 2008. "Meningeal dissemination in primary CNS lymphoma: prospective evaluation of 282 patients." *Neurology* 71:1102-1108.

[7] Grimm, S. A., McCannel, C. A., Omuro, A. M., Ferreri, A. J., Blay, J. Y., Neuwelt, E. A., Siegal, T., et al. 2008. "Primary CNS lymphoma with intraocular involvement: International PCNSL Collaborative Group Report." *Neurology* 71:1355-1360.

[8] Skarin, A. T., Zuckerman, K. S., Pitman, S. W., Rosenthal, D. S., Moloney, W., Frei, E., 3rd, Canellos, G. P. 1977. "High-dose methotrexate with folinic acid in the treatment of advanced non-Hodgkin lymphoma including CNS involvement." *Blood* 50:1039-1047.

[9] Abelson, H. T., Kufe, D. W., Skarin, A. T., Major, P., Ensminger, W., Beardsley, G. P., Canellos, G. P. 1981. "Treatment of central nervous system tumors with methotrexate." *Cancer Treat Rep* 65 Suppl 1:137-140.

[10] Petursson, S. R. 1989. "Primary central nervous system lymphoma: long-term survival following treatment with radiation and methotrexate." *Eur J Surg Oncol* 15:69-72.

[11] Gabbai, A. A., Hochberg, F. H., Linggood, R. M., Bashir, R., Hotleman, K. 1989. "High-dose methotrexate for non-AIDS primary central nervous system lymphoma. Report of 13 cases." *J Neurosurg* 70:190-194.

[12] DeAngelis, L. M., Yahalom, J., Heinemann, M. H., Cirrincione, C., Thaler, H. T., Krol, G. 1990. "Primary CNS lymphoma: combined treatment with chemotherapy and radiotherapy." *Neurology* 40:80-86.

[13] DeAngelis, L. M., Yahalom, J., Thaler, H. T., Kher, U. 1992. "Combined modality therapy for primary CNS lymphoma." *J Clin Oncol* 10:635-643.

[14] Lippens, R. J., Winograd, B. 1988. "Methotrexate concentration levels in the cerebrospinal fluid during high-dose methotrexate infusions: an unreliable prediction." *Pediatr Hematol Oncol* 5:115-124.

[15] Batchelor, T., Carson, K., O'Neill, A., Grossman, S. A., Alavi, J., New, P., Hochberg, F., Priet, R. 2003. "Treatment of primary CNS lymphoma with methotrexate and deferred radiotherapy: a report of NABTT 96-07." *J Clin Oncol* 21:1044-1049.

[16] Abrey, L. E., Yahalom, J., DeAngelis, L. M. 2000. "Treatment for primary CNS lymphoma: the next step." *J Clin Oncol* 18:3144-3150.

[17] Morris, P. G., Correa, D. D., Yahalom, J., Raizer, J. J., Schiff, D., Grant, B., Grimm, S., et al. 2013. "Rituximab, methotrexate, procarbazine, and vincristine followed by consolidation reduced-dose whole-brain radiotherapy and cytarabine in newly diagnosed primary CNS lymphoma: final results and long-term outcome." *J Clin Oncol* 31:3971-3979.

[18] Thiel, E., Korfel, A., Martus, P., Kanz, L., Griesinger, F., Rauch, M., Roth, A., et al. 2010. "High-dose methotrexate with or without whole brain radiotherapy for primary CNS lymphoma (G-PCNSL-SG-1): a phase 3, randomised, non-inferiority trial." *Lancet Oncol* 11:1036-1047.

[19] Ferreri, A. J., Reni, M., Foppoli, M., Martelli, M., Pangalis, G. A., Frezzato, M., Cabras, M. G., et al. 2009. "High-dose cytarabine plus high-dose methotrexate versus high-dose methotrexate alone in patients with primary CNS lymphoma: a randomised phase 2 trial." *Lancet* 374:1512-1520.

[20] Omuro, A. M., Taillandier, L., Chinot, O., Carnin, C., Barrie, M., Hoang-Xuan, K. 2007. "Temozolomide and methotrexate for primary central nervous system lymphoma in the elderly." *J Neurooncol* 85:207-211.

[21] Glantz, M. J., Cole, B. F., Recht, L., Akerley, W., Mills, P., Saris, S., Hochberg, F., Calabresi, P., Egorin, M. J. 1998. "High-dose intravenous methotrexate for patients with nonleukemic leptomeningeal cancer: is intrathecal chemotherapy necessary?" *J Clin Oncol* 16:1561-1567.

[22] Khan, R. B., Shi, W., Thaler, H. T., DeAngelis, L. M., Abrey, L. E. 2002. "Is intrathecal methotrexate necessary in the treatment of primary CNS lymphoma?" *J Neurooncol* 58:175-178.

[23] Omuro, A., Correa, D. D., DeAngelis, L. M., Moskowitz, C. H., Matasar, M. J., Kaley, T. J., Gavrilovic, I. T., et al. 2015. "R-MPV followed by high-dose chemotherapy with TBC and autologous stem-cell transplant for newly diagnosed primary CNS lymphoma." *Blood* 125:1403-1410.

[24] Rubenstein, J. L., Gupta, N. K., Mannis, G. N., Lamarre, A. K., Treseler, P. 2013. "How I treat CNS lymphomas." *Blood* 122:2318-2330.

[25] Bernstein, S. H., Unger, J. M., Leblanc, M., Friedberg, J., Miller, T. P., Fisher, R. I. 2009. "Natural history of CNS relapse in patients with aggressive non-Hodgkin's lymphoma: a 20-year follow-up analysis of SWOG 8516 -- the Southwest Oncology Group." *J Clin Oncol* 27:114-119.

[26] Soussain, C., Suzan, F., Hoang-Xuan, K., Cassoux, N., Levy, V., Azar, N., Belanger, C., et al. 2001. "Results of intensive chemotherapy followed by hematopoietic stem-cell rescue in 22 patients with refractory or recurrent primary CNS lymphoma or intraocular lymphoma." *J Clin Oncol* 19:742-749.

[27] Korfel, A., Elter, T., Thiel, E., Hanel, M., Mohle, R., Schroers, R., Reiser, M., et al. 2013. "Phase II study of central nervous system (CNS)-directed chemotherapy including high-dose chemotherapy with autologous stem cell transplantation for CNS relapse of aggressive lymphomas." *Haematologica* 98:364-370.

In: Diffuse Large B-Cell Lymphoma (DLBCL)
Editor: Haipeng Shao

ISBN: 978-1-63484-402-4

Chapter 7

PRIMARY CUTANEOUS DIFFUSE LARGE B-CELL LYMPHOMA, LEG TYPE

Christa Roe, Frank Glass, Bela Kis and Lubomir Sokol

Departments of Malignant Hematology
H. Lee Moffitt Cancer Center and Research Institute,
Tampa, FL, US

ABSTRACT

Primary cutaneous diffuse large B-cell lymphoma, leg type (PCDLBCL-LT) is a distinct intermediate-grade B-cell lymphoproliferative disorder with a 5-year disease-specific survival rate of approximately fifty percent. Skin biopsies with cytomorphology, immunohistochemistry, and molecular clonality studies are essential for a diagnosis of this disease. Comprehensive lymphoma staging with laboratory tests, imaging studies, and bone marrow aspiration and biopsy (BMAB) are important for estimation of the prognosis and differential diagnosis between PCDLBCL-LT and systemic diffuse large B-cell lymphoma with secondary skin involvement. Anthracycline-based chemotherapy regimens with rituximab are the preferred initial treatment that results in an improvement of outcome. Although no randomized prospective studies have been conducted in patients with PCDLBCL-LT, treatment regimens derived from management of systemic intermediate-grade B-cell lymphomas have shown promising results.

INTRODUCTION

Primary cutaneous diffuse large B-cell lymphoma, leg type (PCDLBCL-LT), is an intermediate grade extra nodal non-Hodgkin lymphoma (NHL) manifesting with skin lesions and no evidence of systemic or extra-cutaneous disease at the time of diagnosis. This rare disease comprises approximately one to three percent of all primary cutaneous lymphomas (PCL) and approximately twenty percent of primary cutaneous B-cell lymphoma (PCBCL)

[1]. In 1987, the first report of nineteen elderly women with tumor lesions on the legs showed a very poor prognosis [2].

Nearly ten years later, PCDLBCL-LT was classified as a unique entity [3], and subsequently the 2005 World Health Organization/European Organization for the Research and Treatment of Cancer (WHO/EORTC) classification and the 2008 World Health Organization (WHO) classification for tumors of hematopoietic and lymphoid tissues included pertinent updates and changes to PCBCL, including PCDLBCL-LT [1, 4]. These new classifications include updates on terminology, staging, and practice that have been adopted by oncologists, hematologists, pathologists, and dermatologists worldwide. The three distinct histologic types of PCBCL are primary cutaneous follicle center lymphoma (PCFCL), primary cutaneous marginal zone lymphoma (PCMZL), and primary cutaneous diffuse large B-cell lymphoma, leg type (PCDLBCL, LT) [5].

Epidemiology

PCLBCL-LT is a rare variant of extranodal DLBCL. This entity accounts for approximately twenty percent of all PCBCL and ranks second next to primary gastrointestinal NHL, as the most common extranodal aggressive B-cell lymphoma. Smith at al reported on the incidence of PCL based on the data at the Surveillance, Epidemiology, and End Results (SEER) registry collected between 1973 and 2001 [6]. The overall incidence rate of PCBCLs was 3.9 per one million people. The study revealed that PCDLBCL-LT is mainly a disease of elderly population, with a median age of seventy-eight years at diagnosis, and it is more common in females than males with M/F ratio of 1.3-4 [3]. The disease has been reported primarily in non-Hispanic white individuals [7].

Etiology

The etiology of PCDLBCL-LT is not well understood. There have been many reports from Europe that have revealed an association between PCBCL including PCDLBCL-LT, with Borrelia burgdorferi. A positive correlation between a history of tick bite or antibodies against Borrelia burgdorferi in serum emerged in literature and was reported in 1,579 patients from one European study. However, overall risk of NHL was not associated with a self-reported history of tick bite or the presence of anti- Borrelia burgdorferi antibodies [8, 9]. Another study reported by Jelić et al. showed that twelve of twenty-two patients with PCBCL had a positive serology for Borrelia burgdorferi [9]. Goodlad et al. detected Borrelia burgdorferi -specific DNA sequences in two of twenty patients with PCDLBCL-LT [10].

Pathology and Molecular Biology

Morphologically, PCDLBCL-LT presents with a diffuse infiltrate of centroblasts or immunoblasts. The lymphoma cells characteristically express MUM1 and BCL2 and show a predisposition to invade the subcutaneous tissue. The recent progress of molecular technology allowed better understanding of the biology of PCBCL. Dijkman et al. studied twelve patients with PCDLBCL-LT using array-based comparative genomic hybridization, fluorescence in situ hybridization, and examination of promoter hypermethylation [11]. The study reported amplification of 18q21.31-q21.33 and small deletions of a region that contain the CDKN2A and CDKN2B genes in patients with PCDLBCL-LT. Gene expression profiling studies of PCDLBCL-LT revealed activated B-cell (ABC) type with constitutive activation of NF-κB pathway and expression of the IRF4/MUM1 B-cell transcription factor [12].

Another study showed that 69% of patients with PCDLCL-LT had a high incidence of recurrent MYD88 L265P mutation [13]. Experimental studies with inhibitors of IRAK4 kinase of the MYD88 signaling complex resulted in inhibition of cell survival of nodal ABC-type cell lines with MYD88 L265P mutation, suggesting a possibility of novel targeted therapy [14].

Clinical Manifestation

PCDLBCL-LT presents most frequently with cutaneous nodules, tumors and infiltrated plaques. They are reddish or bluish in color [15]. They manifest predominantly on the lower extremities and/or trunk. True to the name, around eighty-eight percent of patients diagnosed have lesions on their lower extremities. However, around twelve percent of lesions present on other areas of the skin including head and neck, trunk, and upper extremities [16, 17]. In contrast to other PCBCL, PCDLBCL-LT frequently disseminates to nodal and visceral regions, and the central nervous system (CNS). Bone marrow involvement is not uncommon with advanced disease progression [18, 19] (Table 1).

Diagnosis

A complete history and physical examination, complete blood cell count with differential count (CBC/Diff), chemistry with lactate dehydrogenase (LDH), flow cytometry (FC) on peripheral blood, and imaging studies with computed tomography (CT) scan of the chest, abdomen, and pelvis with contrast or positron emission-tomography/CT (PET/CT) are essential staging tests. Although a contrast CT scan is sufficient for a diagnosis of adenopathy and organomegaly, smaller skin lesions can be missed. Fusion PET/CT on the other side can visualize metabolically active skin lesions that can be missed on physical examination. Skin punch (4–6 mm) or wedge-incisional biopsies, or excisional biopsies of lymph nodes that are greater than 1.5 cm should be performed for the diagnosis of PCDLBCL-LT. Immunohistochemistry (IHC) with a panel of antibodies against B-cell antigens including CD20, CD79a, and CD5, CD10, BCL-2, BCL-6, kappa/lambda, and MUM1/IRF4 is an important diagnostic tool. Clonality studies using Ig heavy-chain and light chain gene rearrangement by polymerase chain reaction (PCR) can be done on paraffin-embedded tissue or by flow cytometry on fresh tissues. Bone marrow biopsy is recommended for all patients with intermediate-grade PCBCL including PCDLBCL-LT [21, 22].

Table1. Features of primary cutaneous diffuse large B-cell lymphoma, leg type

<table>
<tr><td colspan="3">Clinical Features</td></tr>
<tr><td colspan="3">Single or multiple skin plaques and tumors
Primarily on the lower extremities (legs) and occasionally on trunk, upper extremities, and head
Disease of the Elderly (median age, 76 years)
Multiple relapses and extra-cutaneous dissemination</td></tr>
<tr><td colspan="3">Etiology</td></tr>
<tr><td colspan="3">Unknown</td></tr>
<tr><td colspan="3">Histologic Features</td></tr>
<tr><td colspan="3">Diffuse infiltrate
Centroblasts
Immunoblasts</td></tr>
<tr><td colspan="3">Immunophenotype</td></tr>
<tr><td colspan="3">CD20$^+$ and CD79a$^+$
Bcl-2$^+$, Bcl-6$^{+/-}$, and CD10$^-$
MUM1/IRF4$^+$and FOXP1$^+$</td></tr>
<tr><td colspan="3">Molecular Findings</td></tr>
<tr><td colspan="3">Translocations of myc, Bcl-6, or IgH genes [20]
Gains of chromosomes 1, 2, 3, 7, and 12
Losses of 6q, 13, and 14
DNA amplification of 18q21.31- q21.31
Deletions in 9p21.3 (CDKN2A and CDKN2B)</td></tr>
<tr><td>PCDLBCL, LT type and involvement</td><td>Localized Disease</td><td>Generalized Disease</td></tr>
<tr><td>Frontline therapy</td><td>R-CHOP with local RT; local RT or clinical trial</td><td>R-CHOP; or RT to previously unirradiated tumor</td></tr>
<tr><td>Therapy for secondary, relapsed, or refractory disease</td><td>R-CHOP with or without local RT; clinical trial</td><td>Local RT for palliation; radioimmunotherapy</td></tr>
<tr><td colspan="3">5-year Overall Survival</td></tr>
<tr><td colspan="3">Approximately 50%</td></tr>
</table>

Differential Diagnosis

Skin biopsies with histology, immunohistochemistry, and molecular clonality studies integrated with clinical information are essential for a correct diagnosis PCDLBCL-LT [23, 31]. It is important to note that without staging studies, the confirmation of the primary origin of this lymphoma in skin cannot be made. Neither IHC nor histology can differentiate between cutaneous or systemic diffuse large B-cell lymphoma. PCDLBCL-LT shares many features of other lymphomas [24]. Pathological review provides a list of differential rather than definitive diagnoses and final diagnoses can only be made with the completion of staging, history and physical exam including complete skin evaluation. Many academic institutions serve as a referral centers for patients in the community, and a team of experts should be involved in confirmation of the final diagnosis [25].

STAGING

The Ann Arbor staging system used for staging of systemic non-Hodgkin lymphoma (NHL) has only limited prognostic value in PCBCL as patients are classified into only two stages: IE and IVE [26]. Two prognostic systems have been used for PCBCL risk stratification [6, 27]. The International Society for Cutaneous Lymphoma and the Cutaneous Task Force of EORTC (ISCL/EORTC) developed a new TNM staging system for primary cutaneous lymphomas other than mycosis fungoides and Sézary syndrome (Table 2). The National Comprehensive Cancer Network (NCCN) guidelines for NHL created evidence based algorithm of diagnosis and management of PCBCL [27, 28].

Table 2. International Society for Cutaneous Lymphomas/European Organization of Research and Treatment of Cancer (ISCL/EORTC) Proposal on Tumor Node Metastasis (TNM) Classification of Cutaneous Lymphoma Other Than Mycosis Fungoides and Sézary Syndrome

TUMOR	NODE	METASTASIS
T1 Solitary skin involvement **T1a** A solitary lesion less than 5-cm diameter **T1b** A solitary greater than 5-cm diameter	**N0** No clinical or pathologic lymph node involvement	**M0** No evidence of extracutaneous non-lymph node disease
T2 Regional skin involvement multiple lesions limited to 1 body region or 2 contiguous body regions **T2a** All-disease-encompassing in a less than 15-cm diameter circular area	**N1** Involvement of 1 peripheral lymph node region that drains an area of current or prior skin involvement	**M1** Extracutaneous non-lymph node disease present
T2b All-disease-encompassing in a greater than 15- and less than 30-cm diameter circular area **T2c** All-disease-encompassing in a 30-cm diameter circular area	**N2** Involvement of 2 or more peripheral lymph node regions or involvement of any lymph node region that does not drain an area of current or prior skin involvement	
T3 Generalized skin involvement **T3a** Multiple lesions involving 2 noncontiguous body regions **T3b** Multiple lesions involving greater than or equal to 3 body regions	**N3** Involvement of central lymph nodes	

Over the past fifteen years, differences have been recognized in the diagnosis and management of PCBCL along with separate recommendations for this group of B-cell malignancies. The TNM staging systems are based on the number, size, and area of distribution of tumor lesions. For PCDLBDL-LT a history, physical exam, punch biopsy, laboratory studies, imaging and bone marrow biopsy with aspiration are recommended [29].

THERAPY

In PCDLBCL-LT, the standard frontline therapeutic treatment as recommended by NCCN guidelines includes multi-agent anthracycline-based chemotherapy with anti-CD20 monoclonal antibodies [30].

In limited skin disease with solitary or few skin lesions which can be included in a single radiation field, systemic immune-chemotherapy with limited number of cycles is usually followed by involved-field radiation therapy. Patients with disseminated disease are usually treated with systemic chemoimmunotherapy such as cyclophosphamide, doxorubicin, oncovin, and prednisone with rituximab. Since this disease is most prevalent in the elderly population, treatment modifications are recommended in those patients who are at increased risk of developing drug toxicities. Monotherapy with radiation only, is offered to those cases that cannot tolerate any systemic treatment [31]. Based on data from clinical trials with DLBCL the use of oral immunomodulatory agents such as lenalidomide could be potentially effective and relatively well tolerated in elderly patients with relapsed/refractory PCDLBCL-LT [32]. Other targeted agents are currently being studiedin clinical trials in patients with DLBCL such as ofatumumab, lumilixumab, ibrutinib, and dacetuzumab. These agents could have a favorable impact on outcome in patients with intermediate-grade DLBCL including PCDLBCL-LT (Figure 1).

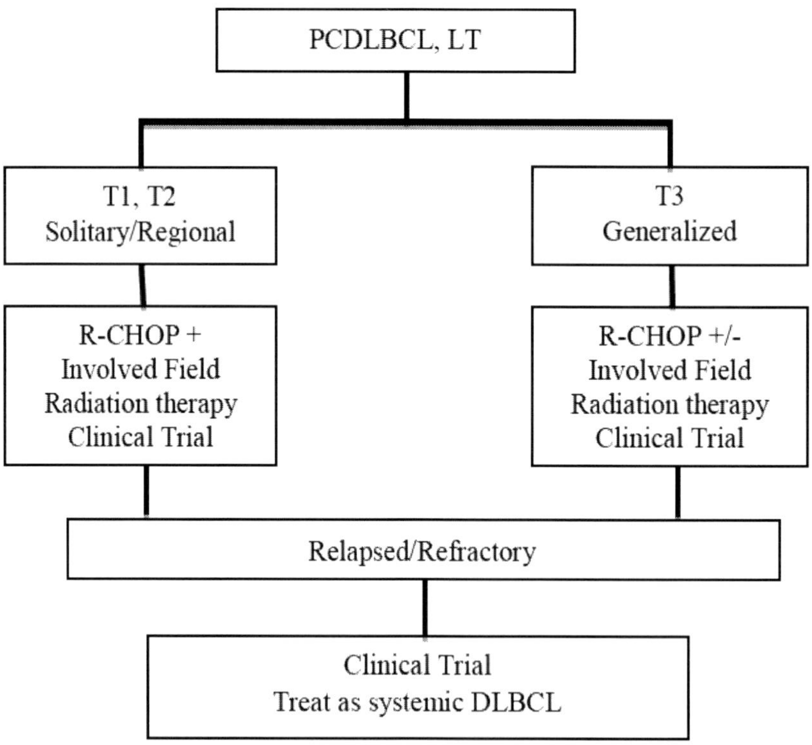

Figure 1. Treatment options for PCDLBCL-LT.

PROGNOSIS

PCDLBCL-LT is the most aggressive for of PCBCL with the worst prognosis among PCBCL [33]. PCDLBCL-LT is characterized by frequent cutaneous relapses and dissemination into extracutaneous anatomic regions. The 5-year disease specific survival is forty-seven percent [34]. A retrospective study showed that despite a high response rate of 91% to radiation therapy or chemotherapy relapse rate was as high as 47% [35]. One particular study showed that the overall survival rate was over thirty percent higher when the lesion presented not on the leg but elsewhere on the body [36]. In another retrospective study, patients treated with combined anthracycline and rituximab-based therapies had a more favorable short-term outcome compared to patients treated with chemotherapy regimens without rituximab [37]. Poor performance status (PS) is independent risk factor in PCDBCL-LT, and is common in patients with aggressive lymphoma and elevated LDH levels. In the study conducted by Dijkman et al. all patients diagnosed with PCDLBCL-LT with deletion of 9p21.3 and complete methylation of CDKN2A died because of lymphoma [11].

CONCLUSION

Since the first description of PCLBCL, LT in 1987, significant progress has been made in the classification, diagnosis, staging, and prognosis of this lymphoma. An increased understanding of the disease and its molecular characteristics, have provided a means for improvement in diagnosis and prognosis. This disease is rare, and the etiology remains unknown. Unfortunately, no randomized prospective clinical trials on PCDLBCL-LT are conducted but therapy with immuno-chemotherapy regimens well established in systemic DLBCL shows promise. Multi-agent anthracycline based chemotherapy regimens with or without radiation have shown significant clinical results in systemic B-cell lymphomas and have provided a strategy for an increased overall survival in PCDLBCL-LT. Novel targeted agents tested in clinical trials in systemic DLBCL might also be useful in PCLBCL-LT and lead to less toxicity and better long-term outcome in patients with this lymphoma.

REFERENCES

[1] Swerdlow SH, Campo E, Harris NL, Jaffe ES, Pileri SA, Stein H. 2008; *WHO classification of tumours of haematopoietic and lymphoid tissues*. IARC, Lyon.

[2] Willemze, R., Meijer, C. J., Sentis, H. J., Scheffer, E., van Vloten, W. A., Toonstra, J., van der Putte, S. C. 1987. "Primary cutaneous large cell lymphomas of follicular center cell origin. A clinical follow-up study of nineteen patients." *J Am Acad Dermatol* 16:518-526.

[3] Vermeer, M. H., Geelen, F. A., van Haselen, C. W., van Voorst Vader, P. C., Geerts, M. L., van Vloten, W. A., Willemze, R. 1996. "Primary cutaneous large B-cell lymphomas of the legs. A distinct type of cutaneous B-cell lymphoma with an intermediate prognosis. Dutch Cutaneous Lymphoma Working Group." *Arch Dermatol* 132:1304-1308.

[4] Willemze, R., Jaffe, E. S., Burg, G., Cerroni, L., Berti, E., Swerdlow, S. H., Ralfkiaer, E., et al. 2005. "WHO-EORTC classification for cutaneous lymphomas." *Blood* 105:3768-3785.
[5] Willemze, R., Kerl, H., Sterry, W., Berti, E., Cerroni, L., Chimenti, S., Diaz-Perez, J. L., et al. 1997. "EORTC classification for primary cutaneous lymphomas: a proposal from the Cutaneous Lymphoma Study Group of the European Organization for Research and Treatment of Cancer." *Blood* 90:354-371.
[6] Smith, B. D., Smith, G. L., Cooper, D. L., Wilson, L. D. 2005. "The cutaneous B-cell lymphoma prognostic index: a novel prognostic index derived from a population-based registry." *J Clin Oncol* 23:3390-3395.
[7] Suarez, A. L., Querfeld, C., Horwitz, S., Pulitzer, M., Moskowitz, A., Myskowski, P. L. 2013. "Primary cutaneous B-cell lymphomas: part II. Therapy and future directions." *J Am Acad Dermatol* 69:343 e341-311; quiz 355-346.
[8] Garbe, C., Stein, H., Dienemann, D., Orfanos, C. E. 1991. "Borrelia burgdorferi-associated cutaneous B cell lymphoma: clinical and immunohistologic characterization of four cases." *J Am Acad Dermatol* 24:584-590.
[9] Jelic, S., Filipovic-Ljeskovic, I. 1999. "Positive serology for Lyme disease borrelias in primary cutaneous B-cell lymphoma: a study in 22 patients; is it a fortuitous finding?" *Hematol Oncol* 17:107-116.
[10] Goodlad, J. R., Davidson, M. M., Hollowood, K., Ling, C., MacKenzie, C., Christie, I., Batstone, P. J., Ho-Yen, D. O. 2000. "Primary cutaneous B-cell lymphoma and Borrelia burgdorferi infection in patients from the Highlands of Scotland." *Am J Surg Pathol* 24:1279-1285.
[11] Dijkman, R., Tensen, C. P., Jordanova, E. S., Knijnenburg, J., Hoefnagel, J. J., Mulder, A. A., Rosenberg, C., et al. 2006. "Array-based comparative genomic hybridization analysis reveals recurrent chromosomal alterations and prognostic parameters in primary cutaneous large B-cell lymphoma." *J Clin Oncol* 24:296-305.
[12] Hoefnagel, J. J., Dijkman, R., Basso, K., Jansen, P. M., Hallermann, C., Willemze, R., Tensen, C. P., Vermeer, M. H. 2005. "Distinct types of primary cutaneous large B-cell lymphoma identified by gene expression profiling." *Blood* 105:3671-3678.
[13] Pham-Ledard, A., Beylot-Barry, M., Barbe, C., Leduc, M., Petrella, T., Vergier, B., Martinez, F., et al. 2014. "High frequency and clinical prognostic value of MYD88 L265P mutation in primary cutaneous diffuse large B-cell lymphoma, leg-type." *JAMA Dermatol* 150:1173-1179.
[14] Ngo, V. N., Young, R. M., Schmitz, R., Jhavar, S., Xiao, W., Lim, K. H., Kohlhammer, H., et al. 2011. "Oncogenically active MYD88 mutations in human lymphoma." *Nature* 470:115-119.
[15] Korgavkar, K., Weinstock, M. A. 2014. "Changing incidence trends of cutaneous B-cell lymphoma." *J Invest Dermatol* 134:840-842.
[16] Senff, N. J., Noordijk, E. M., Kim, Y. H., Bagot, M., Berti, E., Cerroni, L., Dummer, R., et al. 2008. "European Organization for Research and Treatment of Cancer and International Society for Cutaneous Lymphoma consensus recommendations for the management of cutaneous B-cell lymphomas." *Blood* 112:1600-1609.
[17] Senff, N. J., Hoefnagel, J. J., Neelis, K. J., Vermeer, M. H., Noordijk, E. M., Willemze, R., Dutch Cutaneous Lymphoma, Group. 2007. "Results of radiotherapy in 153 primary

cutaneous B-Cell lymphomas classified according to the WHO-EORTC classification." *Arch Dermatol* 143:1520-1526.

[18] Belloni, B., Johansen, N., Glass, L. F., Dummer, R. 2012. "Recent advances in the management of cutaneous lymphomas." *Semin Oncol* 39:150-162.

[19] Salem, A. B., Nfoussi, H., Kchir, N. 2014. "Ureteral spread of a primary cutaneous diffuse large B-cell lymphoma, leg type." *Indian J Urol* 30:222-224.

[20] Hallermann, C., Kaune, K. M., Gesk, S., Martin-Subero, J. I., Gunawan, B., Griesinger, F., Vermeer, M. H., et al. 2004. "Molecular cytogenetic analysis of chromosomal breakpoints in the IGH, MYC, BCL6, and MALT1 gene loci in primary cutaneous B-cell lymphomas." *J Invest Dermatol* 123:213-219.

[21] Quereux, G., Frot, A. S., Brocard, A., Leux, C., Renaut, J. J., Dreno, B. 2009. "Routine bone marrow biopsy in the initial evaluation of primary cutaneous B-cell lymphoma does not appear justified." *Eur J Dermatol* 19:216-220.

[22] Senff, N. J., Kluin-Nelemans, H. C., Willemze, R. 2008. "Results of bone marrow examination in 275 patients with histological features that suggest an indolent type of cutaneous B-cell lymphoma." *Br J Haematol* 142:52-56.

[23] Kempf, W., Sander, C. A. 2010. "Classification of cutaneous lymphomas - an update." *Histopathology* 56:57-70.

[24] Suarez, A. L., Pulitzer, M., Horwitz, S., Moskowitz, A., Querfeld, C., Myskowski, P. L. 2013. "Primary cutaneous B-cell lymphomas: part I. Clinical features, diagnosis, and classification." *J Am Acad Dermatol* 69:329 e321-313; quiz 341-322.

[25] Hristov, A. C. 2012. "Primary cutaneous diffuse large B-cell lymphoma, leg type: diagnostic considerations." *Arch Pathol Lab Med* 136:876-881.

[26] Mian, M., Marcheselli, L., Luminari, S., Federico, M., Cantonetti, M., Sarris, A. H., Rossi, A., et al. 2011. "CLIPI: a new prognostic index for indolent cutaneous B cell lymphoma proposed by the International Extranodal Lymphoma Study Group (IELSG 11)." *Ann Hematol* 90:401-408.

[27] "NCCN Clinical Practice Guidelines in Oncology (NCCN Guidelines®). Non-Hodgkin's Lymphomas. Version 2. 2015. http://www.NCCN.org."

[28] Kim, Y. H., Willemze, R., Pimpinelli, N., Whittaker, S., Olsen, E. A., Ranki, A., Dummer, R., et al. 2007. "TNM classification system for primary cutaneous lymphomas other than mycosis fungoides and Sezary syndrome: a proposal of the International Society for Cutaneous Lymphomas (ISCL) and the Cutaneous Lymphoma Task Force of the European Organization of Research and Treatment of Cancer (EORTC)." *Blood* 110:479-484.

[29] Wilcox, R. A. 2015. "Cutaneous B-cell lymphomas: 2015 update on diagnosis, risk-stratification, and management." *Am J Hematol* 90:73-76.

[30] Fenot, M., Quereux, G., Brocard, A., Renaut, J. J., Dreno, B. 2010. "Rituximab for primary cutaneous diffuse large B-cell lymphoma-leg type." *Eur J Dermatol* 20:753-757.

[31] Pinter-Brown, L. C. 2015. "Diagnosis and Management of Cutaneous B-cell Lymphoma." *Dermatol Clin* 33:835-840.

[32] Sumida, H., Sugaya, M., Miyagaki, T., Minatani, Y., Ohno, Y., Uwajima, Y., Ohmatsu, H., et al. 2013. "Frequent relapse and irradiation strategy in primary cutaneous diffuse large B-cell lymphoma, leg-type." *Acta Derm Venereol* 93:97-98.

[33] Hallermann, C., Niermann, C., Fischer, R. J., Schulze, H. J. 2011. "Survival data for 299 patients with primary cutaneous lymphomas: a monocentre study." *Acta Derm Venereol* 91:521-525.

[34] Vermeer, M. H., Willemze, R. 2014. "Recent advances in primary cutaneous B-cell lymphomas." *Curr Opin Oncol* 26:230-236.

[35] Zinzani, P. L., Quaglino, P., Pimpinelli, N., Berti, E., Baliva, G., Rupoli, S., Martelli, M., et al. 2006. "Prognostic factors in primary cutaneous B-cell lymphoma: the Italian Study Group for Cutaneous Lymphomas." *J Clin Oncol* 24:1376-1382.

[36] Hamilton, S. N., Wai, E. S., Tan, K., Alexander, C., Gascoyne, R. D., Connors, J. M. 2013. "Treatment and outcomes in patients with primary cutaneous B-cell lymphoma: the BC Cancer Agency experience." *Int J Radiat Oncol Biol Phys* 87:719-725.

[37] Grange, F., Beylot-Barry, M., Courville, P., Maubec, E., Bagot, M., Vergier, B., Souteyrand, P., et al. 2007. "Primary cutaneous diffuse large B-cell lymphoma, leg type: clinicopathologic features and prognostic analysis in 60 cases." *Arch Dermatol* 143:1144-1150.

In: Diffuse Large B-Cell Lymphoma (DLBCL)
Editor: Haipeng Shao

ISBN: 978-1-63484-402-4

Chapter 8

Diffuse Large B-Cell Lymphoma Associated with Viral Infections and Immunodeficiency

Julio C. Chavez*
Department of Malignant Hematology,
H. Lee Moffitt Cancer Center and Research Institute, Tampa, FL, US

Abstract

Diffuse large B-cell lymphoma (DLBCL) is a hematological malignancy with genetic and molecular heterogeneity that is responsible for the various responses to standard therapy and survival outcomes. Several predisposing factors have been associated with pathogenesis of DLBCL such as infections (viral), autoimmunity, environmental and genetic factors. The chapter focuses on the viral and immunodeficiency associated DLBCL.

HIV Associated DLBCL

Since the beginning of HIV infection epidemic in early 1980s, cancer represented the most common cause of morbidity and mortality in HIV infected patients, specifically Kaposi's sarcoma (KS) and non-Hodgkin's lymphomas (NHLs) [1, 2]. The introduction of combination of antiretroviral therapy (HAART) improved survival of HIV infected patients and led to a decline of the incidence of lymphomas [3, 4]. Risk of developing lymphomas (particularly CNS lymphomas) is directly linked to levels of CD4 count, with the highest incidence at CD4 count less than 50/μL [4, 5]. The most common type of lymphomas corresponds to B-cell lineage, with DLBCL as the most frequent lymphoma. Following DLBCL in frequency are Burkitt's lymphoma (BL), primary central nervous system lymphoma (PCNSL), primary effusion lymphoma (PEL) and plasmablastic lymphoma (PBL) [6]. Although the incidence of PCNSL, BL and immunoblastic DLBCL have significantly

* Corresponding author: E-mail: Julio.C.Chavez@moffitt.org; Phone: 813-745-8172.

declined with the use of HAART therapy, the impact on the incidence of DLBCL, PEL and PBL have been affected to a lesser extent [7].

Pathogenesis

The current evidence favors the role of HIV related profound immunosuppression of the infected host leading to an altered B-cell homeostasis. There are 2 postulated mechanisms of HIV associated lymphomagenesis: chronic B-cell activation and loss of immune control to oncogenic viruses [8]. *Chronic B-cell activation* occurs as a result of increased cytokines (IL-6, IL-10) and chronic antigenic stimulation. The HIV antigen gp120 has a demonstrated role in B-cell activation and class switching recombination from IgM to IgG, in a process mediated by the activation-induced cytidine deaminase (AID) [8, 9]. Polyclonal hypergammaglobulinemia is commonly seen in HIV infected patients and could be a surrogate marker of highly stimulated B-cell activation. It is postulated that this state of activation perpetuates B-cell proliferation and survival in HIV infected patients [8, 10].

Probably, the most important role of HIV in lymphomagenesis is to predispose the HIV-infected host to reactivation of *oncogenic viruses* such as Epstein Barr virus (EBV) and the Kaposi's sarcoma virus/herpes virus- 8 (KSHV/HHV8). EBV is the most common virus implicated in HIV associated lymphomas and is present in 40 to 80% of cases [5]. Other oncogenic virus increasingly detected in HIV patients, is the human papilloma virus (HPV), which is related to cervical cancer.

There is a loss of the T-cell specific response against EBV in HIV infected patients and development of EBV associated lymphomas (such as DLBCL, BL and classical Hodgkin's lymphoma) seems to be preceded by elevated EBV viral load. This HIV induced impaired response lead to uncontrolled EBV replication and EBV driven lymphomagenesis. In addition to the loss of regulatory immune response to oncogenic viruses, in KSHV/HHV8, the major oncogenic protein, the latency associated nuclear antigen-1 (LANA-1) seems to induce T-cell dysregulation and anergy as a result of decreased HLA class II antigens. Specific mechanisms and related pathways leading to lymphomagenesis by EBV and KSHV/HHV8 will be described below in the sections of EBV-positive diffuse large B-cell lymphoma and KSHV/HHV8 associated lymphomas [11, 12].

Clinical Findings and Diagnosis

Patients with HIV associated aggressive lymphomas should undergo a comprehensive history and physical examination. Past medical history such as history of transfusion, intravenous drug abuse, history of infection by hepatitis B and/or C should be sought in newly diagnosed patients. Physical examination of relevant lymphadenopathy, organomegaly and signs or symptoms of profound immunosuppression (such as oral candidiasis and/or herpes simplex infection) are important [5]. Laboratory studies should include complete blood count and differential, chemistries, LDH, liver function tests, CD4 count levels and assessment of the HIV viral load. Assessment of co-infection with hepatitis B and/or C is relevant, as it will determine concomitant antiviral therapy in addition to chemotherapy. Patients with HIV infection have higher incidence of leptomeningeal involvement by lymphoma, thus a lumbar puncture with cerebral fluid examination through cytology and flow cytometry is strongly recommended [13]. Appropriate referral to a HIV specialist for management of antiretroviral therapy and prophylactic antibiotics are strongly recommended. If risk factors present, HTLV-1 should be assessed [5]. Imaging studies are of paramount importance including CT scanning for appropriate staging. Although positron emission tomography is an important tool in aggressive B-cell lymphomas at diagnosis and response assessment, the role in HIV associated lymphomas is not well established and should be used with appropriate interpretation of findings as increased FDG uptake could be seen in reactive lymphadenopathy commonly present in HIV infected patients [5, 14, 15].

Management

The treatment of HIV associated B-cell aggressive lymphomas have evolved over the past decade. The potential of further immune compromise and infectious complications in HIV patients, in addition to potential interactions with potent antiretroviral therapy by chemotherapy, raised concerns in regards of applying the same intensive chemotherapeutic regimens to this patient population. Currently, it is recommended that HIV patients should be treated with curative intent provided that patients are able to tolerate chemotherapy and have adequate performance status (PS) [5].

Early observations showed that higher dose of chemotherapy was associated with decreased survival in patients due to infectious complications [16]. In a Phase III study, low dose chemotherapy (m-BACOD- methotrexate, bleomycin, doxorubicin, cyclophosphamide, vincristine, and dexamethasone) was compared with standard dose m-BACOD with and without growth factor support in 192 HIV patients with NHLs [17]. There were no differences in response rates and survival, and low intensity chemotherapy was associated with lower hematologic toxicity; however the study did not include patients with CD4 >500/μL. Given that CHOP (cyclophosphamide, doxorubicin, vincristine and prednisone) showed similar survival outcomes with better toxicity profile than m-BACOD, it became the preferred regimen in HIV patients with lymphoma in the post CART era [18].

Although the addition of rituximab improved the survival of HIV- negative DLCBL, its efficacy in HIV+ DLBCL has been questioned initially [19]. This was based on early data of phase II and III studies that showed that rituximab increased rate of infectious complications with no clear benefit in overall survival [20]. Later studies showed that the addition of rituximab to CHOP (R-CHOP) was beneficial without increased rate of infectious deaths [21]. In a pool analysis of prospective trials of CHOP vs. R-CHOP in HIV+ DLBCL; the latter was associated with increased CR rates and OS [22]. It appears that earlier poor outcomes with rituximab were observed in patients with very low CD4 counts (<50/μL) [5, 22].

Rituximab was also administered concurrently or sequentially with infusional chemotherapy with EPOCH (etoposide, cyclophosphamide, doxorubicin, vincristine and prednisone) in HIV+ DLBCL, a regimen that was shown to be effective in the HIV negative counterpart setting [23-25]. No increased infectious complications were seen with the concurrent administration of rituximab and DA-EPOCH [24]. A retrospective comparison of R-CHOP and DA-EPOCH-R in HIV patients with DLBCL performed by the AIDS Malignancy Consortium (AMC), showed that DA-EPOCH-R was significantly superior in terms of CR rates, event free survival (EFS) and OS, regardless the initial stage and IPI score. DA-EPOCH-R was associated with 60-62% reduction of likelihood of death and progression of lymphoma. Treatment-related deaths were significantly associated with CD4 <50/μL [26]. These findings were confirmed by the largest pool analysis of HIV associated DLBCL in over 1500 patients where DA-EPOCH was associated with survival benefit (HR: 0.34; p = 0.03) [27].

Despite evidence of potential interaction of CART with chemotherapy [28], the current evidence suggests that continuation of effective antiretroviral therapy against HIV contributes to control viral replication, effective increase of $CD4^+$ T-cells and decrease further compromise of the immune system; which has been translated into clinical benefit and improved overall survival [22, 26, 27]. Most experts agree on continuation of CART while HIV associated DLBCL patients are undergoing intensive chemotherapy. Although short course chemotherapy with DA-EPOCH for 3 cycles (SC-EPOCH-R) while CART is suspended has shown similar efficacy and clinical outcomes; the small size sample in the study and the general concern and knowledge of generating HIV resistance, makes this protocol less popular, but deserves further investigation [25, 29].

EBV Positive DLBCL of the Elderly

Epstein Barr virus (EBV) positive DLBCL of the elderly is a relatively recent category included in the World Health Organization (WHO) Classification of Haematopietic Tumors [30, 31]. The first description of this condition reported 22 patients with DLBCL that expressed EBV encoded-RNA (EBER) integrated into the malignant cells, later called Oyama cells [30, 32].

Prevalence

The prevalence EBV positive DLBCL of the elderly is variable. It is infrequently reported in Western countries (2-5%) but it is most commonly reported in Latin and Asian countries (8-14%). However there are concerns in regard to the diagnostic criteria for EBV+ DLBCL in the elderly. First, the age 50 and older was developed arbitrarily; in fact, most reports consider elderly in patients older than 60. Second, there is lack of consensus criteria of a positive EBER in DLBCL as many consider a cutoff of 20% while others reported positive cases with cutoff of 30 or 50%.

Pathogenesis

One of the most important factors associated with development of EBV+ DLBCL of the elderly is immunosenescence. Immunosenescence is characterized by progressive decline in humoral response by decreases in antibody producing B-cells and B-cell diversity [33]. There is also a decline in cellular immune response by T-cell functional dysregulation, decreased

CD8$^+$ cytotoxic T-cells, decreased antigen recognition by CD4$^+$ T-cells and decreased activity in cytotoxic activity of NK/T cells [34].

Persistence of EBV infection is another important factors in the pathogenesis of EBV+ DBCL of the elderly (and other EBV associated malignancies), and can occur by evading the host immune system [35, 36]. EBV maintains its genome with minimal amount of genes (latency) [35]. There are three types of latency in EBV associated lymphomas. In latency type 1 there is expression of the EBV nuclear antigen 1 (EBNA1) and EBER. Latency type 1 is seen in Burkitt lymphoma and some cases of gastric cancer. Expression of the latent membrane protein 1 (LMP1) in addition to EBNA1 and EBER is characteristic of latency type 2, which is observed in NK/T cell lymphomas and Hodgkin's lymphoma. Latency type 3 is characterized by the expression of all 6 EBNA proteins (EBNA1, EBNA2, EBNA3a, 3b, 3c and LP) in addition to LMP1, LMP2A and LMP2B. The counterpart malignancy associated with latency type 3 EBV is the posttransplant lymphoproliferative disorder (PTLD). The patterns associated with EBV+ DLBCL in the elderly are latency type 2 and type 3 [36-38].

LMP1 is the best-known oncoprotein that has been studied in EBV associated malignancies. This protein is activated by self-aggregation and oligomerization [39]. LMP1 promotes proliferation by activating several signaling pathways including the NF-κB pathway, the Janus kinase 2/signal transducer and activation pathway (JAK/STAT), the mitogen-activated protein kinase (MAPK/MEK) and the phophoinositide-3 kinase (PI3K) pathway [40]. It also promotes cell cycle progression and inhibits apoptosis by upregulating the cyclin dependent kinase-2 and increasing the expression of the oncoprotein 2, respectively. LMP2A is associated with B-cell survival through the activation and increased expression of Syk and Lyn molecules signaling pathways and Bcl-Xl [41].

Another implicated factor contributing to the EBV+ DLBCL pathogenesis is the increased frequency of microRNAs (miRNAs) [42]. MicroRNAs are small non-coding molecules of RNA that result from cleavage of long non-coding RNAs. These small molecules have been implicated in differentiation, proliferation, cell survival and inhibition of apoptosis in cancer. In the case of EBV+ DLBCL, it appears that miRNAs influence immune evasion, dysregulation of the immune system and prolongs the EBV latency phase [42]. It has been reported that a unique differential expression of miRNAs in EBV+ DBCL that seems to be associated with poor prognosis [43].

Clinical Features and Prognosis

EBV+ DLBCL of the elderly is an aggressive lymphoma with poor prognosis (median overall survival of 2 years) that tends to occur in older patients. Although 70% of patients present with nodal disease, extranodal involvement is frequent (in comparison to EBV negative DLBCL) with the most common organs affected being the skin, soft tissues, bones, nasal cavities, lungs, tonsils, lungs, liver, peritoneum and bone marrow. Patients also have higher international prognostic index (IPI), advanced stage and B symptoms. Patients with EBV+ DLBCL also have poor response to anthracycline-based chemotherapy, in contrast with their EBV negative DLBCL counterparts.

Several prognostic factors have been studied in EBV+ DLBCL. A prognostic score was developed by Oyama et al., which seemed to discriminate three risk groups. It included two factors: age older than 70 and presence of B symptoms. Patients with 0, 1 or 2 factors had an

OS of 59, 25 and 9 months. In addition, EBV+ DLBCL with expression of CD30 was associated with worse overall survival and progression free survival [44]. Lastly, Beltran et al. reported that lymphopenia at diagnosis (cutoff of less than $1.0x10^9$/L), was associated with poor outcomes in a multivariate analysis of Peruvian patients with EBV+ DLBCL of the elderly [45].

Pathologic Features

Two morphologic subtypes of EBV+ DLBCL of the elderly have been described: polymorphic and monomorphic subtypes. The polymorphic subtype is characterized by variable presence of B-cells in different degrees of maturation, plasmablasts, Hodgkin and Reed-Stenberg (HRS) like cells, and immunoblasts. The polymorphic subtype has been subdivided additionally into 3 sub-entities based on the proportion of HRS cells and large transformed B-cells in the neoplastic lesion, with some features similar to Hodgkin lymphoma [46]. The monomorphic subtype EBV+ DLBCL is characterized by the presence of diffuse sheets of large transformed B-cells not different from EBV negative DLBCL [31].

EBV+ DLBCL is a lymphoma that expresses typical B-cell lineage markers such as: CD19, CD20, CD22, CD79a and PAX-5 and negative for T-cell specific markers. Per immunohistochemical analysis, EBV+DLBCL usually shows a profile of non-germinal center (non-GCB) subtype such as CD10 negative, BCL6 negative and expression of MUM1/IRF4 [31]. There is increased expression of CD30 and BCL2. This is in concordance with the increased frequency of activated B-cell subtype DLBCL (ABC-DLBCL) in elderly patients [30, 32].

Management

As mentioned above, the prognosis of EBV+ DLBCL of the elderly is generally poor with the administration of anthracycline-based chemotherapy (i.e., CHOP). While the addition of anti CD20 monoclonal antibodies such as rituximab to chemotherapy (R-CHOP) has improved outcomes in patients with DLBCL in different settings, the efficacy in EBV+ DLBCL of the elderly has been challenged [19, 47]. Data from small reports showed improved outcomes with the addition of rituximab but does not match the outcomes of the EBV negative DLBCL [48, 49]. Due to the lack of standard therapies, most clinicians still consider R-CHOP as the first line of treatment for EBV+ DLBCL of the elderly.

Thus, targeting EBV and/or specific molecular markers in DLBCL offered several opportunities of investigation. Antiviral therapy has been attempted without success, as the virus needs to be in lytic (active phase) in order for standard antiherpes drugs to have a killing effect [39]. The addition of drugs such as histone deacetylase inhibitors (HDACs) has shown induction of latent EBV into lytic phase increasing antiviral effect and clinical response [50, 51].

More interesting is the development of immunotherapy against EBV+ DLBCL based on the high immunogenicity of the virus (especially in latency 3). The initial experience of administering serum from EBV positive donors showed efficacy in EBV associated lymphoproliferative disorders (LPD) post organ and bone marrow transplant [52]. In order to achieve more specificity and with less risk of developing undesirable side effects autologous cytotoxic T-cells against EBV were developed using in vitro EBV transformed cell lines [53]. However, the prolonged time (6 to 12 weeks) required to manufacture these cells constitute hindrance for treating an aggressive lymphoma. Modern technology has been developed in order to generate EBV-CTLs in a more rapid manner. Reports of these studies showed promising efficacy in EBV related lymphoproliferative malignancies [54, 55].

Plasmablastic Lymphoma

Plasmablastic lymphoma (PBL) is a rare type of B-cell malignancy that was initially reported as oral and mucosal lymphoid neoplasms in HIV positive patients, however it can affect individuals with chronic T-cell immunosuppression, such as organ and marrow transplant and elderly/debilitated patients [56, 57]. Almost 100% of cases are associated with EBV infection. PBL represents approximately 2% of all HIV-related lymphomas [58].

Pathogenesis

The pathogenesis of PBL is not well understood. Due to its relation to HIV infection and association with EBV, immunosuppression (or immunosenescense) might be implicated. The frequent presence of MYC rearrangements gives clues of its pathogenesis and frequent resistance to standard chemotherapy. The cell of origin of PBL is thought to be a plasmablast, which is an activated B-cell that has undergone somatic hypermutation and class switching recombination. Thus, activated NF-κB pathway is present in PBL, with consequent increased survival of malignant B-cells. The presence of MYC rearrangements is associated with DNA replication, proliferation, and survival and cell growth [58].

Clinical Features and Prognosis

HIV associated PBL usually affects younger population (median age of 38) with significant male predominance. In half of the cases there is advanced stage of disease (stage III/IV). The oral cavity is affected in more than 50% of cases [59]. HIV negative PBL tends to occur at older age (median age of 57), the male to female ratio of 1.7:1. Advanced stage is present in 60% of cases with extranodal involvement in 80%. GI tract is the second most common area affected. In HIV negative PBL there is usually a history of coexistent immunosuppressive condition such as concurrent malignancy, autoimmune disease or organ transplantation in 30% of cases [60, 61]. PBL as transformation from a prior hematologic malignancy has been described, most commonly in patients with follicular lymphoma and chronic lymphocytic leukemia.

The prognosis of PBL is generally poor with reported median OS between 9-15 months. Response to chemotherapy ranges between 50-80% with CR rates in the range of 41-52%. It appears that HIV positive status is associated with better outcomes, but results have not been consistent in all reports. Other adverse prognostic factors include higher IPI score, advanced stage, poor performance status, a CD4 count less than 200/µl and presence of MYC rearrangements [57, 62-64].

Pathologic Features

Neoplastic cells have round to oval shape with prominent central nucleolus. The presence of tingible body macrophages and abundant mitotic figures in the background can give a "starry-sky" pattern. PBL is a B-cell malignancy but does not express common B-cell lineage markers such as CD19, CD20 and PAX-5. It sometimes expresses CD79a. Additionally it expresses markers of plasmacytic differentiation such as CD38, CD138 and MUM/IRF4. The Ki67 proliferation index is very high (usually >90%). Genetic studies showed the presence of MYC rearrangements in 40% of cases of PBL [64]. EBV infection (latency type 1) detected by EBER has been demonstrated in 80% of HIV associated PBL, 67% of post-transplant PBL and 50% in immunocompetent PBL cases [58, 59].

Management

Since the prognosis is dismal, there is no established standard of care for PBL. As highly aggressive lymphoma, the use of CHOP regimen is considered suboptimal per current guidelines and more intensive therapies are recommended. The following regimens are recommended: dose adjusted infusional etoposide, doxorubicin, vincristine, cyclophosphamide and prednisone (EPOCH), doxorubicin, methotrexate, vincristine and cyclophosphamide alternating with ifosfamide, etoposide and cytarabine (CODOX/IVAC) and hyperfractionated cyclophosphamide, doxorubicin, vincristine and dexamethasone alternating with methotrexate (hyperCVAD) [58]. Small series of cases have shown prolonged OS and PFS with autologous hematopoietic stem cell transplantation (HSCT) in first remission but limited utility in the relapse setting [65].

Given the plasmacytic nature of PBL, the use of standard targeted antimyeloma therapy has been advocated but experience is limited to case reports. Combination of bortezomib with chemotherapy has shown anti-tumor activity in the relapse and frontline settings [66, 67]. Lenalidomide as single agent elicited temporary response in a report of relapsed PBL [68].

HHV8/KSHV Associated Primary Effusion LymphomA (PEL)

The herpes virus 8/Kaposi sarcoma herpesvirus (HHV8/KSHV) has been implicated in the development of three well-described neoplastic conditions: primary effusion lymphoma (PEL), Kaposi sarcoma (KS) and multicentric Castleman disease (MCD). PEL is a an aggressive B-cell lymphoma that was initially described in HIV infected patients and characterized by involvement of body cavities without the presence of a detectable mass [69, 70]. In the seminal work of Cesarman et al., in a study of HIV associated lymphomas, the DNA sequences of KSHV/HHV8 virus were found in PEL specifically, establishing the link between the virus and this type lymphoma, and making the presence of HHV8/KSHV virus in neoplastic tissue an essential feature for the diagnosis of PEL. Although first described in HIV infected patients in advanced stage, PEL can also occur in post solid organ transplant and elderly patients with comorbidities [71].

Pathogenesis

The HHV8/KSHV is a gamma herpesvirus and similar to EBV, infects B-cells and persists lifelong in a latent form in order to evade the immune system response [72]. It has 5 latent genes that are postulated to be associated with the development of PEL: latency associated nuclear antigen-1 (LANA-1), LANA-2/v-IRF3, viral cyclin (v Cyclin), viral FLICE inhibitory protein (v-FLIP) and Kaposin (K12). These gene products are actively implicated in inhibition of apoptosis of HHV8 infected cells and blocking TNF mediated activation of caspases. They also activate the NF-κB, JAK/STAT and AKT/mTOR signaling pathways that are associated with cell survival [71, 73].

Clinical Features and Prognosis

PEL represents 2-4% of all HIV associated lymphomas and is commonly diagnosed in patients with advanced HIV infection, owing to the profound immunosuppression at these stages of infection. It can concomitantly present with other HHV8 associated disease such as KS and MCD.

PEL is characterized by the presence of malignant effusion in the pleural, pericardial or peritoneal spaces without evident tumor or mass. Thus, patients can presents with chest pain, dyspnea, abdominal pain, abdominal distension and symptoms of cardiac tamponade [71, 74]. The pleural space is involved in 70% of cases. PEL with solid mass (extracavitary PEL) has also been described [75, 76]. Extracavitary PEL usually affects the gastrointestinal (GI), but it also has been reported in the skin, lymph nodes, lungs and central nervous system (CNS) [75, 77].

The prognosis of PEL is generally poor with survival times ranging from 4 to 9 months. The largest series of PEL showed that predictors of survival were lack of HAART at diagnosis and poor performance status [78]. It appears that the number of body cavities affected by lymphoma impacts on survival outcomes [79]. The IPI score has not yet been validated in PEL, however, given the nature and clinical presentation of this disease, it might warrant a specific prognostic system.

Pathologic Findings

The diagnosis of PEL is based on morphologic and specific phenotypic findings. The immunohistochemical demonstration of KSHV/HHV8 virus in tumor cells by detection of the LANA-1 antigen is essential for diagnosis. PEL cells are large cells with prominent nucleoli that sometimes resemble plasmablasts or immunoblasts. Classically, PEL has a "B-cell null" immunophenotype with no expression of typical B-cell markers. It expresses markers of plasma cell differentiation such as CD138 and MUM1/IRF4. It frequently expresses markers of lymphocyte activation such as CD30 and CD38 [57, 69].

Management

The standard therapy for PEL has yet to be determined. Standard CHOP regimen has been associated with 40% response rates and median OS of 6 months [80]. Variable response rates have been seen with doxorubicin, cyclophosphamide, vindesine, bleomycin and prednisone (ACVBP) and CHOP plus methotrexate [57]. The dose adjusted-EPOCH has also been used with success in case reports of PEL and, since its efficacy seems to be greater than CHOP in HIV associated lymphomas, it has been considered as frontline therapy [26, 81]. Prolonged remission has been reported in cases of PEL after autologous HSCT, and should be considered in selected cases, especially in patients able to tolerate the procedure [82]. The initiation (or continuation) of effective HAART therapy is essential at diagnosis of PEL due to its impact in prognosis and survival [57, 71].

POST-TRANSPLANT LYMPHOPROLIFERATIVE DISORDER (PTLD)/DLBCL

PTLD comprises a heterogeneous group of lymphoid and plasmacytic proliferation that occurs in the post-solid organ (SOT) and/or allogeneic hematopoietic stem cell transplant (HSCT) settings. Since SOT and HSCT are increasingly used and immunosuppressive techniques improve in order to prevent rejection, the incidence of PTLD is expected to increase. The morphology varies from early polyclonal lesions to monomorphic lymphoma. The latest WHO classification in 2008 has divided PTLD into four histological types: a) early lesions; b) polymorphic PTLD; c) monomorphic PTLD such as DLBCL and d) classical Hodgkin lymphoma [83].

Epidemiology and Incidence

The incidence of PTLD is variable and ranges from 1-20% with the highest risk associated with intestinal and visceral transplants (5-20%), followed by lung and heart transplants (5-10%), and with the lowest incidence in liver and kidney transplants (0.5-5%) [84]. Incidence of PTLD increases with time with 0.7% and 1.4% at 5 and 10 years, respectively according to the French Registry [84, 85]. Early onset PTLD tends to be monomorphic and polymorphic in 48 vs. 42% of cases, but monomorphic PTLD seems to be more frequent in the late onset setting (56%) [85]. In patients with risks factors, PTLD usually peak at 2-3 months post allogeneic HSCT and usually within the first 6 months post-transplant. PTLD after allogeneic HSCT usually has a poor prognosis [86].

The risk of immunosuppression varies with the transplanted organ involved, timing from SOT and intensity, duration and type of immunosuppression. Risks factors for development of PTLD include: seronegative EBV status in recipient (EBV naïve), use of anti-lymphocyte antibodies (thymoglobulin) or T-cell depleting agents (OKT3), long-term chronic immunosuppression (especially tacrolimus) and age older than 60 [87, 88]. As mentioned above, PTLD is also an important complication after allogeneic HSCT and identified risk factors are T-cell depletion, mismatch HLA donor, anti-thymocyte globulin use, older than 50 years and second transplant [89].

Pathogenesis

The Epstein Barr virus (EBV) plays a major role in the pathogenesis of PTLD. Approximately 60-80% of PTLD cases are EBV-driven. The presence of the EBV genome varies depending of the type of PTLD with the highest incidence during the first year after transplantation (90-100%) and lower frequencies in late onset PTLD (50-60%) [90]. As mentioned above, maintaining an EBV latent phase is critical for the virus to infect B-lymphoid cells and to promote lymphomagenesis [35, 36]. As discussed in prior section, EBV related PTLD are associated with type 3 latency (expression of all 6 EBNA proteins in addition to LMP1, LMP2A and LMPB). The lytic phase of EBV also seems to be important, as it appears to induce transformation and proliferation of B-cell infected cells dependent of cytokines and growth factors such as IL-6, cIL-10 and vIL-10 [91]. These cytokines, in addition to interferon-alpha and tumor necrosis factor (TNF), are also generated by chronic B-cell activation seen in patients with EBV infection. Levels of EBV viral load have also been linked to increased activated B-cells, a theory that is supported by the direct correlation of EBV viremia and risk of developing PTLD [92].

Clinical Features and Prognosis

Patients with PTLD present with unspecific symptoms such as fevers, generalized or localized lymphadenopathy, weight loss and symptoms of sepsis. Extranodal involvement to the liver, lungs, gastrointestinal tract, tonsils and bone marrow can occur. Central nervous system (CNS) involvement could be as high as 30%. In some cases PTLD has been described in the transplanted organ especially in the early onset type, thus patients can present with hepatitis, nephritis and pneumonitis [93]. Patients can present with abnormal liver tests and increasingly elevated LDH. These symptoms can also be seen in patients with other transplant related infections such as CMV, adenovirus and *pneumocystis jiroveci* pneumonia.

Accurate staging is important and PTLD patients should be staged using the same imaging techniques as other non-Hodgkin's lymphomas using current criteria [15]. F-FDG-PET/CT has shown to be highly sensitive and specific in PTLD and should be considered for initial staging and response assessment [94].

As noted above, most PTLD are associated to EBV and screening for early detection of EBV has been investigated and proven to be effective. EBV viral load be measured by polymerase chain reaction (PCR) technology has been shown to be a warning sign of PTLD and preemptive therapy has been recommended based of early EBV detection; however a specific cutoff of viral load has not been determined and approaches for preemptive treatment should take into account the clinical features and risk factors [95, 96]. It is important to note that in cases of EBV negative PTLD, EBV viral load may not be detected.

The prognosis of PTLD is poor when compared with a similar condition such as DLBCL with an overall survival at 5 years of 40-50% with most of death due to progressive disease but with an important proportion of patients dying of complications related to transplant (infections or toxicity). There is no consensus in regards to a prognostic scoring system; however it appears that advanced age, poor performance status, CNS involvement and elevated LDH have been consistently noted as poor prognostic indicators [97, 98].

Management

The most important first step in the treatment of PTLD is reduction of immunosuppression (RIS) to the minimum tolerated dose without causing transplanted organ rejection. RIS appears to be effective in achieving remission in 25-50% of cases, especially in early onset PTLD; however, often times, additional therapy is needed [99]. In patients with no response to RIS, the use of immunotherapy with rituximab appears to be also effective with response rates of 40-70& as reported across the series, but CR rates are 35% with common relapses [100]. Extended rituximab use can increase efficacy but with no proven effect on overall survival [101]. Responses rates could be as high as 90% if rituximab is used in the preemptive setting [84, 100].

Chemotherapy as first line approach has been attempted with several regimens at cost of increased treatment-related mortality (TRM) [88]. R-CHOP and CHOP were used in PTLD with a CR rate of 53%, median OS of 42 months and TRM of 26% [102]. The more aggressive regimen ACVBP yielded a response rate of 73%, a long-term survival with 5-year OS of 60% and TRM 9% but increased hematologic toxicity [103]. In order to minimize toxicity from chemotherapy a multicenter trial was carried out by the European PTLD Network (PTLD-1 trial) that consisted in sequential therapy of 4 weekly standard doses of rituximab followed by 4 weeks without treatment. Patients not achieving response received 4 cycles of R-CHOP every three weeks. Seventy patients were included and 66 underwent sequential therapy with R-CHOP. The response rate was 90% with CR of 67% and the median overall survival was 6.6 years. There were improvements in response rates and overall survival regardless of the PTLD EBV status. The TRM was 10.6% but lower in rituximab responders (4.2%) [104].

Since antiviral drugs have proven to be ineffective to suppress EBV replication, restoring antiviral immunity was the next best logic step in the treatment of EBV-PTLD [39]. Adoptive immunotherapy by transfer of EBV-specific cytotoxic T-cells (CTLs) has been investigated for many years [105]. The first approach was to administer EBV seropositive donor lymphocytes infusions (DLI) in PTLD post allogeneic HSCT, however it was associated with increased risk of GVHD [106]. Another common approach was to generate autologous EBV-CTLs by using EBV infected lymphoblastic cell lines, a process that takes approximately 6-12 weeks [105, 107]. Using a cytokine secreting system, EBNA1 specific EBV-CTLs could be generated in 3-5 days, allowing a more rapid availability of CTLs [108]. In general, response rates of adoptive therapy in refractory EBV-PTLD were impressive with rates between 50-70%, however this technology is not widely available [108]. In SOT, generating donor derived CTLs is more challenging since the donor is not often available and the recipient and donor are not usually HLA-matched. Although EBV-CTLs in PTLD post SOT were not able to decrease EBV viral load it prevented the development of PTLD in 11 out of

13 patients [53]. Future development of EBV-CTLs includes the development of faster system to generate CTLs, having a bank of HLA specific EBV-CTLs and prolonging the persistence of EBV-CTLs by genetically modifying CTLs in order to be resistant to common immunosuppressive drugs.

REFERENCES

[1] Engels, E. A., Pfeiffer, R. M., Goedert, J. J., Virgo, P., McNeel, T. S., Scoppa, S. M., Biggar, R. J., Study, Hiv Aids Cancer Match. 2006. "Trends in cancer risk among people with AIDS in the United States 1980-2002." *AIDS* 20:1645-1654.

[2] Coghill, A. E., Shiels, M. S., Suneja, G., Engels, E. A. 2015. "Elevated Cancer-Specific Mortality Among HIV-Infected Patients in the United States." *J Clin Oncol* 33:2376-2383.

[3] Detels, R., Munoz, A., McFarlane, G., Kingsley, L. A., Margolick, J. B., Giorgi, J., Schrager, L. K., Phair, J. P. 1998. "Effectiveness of potent antiretroviral therapy on time to AIDS and death in men with known HIV infection duration. Multicenter AIDS Cohort Study Investigators." *JAMA* 280:1497-1503.

[4] Besson, C., Goubar, A., Gabarre, J., Rozenbaum, W., Pialoux, G., Chatelet, F. P., Katlama, C., et al., 2001. "Changes in AIDS-related lymphoma since the era of highly active antiretroviral therapy." *Blood* 98:2339-2344.

[5] Dunleavy, K., Wilson, W. H. 2012. "How I treat HIV-associated lymphoma." *Blood* 119:3245-3255.

[6] Little, R. F., Dunleavy, K. 2013. "Update on the treatment of HIV-associated hematologic malignancies." *Hematology Am Soc Hematol Educ Program* 2013:382-388.

[7] Aboulafia, D. M., Pantanowitz, L., Dezube, B. J. 2004. "AIDS-related non-Hodgkin lymphoma: still a problem in the era of HAART." *AIDS Read* 14:605-617.

[8] Gloghini, A., Dolcetti, R., Carbone, A. 2013. "Lymphomas occurring specifically in HIV-infected patients: from pathogenesis to pathology." *Semin Cancer Biol* 23:457-467.

[9] He, B., Qiao, X., Klasse, P. J., Chiu, A., Chadburn, A., Knowles, D. M., Moore, J. P., Cerutti, A. 2006. "HIV-1 envelope triggers polyclonal Ig class switch recombination through a CD40-independent mechanism involving BAFF and C-type lectin receptors." *J Immunol* 176:3931-3941.

[10] Breen, E. C., Hussain, S. K., Magpantay, L., Jacobson, L. P., Detels, R., Rabkin, C. S., Kaslow, R. A., et al., 2011. "B-cell stimulatory cytokines and markers of immune activation are elevated several years prior to the diagnosis of systemic AIDS-associated non-Hodgkin B-cell lymphoma." *Cancer Epidemiol Biomarkers Prev* 20:1303-1314.

[11] Sabbah, S., Jagne, Y. J., Zuo, J., de Silva, T., Ahasan, M. M., Brander, C., Rowland-Jones, S., Flanagan, K. L., Hislop, A. D. 2012. "T-cell immunity to Kaposi sarcoma-associated herpesvirus: recognition of primary effusion lymphoma by LANA-specific CD4+ T cells." *Blood* 119:2083-2092.

[12] Carbone, A., Vaccher, E., Gloghini, A., Pantanowitz, L., Abayomi, A., de Paoli, P., Franceschi, S. 2014. "Diagnosis and management of lymphomas and other cancers in HIV-infected patients." *Nat Rev Clin Oncol* 11:223-238.

[13] Hegde, U., Filie, A., Little, R. F., Janik, J. E., Grant, N., Steinberg, S. M., Dunleavy, K., et al., 2005. "High incidence of occult leptomeningeal disease detected by flow cytometry in newly diagnosed aggressive B-cell lymphomas at risk for central nervous system involvement: the role of flow cytometry versus cytology." *Blood* 105:496-502.

[14] Dunleavy, K., Mikhaeel, G., Sehn, L. H., Hicks, R. J., Wilson, W. H. 2010. "The value of positron emission tomography in prognosis and response assessment in non-Hodgkin lymphoma." *Leuk Lymphoma* 51 Suppl 1:28-33.

[15] Barrington, S. F., Mikhaeel, N. G., Kostakoglu, L., Meignan, M., Hutchings, M., Mueller, S. P., Schwartz, L. H., et al., 2014. "Role of imaging in the staging and response assessment of lymphoma: consensus of the International Conference on Malignant Lymphomas Imaging Working Group." *J Clin Oncol* 32:3048-3058.

[16] Kaplan, L. D., Abrams, D. I., Feigal, E., McGrath, M., Kahn, J., Neville, P., Ziegler, J., Volberding, P. A. 1989. "AIDS-associated non-Hodgkin's lymphoma in San Francisco." *JAMA* 261:719-724.

[17] Kaplan, L. D., Straus, D. J., Testa, M. A., Von Roenn, J., Dezube, B. J., Cooley, T. P., Herndier, B., et al., 1997. "Low-dose compared with standard-dose m-BACOD chemotherapy for non-Hodgkin's lymphoma associated with human immunodeficiency virus infection. National Institute of Allergy and Infectious Diseases AIDS Clinical Trials Group." *N Engl J Med* 336:1641-1648.

[18] Fisher, R. I., Gaynor, E. R., Dahlberg, S., Oken, M. M., Grogan, T. M., Mize, E. M., Glick, J. H., Coltman, C. A., Jr., Miller, T. P. 1993. "Comparison of a standard regimen (CHOP) with three intensive chemotherapy regimens for advanced non-Hodgkin's lymphoma." *N Engl J Med* 328:1002-1006.

[19] Coiffier, B., Lepage, E., Briere, J., Herbrecht, R., Tilly, H., Bouabdallah, R., Morel, P., et al., 2002. "CHOP chemotherapy plus rituximab compared with CHOP alone in elderly patients with diffuse large-B-cell lymphoma." *N Engl J Med* 346:235-242.

[20] Kaplan, L. D., Lee, J. Y., Ambinder, R. F., Sparano, J. A., Cesarman, E., Chadburn, A., Levine, A. M., Scadden, D. T. 2005. "Rituximab does not improve clinical outcome in a randomized phase 3 trial of CHOP with or without rituximab in patients with HIV-associated non-Hodgkin lymphoma: AIDS-Malignancies Consortium Trial 010." *Blood* 106:1538-1543.

[21] Boue, F., Gabarre, J., Gisselbrecht, C., Reynes, J., Cheret, A., Bonnet, F., Billaud, E., et al., 2006. "Phase II trial of CHOP plus rituximab in patients with HIV-associated non-Hodgkin's lymphoma." *J Clin Oncol* 24:4123-4128.

[22] Castillo, J. J., Echenique, I. A. 2012. "Rituximab in combination with chemotherapy versus chemotherapy alone in HIV-associated non-Hodgkin lymphoma: a pooled analysis of 15 prospective studies." *Am J Hematol* 87:330-333.

[23] Wilson, W. H., Grossbard, M. L., Pittaluga, S., Cole, D., Pearson, D., Drbohlav, N., Steinberg, S. M., et al., 2002. "Dose-adjusted EPOCH chemotherapy for untreated large B-cell lymphomas: a pharmacodynamic approach with high efficacy." *Blood* 99:2685-2693.

[24] Sparano, J. A., Lee, J. Y., Kaplan, L. D., Levine, A. M., Ramos, J. C., Ambinder, R. F., Wachsman, W., et al., 2010. "Rituximab plus concurrent infusional EPOCH

chemotherapy is highly effective in HIV-associated B-cell non-Hodgkin lymphoma." *Blood* 115:3008-3016.

[25] Dunleavy, K., Little, R. F., Pittaluga, S., Grant, N., Wayne, A. S., Carrasquillo, J. A., Steinberg, S. M., et al., 2010. "The role of tumor histogenesis, FDG-PET, and short-course EPOCH with dose-dense rituximab (SC-EPOCH-RR) in HIV-associated diffuse large B-cell lymphoma." *Blood* 115:3017-3024.

[26] Barta, S. K., Lee, J. Y., Kaplan, L. D., Noy, A., Sparano, J. A. 2012. "Pooled analysis of AIDS malignancy consortium trials evaluating rituximab plus CHOP or infusional EPOCH chemotherapy in HIV-associated non-Hodgkin lymphoma." *Cancer* 118:3977-3983.

[27] Barta, S. K., Xue, X., Wang, D., Tamari, R., Lee, J. Y., Mounier, N., Kaplan, L. D., et al., 2013. "Treatment factors affecting outcomes in HIV-associated non-Hodgkin lymphomas: a pooled analysis of 1546 patients." *Blood* 122:3251-3262.

[28] Ratner, L., Lee, J., Tang, S., Redden, D., Hamzeh, F., Herndier, B., Scadden, D., et al., 2001. "Chemotherapy for human immunodeficiency virus-associated non-Hodgkin''s lymphoma in combination with highly active antiretroviral therapy." *J Clin Oncol* 19:2171-2178.

[29] Hirsch, M. S., Brun-Vezinet, F., Clotet, B., Conway, B., Kuritzkes, D. R., D'Aquila, R. T., Demeter, L. M., et al., 2003. "Antiretroviral drug resistance testing in adults infected with human immunodeficiency virus type 1: 2003 recommendations of an International AIDS Society-USA Panel." *Clin Infect Dis* 37:113-128.

[30] Ok, C. Y., Papathomas, T. G., Medeiros, L. J., Young, K. H. 2013. "EBV-positive diffuse large B-cell lymphoma of the elderly." *Blood* 122:328-340.

[31] Nakamura, S, Jaffe, ES, Swerdlow, SH. 2008. "EBV positive diffuse large B-cell lymphoma of the elderly." *WHO classification of tumours of haematopoietic and lymphoid tissues. Lyon: IARC* 243-244.

[32] Oyama, T., Yamamoto, K., Asano, N., Oshiro, A., Suzuki, R., Kagami, Y., Morishima, Y., et al., 2007. "Age-related EBV-associated B-cell lymphoproliferative disorders constitute a distinct clinicopathologic group: a study of 96 patients." *Clin Cancer Res* 13:5124-5132.

[33] Gibson, K. L., Wu, Y. C., Barnett, Y., Duggan, O., Vaughan, R., Kondeatis, E., Nilsson, B. O., et al., 2009. "B-cell diversity decreases in old age and is correlated with poor health status." *Aging Cell* 8:18-25.

[34] Lefebvre, J. S., Maue, A. C., Eaton, S. M., Lanthier, P. A., Tighe, M., Haynes, L. 2012. "The aged microenvironment contributes to the age-related functional defects of CD4 T cells in mice." *Aging Cell* 11:732-740.

[35] Thorley-Lawson, D. A., Gross, A. 2004. "Persistence of the Epstein-Barr virus and the origins of associated lymphomas." *N Engl J Med* 350:1328-1337.

[36] Ok, C. Y., Li, L., Young, K. H. 2015. "EBV-driven B-cell lymphoproliferative disorders: from biology, classification and differential diagnosis to clinical management." *Exp Mol Med* 47:e132.

[37] Hong, J. Y., Ko, Y. H., Kim, S. J., Kim, W. S. 2015. "Epstein-Barr virus-positive diffuse large B-cell lymphoma of the elderly: a concise review and update." *Curr Opin Oncol* 27:392-398.

[38] Nguyen-Van, D., Keane, C., Han, E., Jones, K., Nourse, J. P., Vari, F., Ross, N., et al., 2011. "Epstein-Barr virus-positive diffuse large B-cell lymphoma of the elderly expresses EBNA3A with conserved CD8 T-cell epitopes." *Am J Blood Res* 1:146-159.

[39] Liebowitz, D. 1998. "Epstein-Barr virus and a cellular signaling pathway in lymphomas from immunosuppressed patients." *N Engl J Med* 338:1413-1421.

[40] Dawson, C. W., Tramountanis, G., Eliopoulos, A. G., Young, L. S. 2003. "Epstein-Barr virus latent membrane protein 1 (LMP1) activates the phosphatidylinositol 3-kinase/Akt pathway to promote cell survival and induce actin filament remodeling." *J Biol Chem* 278:3694-3704.

[41] Brinkmann, M. M., Schulz, T. F. 2006. "Regulation of intracellular signalling by the terminal membrane proteins of members of the Gammaherpesvirinae." *J Gen Virol* 87:1047-1074.

[42] Imig, J., Motsch, N., Zhu, J. Y., Barth, S., Okoniewski, M., Reineke, T., Tinguely, M., et al., 2011. "microRNA profiling in Epstein-Barr virus-associated B-cell lymphoma." *Nucleic Acids Res* 39:1880-1893.

[43] Andrade, T. A., Evangelista, A. F., Campos, A. H., Poles, W. A., Borges, N. M., Camillo, C. M., Soares, F. A., et al., 2014. "A microRNA signature profile in EBV+ diffuse large B-cell lymphoma of the elderly." *Oncotarget* 5:11813-11826.

[44] Ok, C. Y., Li, L., Xu-Monette, Z. Y., Visco, C., Tzankov, A., Manyam, G. C., Montes-Moreno, S., et al., 2014. "Prevalence and clinical implications of epstein-barr virus infection in de novo diffuse large B-cell lymphoma in Western countries." *Clin Cancer Res* 20:2338-2349.

[45] Beltran, B. E., Castillo, J. J., Morales, D., de Mendoza, F. H., Quinones, P., Miranda, R. N., Gallo, A., et al., 2011. "EBV-positive diffuse large B-cell lymphoma of the elderly: a case series from Peru." *Am J Hematol* 86:663-667.

[46] Montes-Moreno, S., Odqvist, L., Diaz-Perez, J. A., Lopez, A. B., de Villambrosia, S. G., Mazorra, F., Castillo, M. E., et al., 2012. "EBV-positive diffuse large B-cell lymphoma of the elderly is an aggressive post-germinal center B-cell neoplasm characterized by prominent nuclear factor-kB activation." *Mod Pathol* 25:968-982.

[47] Ahn, J. S., Yang, D. H., Duk Choi, Y., Jung, S. H., Yhim, H. Y., Kwak, J. Y., Sung Park, H., et al., 2013. "Clinical outcome of elderly patients with Epstein-Barr virus positive diffuse large B-cell lymphoma treated with a combination of rituximab and CHOP chemotherapy." *Am J Hematol* 88:774-779.

[48] Sato, A., Nakamura, N., Kojima, M., Ohmachi, K., Carreras, J., Kikuti, Y. Y., Numata, H., et al., 2014. "Clinical outcome of Epstein-Barr virus-positive diffuse large B-cell lymphoma of the elderly in the rituximab era." *Cancer Sci* 105:1170-1175.

[49] Lu, T. X., Liang, J. H., Miao, Y., Fan, L., Wang, L., Qu, X. Y., Cao, L., et al., 2015. "Epstein-Barr virus positive diffuse large B-cell lymphoma predict poor outcome, regardless of the age." *Sci Rep* 5:12168.

[50] Ghosh, S. K., Perrine, S. P., Faller, D. V. 2012. "Advances in Virus-Directed Therapeutics against Epstein-Barr Virus-Associated Malignancies." *Adv Virol* 2012:509296.

[51] Ghosh, S. K., Perrine, S. P., Williams, R. M., Faller, D. V. 2012. "Histone deacetylase inhibitors are potent inducers of gene expression in latent EBV and sensitize lymphoma cells to nucleoside antiviral agents." *Blood* 119:1008-1017.

[52] Papadopoulos, E. B., Ladanyi, M., Emanuel, D., Mackinnon, S., Boulad, F., Carabasi, M. H., Castro-Malaspina, H., et al., 1994. "Infusions of donor leukocytes to treat Epstein-Barr virus-associated lymphoproliferative disorders after allogeneic bone marrow transplantation." *N Engl J Med* 330:1185-1191.

[53] Savoldo, B., Goss, J. A., Hammer, M. M., Zhang, L., Lopez, T., Gee, A. P., Lin, Y. F., et al., 2006. "Treatment of solid organ transplant recipients with autologous Epstein Barr virus-specific cytotoxic T lymphocytes (CTLs)." *Blood* 108:2942-2949.

[54] Bollard, C. M., Straathof, K. C., Huls, M. H., Leen, A., Lacuesta, K., Davis, A., Gottschalk, S., et al., 2004. "The generation and characterization of LMP2-specific CTLs for use as adoptive transfer from patients with relapsed EBV-positive Hodgkin disease." *J Immunother* 27:317-327.

[55] Bollard, C. M., Gottschalk, S., Torrano, V., Diouf, O., Ku, S., Hazrat, Y., Carrum, G., et al., 2014. "Sustained complete responses in patients with lymphoma receiving autologous cytotoxic T lymphocytes targeting Epstein-Barr virus latent membrane proteins." *J Clin Oncol* 32:798-808.

[56] Delecluse, H. J., Anagnostopoulos, I., Dallenbach, F., Hummel, M., Marafioti, T., Schneider, U., Huhn, D., et al., 1997. "Plasmablastic lymphomas of the oral cavity: a new entity associated with the human immunodeficiency virus infection." *Blood* 89:1413-1420.

[57] Castillo, J. J., Chavez, J. C., Hernandez-Ilizaliturri, F. J., Montes-Moreno, S. 2015. "CD20-negative diffuse large B-cell lymphomas: biology and emerging therapeutic options." *Expert Rev Hematol* 8:343-354.

[58] Castillo, J. J., Bibas, M., Miranda, R. N. 2015. "The biology and treatment of plasmablastic lymphoma." *Blood* 125:2323-2330.

[59] Morscio, J., Dierickx, D., Nijs, J., Verhoef, G., Bittoun, E., Vanoeteren, X., Wlodarska, I., Sagaert, X., Tousseyn, T. 2014. "Clinicopathologic comparison of plasmablastic lymphoma in HIV-positive, immunocompetent, and posttransplant patients: single-center series of 25 cases and meta-analysis of 277 reported cases." *Am J Surg Pathol* 38:875-886.

[60] Liu, J. J., Zhang, L., Ayala, E., Field, T., Ochoa-Bayona, J. L., Perez, L., Bello, C. M., et al., 2011. "Human immunodeficiency virus (HIV)-negative plasmablastic lymphoma: a single institutional experience and literature review." *Leuk Res* 35:1571-1577.

[61] Castillo, J. J., Winer, E. S., Stachurski, D., Perez, K., Jabbour, M., Milani, C., Colvin, G., Butera, J. N. 2010. "Clinical and pathological differences between human immunodeficiency virus-positive and human immunodeficiency virus-negative patients with plasmablastic lymphoma." *Leuk Lymphoma* 51:2047-2053.

[62] Castillo, J. J., Winer, E. S., Stachurski, D., Perez, K., Jabbour, M., Milani, C., Colvin, G., Butera, J. N. 2010. "Prognostic factors in chemotherapy-treated patients with HIV-associated Plasmablastic lymphoma." *Oncologist* 15:293-299.

[63] Schommers, P., Wyen, C., Hentrich, M., Gillor, D., Zoufaly, A., Jensen, B., Bogner, J. R., et al., 2013. "Poor outcome of HIV-infected patients with plasmablastic lymphoma: results from the German AIDS-related lymphoma cohort study." *AIDS* 27:842-845.

[64] Valera, A., Balague, O., Colomo, L., Martinez, A., Delabie, J., Taddesse-Heath, L., Jaffe, E. S., Campo, E. 2010. "IG/MYC rearrangements are the main cytogenetic alteration in plasmablastic lymphomas." *Am J Surg Pathol* 34:1686-1694.

[65] Al-Malki, M. M., Castillo, J. J., Sloan, J. M., Re, A. 2014. "Hematopoietic cell transplantation for plasmablastic lymphoma: a review." *Biol Blood Marrow Transplant* 20:1877-1884.
[66] Yan, M., Dong, Z., Zhao, F., Chauncey, T., Deauna-Limayo, D., Wang-Rodriguez, J., Liu, D., Wang, H. Y., Pilz, R. 2014. "CD20-positive plasmablastic lymphoma with excellent response to bortezomib combined with rituximab." *Eur J Haematol* 93:77-80.
[67] Castillo, J. J., Reagan, J. L., Sikov, W. M., Winer, E. S. 2015. "Bortezomib in combination with infusional dose-adjusted EPOCH for the treatment of plasmablastic lymphoma." *Br J Haematol* 169:352-355.
[68] Bibas, M., Grisetti, S., Alba, L., Picchi, G., Del Nonno, F., Antinori, A. 2010. "Patient with HIV-associated plasmablastic lymphoma responding to bortezomib alone and in combination with dexamethasone, gemcitabine, oxaliplatin, cytarabine, and pegfilgrastim chemotherapy and lenalidomide alone." *J Clin Oncol* 28:e704-708.
[69] Said, J, Cesarman, E. 2008. "Primary effusion lymphoma." *WHO classification of tumours of haematopoietic and lymphoid tissues* 4:260-261.
[70] Cesarman, E., Chang, Y., Moore, P. S., Said, J. W., Knowles, D. M. 1995. "Kaposi's sarcoma-associated herpesvirus-like DNA sequences in AIDS-related body-cavity-based lymphomas." *N Engl J Med* 332:1186-1191.
[71] Riva, G., Luppi, M., Barozzi, P., Forghieri, F., Potenza, L. 2012. "How I treat HHV8/KSHV-related diseases in posttransplant patients." *Blood* 120:4150-4159.
[72] Carbone, A., Cesarman, E., Spina, M., Gloghini, A., Schulz, T. F. 2009. "HIV-associated lymphomas and gamma-herpesviruses." *Blood* 113:1213-1224.
[73] Okada, S., Goto, H., Yotsumoto, M. 2014. "Current status of treatment for primary effusion lymphoma." *Intractable Rare Dis Res* 3:65-74.
[74] Kaplan, L. D. 2013. "Human herpesvirus-8: Kaposi sarcoma, multicentric Castleman disease, and primary effusion lymphoma." *Hematology Am Soc Hematol Educ Program* 2013:103-108.
[75] Carbone, A., Gloghini, A., Vaccher, E., Cerri, M., Gaidano, G., Dalla-Favera, R., Tirelli, U. 2005. "Kaposi's sarcoma-associated herpesvirus/human herpesvirus type 8-positive solid lymphomas: a tissue-based variant of primary effusion lymphoma." *J Mol Diagn* 7:17-27.
[76] Pan, Z. G., Zhang, Q. Y., Lu, Z. B., Quinto, T., Rozenvald, I. B., Liu, L. T., Wilson, D., et al., 2012. "Extracavitary KSHV-associated large B-Cell lymphoma: a distinct entity or a subtype of primary effusion lymphoma? Study of 9 cases and review of an additional 43 cases." *Am J Surg Pathol* 36:1129-1140.
[77] Chadburn, A., Hyjek, E., Mathew, S., Cesarman, E., Said, J., Knowles, D. M. 2004. "KSHV-positive solid lymphomas represent an extra-cavitary variant of primary effusion lymphoma." *Am J Surg Pathol* 28:1401-1416.
[78] Boulanger, E., Gerard, L., Gabarre, J., Molina, J. M., Rapp, C., Abino, J. F., Cadranel, J., Chevret, S., Oksenhendler, E. 2005. "Prognostic factors and outcome of human herpesvirus 8-associated primary effusion lymphoma in patients with AIDS." *J Clin Oncol* 23:4372-4380.
[79] Castillo, J. J., Shum, H., Lahijani, M., Winer, E. S., Butera, J. N. 2012. "Prognosis in primary effusion lymphoma is associated with the number of body cavities involved." *Leuk Lymphoma* 53:2378-2382.

[80] Simonelli, C., Spina, M., Cinelli, R., Talamini, R., Tedeschi, R., Gloghini, A., Vaccher, E., Carbone, A., Tirelli, U. 2003. "Clinical features and outcome of primary effusion lymphoma in HIV-infected patients: a single-institution study." *J Clin Oncol* 21:3948-3954.

[81] El-Ayass, W., Yu, E. M., Karcher, D. S., Aragon-Ching, J. B. 2012. "Complete response to EPOCH in a patient with HIV and extracavitary primary effusion lymphoma involving the colon: a case report and review of literature." *Clin Lymphoma Myeloma Leuk* 12:144-147.

[82] Won, J. H., Han, S. H., Bae, S. B., Kim, C. K., Lee, N. S., Lee, K. T., Park, S. K., et al., 2006. "Successful eradication of relapsed primary effusion lymphoma with high-dose chemotherapy and autologous stem cell transplantation in a patient seronegative for human immunodeficiency virus." *Int J Hematol* 83:328-330.

[83] Harris, NL, Swerdlow, SH, Frizzera, G, Knowles, DM. "Posttransplant lymphoproliferative disorders In: Jaffe ES, Harris NL, Stein H, Vardiman JW, eds." *World Health Organization Classification of Tumours. Pathology and Genetics of Tumours of Haematopoietic and Lymphoid Tissues.*

[84] Petrara, M. R., Giunco, S., Serraino, D., Dolcetti, R., De Rossi, A. 2015. "Post-transplant lymphoproliferative disorders: From epidemiology to pathogenesis-driven treatment." *Cancer Lett* 369:37-44.

[85] Quinlan, S. C., Pfeiffer, R. M., Morton, L. M., Engels, E. A. 2011. "Risk factors for early-onset and late-onset post-transplant lymphoproliferative disorder in kidney recipients in the United States." *Am J Hematol* 86:206-209.

[86] Rasche, L., Kapp, M., Einsele, H., Mielke, S. 2014. "EBV-induced post transplant lymphoproliferative disorders: a persisting challenge in allogeneic hematopoetic SCT." *Bone Marrow Transplant* 49:163-167.

[87] van Leeuwen, M. T., Grulich, A. E., Webster, A. C., McCredie, M. R., Stewart, J. H., McDonald, S. P., Amin, J., et al., 2009. "Immunosuppression and other risk factors for early and late non-Hodgkin lymphoma after kidney transplantation." *Blood* 114:630-637.

[88] Zimmermann, H., Trappe, R. U. 2013. "EBV and posttransplantation lymphoproliferative disease: what to do?" *Hematology Am Soc Hematol Educ Program* 2013:95-102.

[89] Landgren, O., Gilbert, E. S., Rizzo, J. D., Socie, G., Banks, P. M., Sobocinski, K. A., Horowitz, M. M., et al., 2009. "Risk factors for lymphoproliferative disorders after allogeneic hematopoietic cell transplantation." *Blood* 113:4992-5001.

[90] Izadi, M., Taheri, S. 2011. "Features, predictors and prognosis of lymphoproliferative disorders post-liver transplantation regarding disease presentation time: report from the PTLD.Int. survey." *Ann Transplant* 16:39-47.

[91] Hong, G. K., Gulley, M. L., Feng, W. H., Delecluse, H. J., Holley-Guthrie, E., Kenney, S. C. 2005. "Epstein-Barr virus lytic infection contributes to lymphoproliferative disease in a SCID mouse model." *J Virol* 79:13993-14003.

[92] Kimura, H., Ito, Y., Suzuki, R., Nishiyama, Y. 2008. "Measuring Epstein-Barr virus (EBV) load: the significance and application for each EBV-associated disease." *Rev Med Virol* 18:305-319.

[93] Vegso, G., Hajdu, M., Sebestyen, A. 2011. "Lymphoproliferative disorders after solid organ transplantation-classification, incidence, risk factors, early detection and treatment options." *Pathol Oncol Res* 17:443-454.

[94] Dierickx, D., Tousseyn, T., Requile, A., Verscuren, R., Sagaert, X., Morscio, J., Wlodarska, I., et al., 2013. "The accuracy of positron emission tomography in the detection of posttransplant lymphoproliferative disorder." *Haematologica* 98:771-775.

[95] Weinstock, D. M., Ambrossi, G. G., Brennan, C., Kiehn, T. E., Jakubowski, A. 2006. "Preemptive diagnosis and treatment of Epstein-Barr virus-associated post transplant lymphoproliferative disorder after hematopoietic stem cell transplant: an approach in development." *Bone Marrow Transplant* 37:539-546.

[96] Ahmad, I., Cau, N. V., Kwan, J., Maaroufi, Y., Meuleman, N., Aoun, M., Lewalle, P., et al., 2009. "Preemptive management of Epstein-Barr virus reactivation after hematopoietic stem-cell transplantation." *Transplantation* 87:1240-1245.

[97] Leblond, V., Dhedin, N., Mamzer Bruneel, M. F., Choquet, S., Hermine, O., Porcher, R., Nguyen Quoc, S., et al., 2001. "Identification of prognostic factors in 61 patients with posttransplantation lymphoproliferative disorders." *J Clin Oncol* 19:772-778.

[98] Dierickx, D., Tousseyn, T., Gheysens, O. 2015. "How we diagnose and treat posttransplant lymphoproliferative disorders." *Blood*.

[99] Hatton, O., Martinez, O. M., Esquivel, C. O. 2012. "Emerging therapeutic strategies for Epstein-Barr virus+ post-transplant lymphoproliferative disorder." *Pediatr Transplant* 16:220-229.

[100] Choquet, S., Leblond, V., Herbrecht, R., Socie, G., Stoppa, A. M., Vandenberghe, P., Fischer, A., et al., 2006. "Efficacy and safety of rituximab in B-cell post-transplantation lymphoproliferative disorders: results of a prospective multicenter phase 2 study." *Blood* 107:3053-3057.

[101] Gonzalez-Barca, E., Domingo-Domenech, E., Capote, F. J., Gomez-Codina, J., Salar, A., Bailen, A., Ribera, J. M., et al., 2007. "Prospective phase II trial of extended treatment with rituximab in patients with B-cell post-transplant lymphoproliferative disease." *Haematologica* 92:1489-1494.

[102] Elstrom, R. L., Andreadis, C., Aqui, N. A., Ahya, V. N., Bloom, R. D., Brozena, S. C., Olthoff, K. M., et al., 2006. "Treatment of PTLD with rituximab or chemotherapy." *Am J Transplant* 6:569-576.

[103] Fohrer, C., Caillard, S., Koumarianou, A., Ellero, B., Woehl-Jaegle, M. L., Meyer, C., Epailly, E., et al., 2006. "Long-term survival in post-transplant lymphoproliferative disorders with a dose-adjusted ACVBP regimen." *Br J Haematol* 134:602-612.

[104] Trappe, R., Oertel, S., Leblond, V., Mollee, P., Sender, M., Reinke, P., Neuhaus, R., et al., 2012. "Sequential treatment with rituximab followed by CHOP chemotherapy in adult B-cell post-transplant lymphoproliferative disorder (PTLD): the prospective international multicentre phase 2 PTLD-1 trial." *Lancet Oncol* 13:196-206.

[105] Bollard, C. M., Rooney, C. M., Heslop, H. E. 2012. "T-cell therapy in the treatment of post-transplant lymphoproliferative disease." *Nat Rev Clin Oncol* 9:510-519.

[106] Heslop, H. E., Brenner, M. K., Rooney, C. M. 1994. "Donor T cells to treat EBV-associated lymphoma." *N Engl J Med* 331:679-680.

[107] Wilkie, G. M., Taylor, C., Jones, M. M., Burns, D. M., Turner, M., Kilpatrick, D., Amlot, P. L., Crawford, D. H., Haque, T. 2004. "Establishment and characterization of

a bank of cytotoxic T lymphocytes for immunotherapy of epstein-barr virus-associated diseases." *J Immunother* 27:309-316.

[108] Icheva, V., Kayser, S., Wolff, D., Tuve, S., Kyzirakos, C., Bethge, W., Greil, J., et al., 2013. "Adoptive transfer of epstein-barr virus (EBV) nuclear antigen 1-specific t cells as treatment for EBV reactivation and lymphoproliferative disorders after allogeneic stem-cell transplantation." *J Clin Oncol* 31:39-48.

In: Diffuse Large B-Cell Lymphoma (DLBCL)
Editor: Haipeng Shao
ISBN: 978-1-63484-402-4

Chapter 9

"Double Hit" Diffuse Large B-Cell Lymphoma, from Biology to Clinical Outcome, Management and Future Direction

Sarah Jewell, Shebli Atrash, Rebecca Levy, Appalanaidu Sasapu, Konstantinos Arnaoutakis and Pooja Motwani***

Division of Hematology/Oncology, Winthrop P Rockefeller Cancer Institute, University of Arkansas for Medical Sciences, Little Rock, AR, US

Abstract

Diffuse Large B-Cell Lymphoma (DLBCL) is the most common lymphoma in the United States. It is a heterogeneous disease in terms of morphology, genetics, and biological behavior. Clinical response with standard chemotherapy is variable. In this chapter, we focus on a subset of DLBCL with concurrent rearrangement of MYC and BCL2 or, occasionally, BCL6; an entity commonly described as "double hit" DLBCL. These lymphomas are relatively uncommon, and associated with poorer prognosis. We discuss the diagnosis and current treatment strategies as well as new approaches and novel agents. Diagnosis of double hit lymphomas can be challenging. We discuss the role of cytogenetics by karyotyping and fluorescent-in-situ-hybridization (FISH), immunohistochemistry and flow cytometry, and how these tests are collectively used to identify this subgroup of high-risk lymphoma. Treatment of double hit lymphomas is often challenging for several reasons. As a general rule, intensive induction is associated with improved progression-free survival. Several series using regimens other than rituxan, cyclophosphamide, hydroxy-adriamycin, onco-vincristine, and prednisone (R-CHOP) are discussed. Dose adjusted rituxan, etoposide, prednisone, onco-vincristine, cyclophosphamide, hydroxy-adriamycin (R-EPOCH) appears to do better than other chemotherapy regimens for patients who can tolerate it. Unfortunately, a lot of these

* Corresponding author: Email: PMotwani@uams.edu; Phone: (501) 526-6990 x 8051

patients are older and may not tolerate an aggressive treatment regimen. Autologous transplant may not be associated with improved overall survival.

INTRODUCTION

Diffuse large B cell lymphoma is the most frequently occurring lymphoma in the United States [1]. It is a heterogeneous disease in regard to pathology and treatment outcomes. Using FISH, up to 14% of DLBCL has MYC gene rearrangement. MYC rearrangement is the hallmark cytogenetic change in Burkitt lymphoma. However, in contrast to Burkitt lymphoma (BL), the MYC gene is frequently rearranged with non-immunoglobulin genes in DLBCL. Additionally, it tends to control anti-apoptotic cascades as opposed to controlling proliferative genes in Burkitt lymphoma [2].

Single hit lymphoma is described as DLBCL with MYC rearrangements without additional breaks in BCL2 or BCL6 gene. MYC rearrangement, in combination with either BCL2 and/or BCL6 gene rearrangement, defines a subgroup of DLBCL as double hit lymphomas (DHL). These rearrangements have a major impact on tumor aggressiveness and predict poor clinical outcome. Triple hit lymphomas (THL) are defined by the rearrangement of all three genes: MYC, BCL2, and BCL6. Additionally, double expression lymphoma, defined as coexpression of both MYC and BCL2 proteins by immunohistochemistry, is a recognized entity as well, and is associated with poor prognosis even within international prognostication index subgroups [3].

In the last two decades, two year survival rate for DLBCL has improved from 51% to 69% due to addition of rituximab to the CHOP regimen. However, DLBCL with MYC rearrangement is still associated with dismal outcome of about 35% overall survival rate at 2 years when compared to 61% overall survival rate in patients without MYC rearrangement.

Taking into account the relative frequency of lymphomas, there are more patients diagnosed with double hit DLBCL than with BL every year in the United States, which makes double hit lymphoma an important group in malignant hematology. Treatment of double hit lymphomas is often therapeutically challenging. Understanding of the regulatory network of MYC protein may help in identifying new targets for novel treatment.

This chapter provides detailed discussion of the epidemiology, clinical presentation, biology, pathology and treatment options for double hit lymphoma.

CLINICAL PRESENTATION

Patients with double hit lymphoma often present with a rapidly enlarging symptomatic mass, most commonly in the neck or abdomen [4]. The majority of patients present with advanced stage of disease and elevated lactate dehydrogenase (LDH) [3, 5]. B symptoms (fever, weight loss, and night sweats) are present in about 40% cases. Based on previous clinical observation, the presence of MYC translocation by cytogenetics might be associated with increased risk of central nervous system involvement at presentation [5, 6], but this association has not been shown to be statistically significant when compared to cases without MYC translocation. The incidence of CNS relapse is also higher in DLBCL with MYC rearrangement. Extranodal involvement (bone marrow, sinuses, gastrointestinal, kidney, and liver) in two or more sites is reported in about a third of patients [7,8]. The presence of BCL6 rearrangement correlates with higher likelihood of extranodal involvement. Bone marrow involvement by lymphoma is variable and reported to be between 40% and 84%. About 80% of cases have germinal center type immunophenotype, with Ki-67 reported to be between 75-95% [9, 10].

EPIDEMIOLOGY

The median age of patients with DHL at diagnosis is 60 years old with male: female ratio of 2:1 [11]. DHL occurs in 5-16% of patients with DLBCL [8], with the most common form being MYC/BCL2 DHL [12], and THL occurs in 3% DLBCL [3]. In contrast, approximately a third DLBCL has coexpression of MYC/BCL2 by immunohistochemistry (IHC) [7, 13].

Table 1. Characteristics of double hit lymphoma at presentation from pooled data of multiple clinical trials [3-6, 9, 11, 14, 15]

Presentation	Median %	Range %
Male	55.5	43-67
Age	62 years	51-68.5
EN involvement	48	28-89
CNS involvement	9	4 – 44
Elevated LDH	82	50-100
Prior indolent lymphoma	26	11 – 42
Stage III/IV	83.5	69-100
Bone marrow involvement	59	24-84
Ki-67	78	70-95

BIOLOGY OF DOUBLE HIT LYMPHOMA

The MYC oncogene has an important role in the pathogenesis of double hit lymphomas. MYC is known to be deregulated by the t(8;14)(q24:q32) translocation in Burkitt lymphoma. However, it has been found to be rearranged in other lymphoid neoplasms with aggressive behavior [16]. It is estimated that MYC regulates 10% of all human genes [17]. MYC oncogene encodes an important DNA-binding transcriptional factor. It plays roles in cell cycle progression, especially in the transition from G0 to S phase, differentiation and apoptosis. It also controls DNA replication independent of its transcriptional activity promoting genomic instability. It increases the expression of Aurora A and B kinases (members of a family of mitotic serine/threonine kinases). MYC protein forms a functional heterodimer with its binding factor (MAX). This heterodimer helps the recruitment and function of several other important proteins involved in transcription and its stability is further facilitated by PIM kinases, another member of the family of serine/threonine kinases. MYC expression seems to vary throughout the lymphocyte development and is important in the development of germinal centers [18].

There are important differences in the biology of Burkitt lymphoma compared with that of MYC-rearranged non-Burkitt lymphomas. In 80% of Burkitt lymphoma, the translocation partner is the immunoglobulin heavy chain gene locus on chromosome 14q21, and less commonly, the immunoglobulin light chain gene loci on chromosomes 2p22 and 22q11. In non-Burkitt lymphomas, the translocation partner is a non-immunoglobulin (IG) gene such as PAX5, BCL2, BCL6, IKZF1 [17, 19]. It appears that the non-IG partners exert different regulatory effect at the MYC breakpoint. In addition, in non-Burkitt lymphomas, MYC-rearrangement is often associated with additional complex chromosomal abnormalities which probably also increase their genomic instability.

Although MYC translocation is the predominant mechanism of lymphomagenesis in DHL, gene amplification without translocation is seen in a subset of cases. Other mechanisms such as mutations or miRNA deregulations could possibly be present, while the mechanism is unknown in some cases. These events probably explain the FISH negative cases with double expression of MYC/BCL2 and underscore the importance of MYC protein overexpression regardless of the genetic cause.

Gene expression profiling studies have shown distinct differences between Burkitt lymphoma and other MYC-rearranged lymphoid neoplasms, with the former involving genes related to cell proliferation and the latter involving genes related to the nuclear factor kappa-B and anti-apoptosis pathways [17]. This information could have a therapeutic potential.

BCL2 gene, the most frequently rearranged in DHL in addition to MYC gene rearrangement, encodes an important anti-apoptotic protein. BCL2 is most frequently overexpressed in follicular lymphoma due to the characteristic t(14;18)(q32;q21) and has been associated with poor prognosis in patients with DLBCL [20]. BCL-6 gene is the other frequently rearranged gene in DHL. It is a zinc finger transcription factor consisting of DNA binding and POZ domains. BCL6 acts as a sequence-specific repressor of transcriptional activity. Microarray analysis has shown BCL6 to be an important and distinct upregulated gene in the germinal center B cell-like DLBCL [21].

It appears that MYC protein is most important in the biology of double and triple hit lymphomas. However, the partner genes in DHL also play a role in the clinical presentation, and therefore it is important to identify and further study the potential partner genes. For example, it seems that MYC/BCL6 DHL usually presents with extranodal disease and is usually CD10 negative, while MYC/BCL2 DHL is typically CD10 positive and has predominantly nodal disease. Little is known, however, about the interaction of the other partner genes and how they contribute to the pathogenesis of double expression lymphomas.

There is controversy regarding whether MYC is a primary or secondary event in the pathogenesis of DHL [19]. In many cases, BCL2 and MYC rearrangements are seen only in a small number of cells by FISH in patients with low-grade lymphomas at the time of transformation, suggesting a secondary role in promoting transformation However, others argue that MYC could be a primary genetic event in some cases.

In summary, MYC appears to be essential in the pathogenesis of many aggressive lymphomas, including DHL. The overexpression of MYC/BCL2 proteins is prognostically important, regardless of the underlying genetic alterations. Understanding the MYC function and regulation could be helpful in designing novel and targeted therapies.

PATHOLOGY

Morphology

Burkitt lymphoma (BL) commonly displays a starry sky pattern consisting of dense sheets of lymphoma cells with scattered tingible body macrophages. However, this pattern is not unique to Burkitt lymphoma, as it is often seen in any lymphoma with a high proliferation index. BL consists of a population of monomorphic intermediate sized lymphoid cells with minimal cytoplasm, small nucleoli and frequent apoptotic figures (Figure 1). The classic immunophenotype of BL is CD20+, CD10+ and negative for BCL2 by IHC. There is a very high proliferation index with Ki-67 stain positive in almost 100% of the lymphoma cells.

In contrast, DHL displays a slightly different morphology. By pathologic standards published in the 2008 WHO classification, these lymphomas are defined as B-cell lymphoma unclassifiable (BCLU) with concurrent rearrangement of MYC and BCL2 or BCL6 identified by FISH or karyotyping [4, 22]. The histologic pattern is similar to BL, however, the cell size is more variable with less morphologic monotony. Some of the lymphoma cells may be larger, have a blastoid nuclear appearance, irregular nuclei or prominent nucleoli (Figure 1). The MYC/BCL2 DHL commonly displays a germinal center type phenotype (CD10+, BCL6+/-, and IRF4/MUM1 negative). However, MYC/BCL6 DHL is more often CD10 negative and expresses MUM1, consistent with an activated B cell type [22]. The Ki-67 proliferation index is commonly increased (>80%) in DHL. However, published reports have shown a range of Ki-67 proliferation index (60-90%) [22]. MYC and BCL2 expression by IHC is variable in cases of DHL and THL, and multiple studies have set different standards of positive staining, ranging from >30%, >40% or >50% of lymphoma cells [4]. The studies agree that protein expression by IHC can be used as a screening tool, as the gene rearrangements by FISH are necessary for the diagnosis of DHL [16].

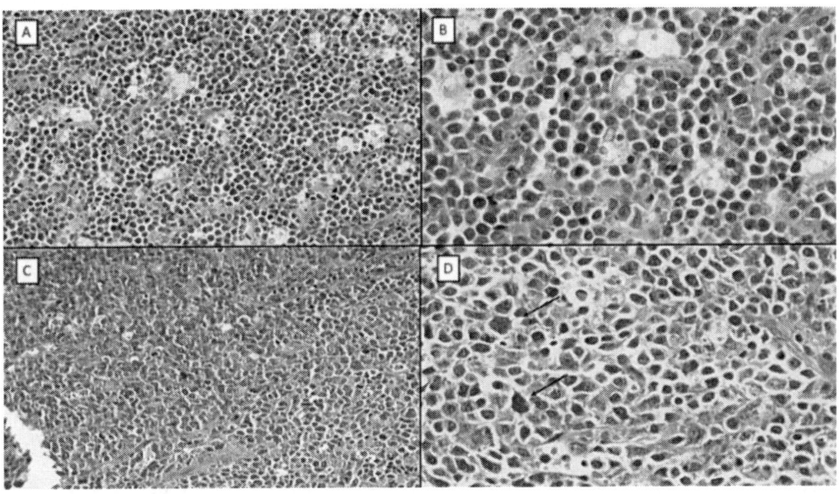

Figure 1. (A). Burkitt Lymphoma displays a starry sky pattern. (B). Burkitt Lymphoma shows monomorphic intermediate-sized lymphoma cells with high nuclear/cytoplasmic ratio, rare nucleoli and frequent apoptotic cells. (C). Double hit lymphoma shows dense sheets of lymphoma cells with rare tingible body macrophages. (D). Double hit Lymphoma shows variable cell size, with some large cells (black arrows), irregular nuclei and rare prominent nucleoli.

Cytogenetics

The most frequent translocation in DLBCL is t(3;14)(q27;q32) BCL6/IgH. BL display MYC gene rearrangements with IgH, kappa or lambda genes: t(8;14)(q34,q32) MYC/IgH, t(2;8)(p12,q34) MYC/Kappa or t(8;22)(q34,q11) MYC/Lambda. Most of the DHL display a complex karyotype by chromosome analysis [4]. The small percentage of case with MYC/BCL6 have been reported in recent studies to have a less complex karyotype than MYC/BCL2 [23]. Gene rearrangement by FISH is illustrated in Figure 2.

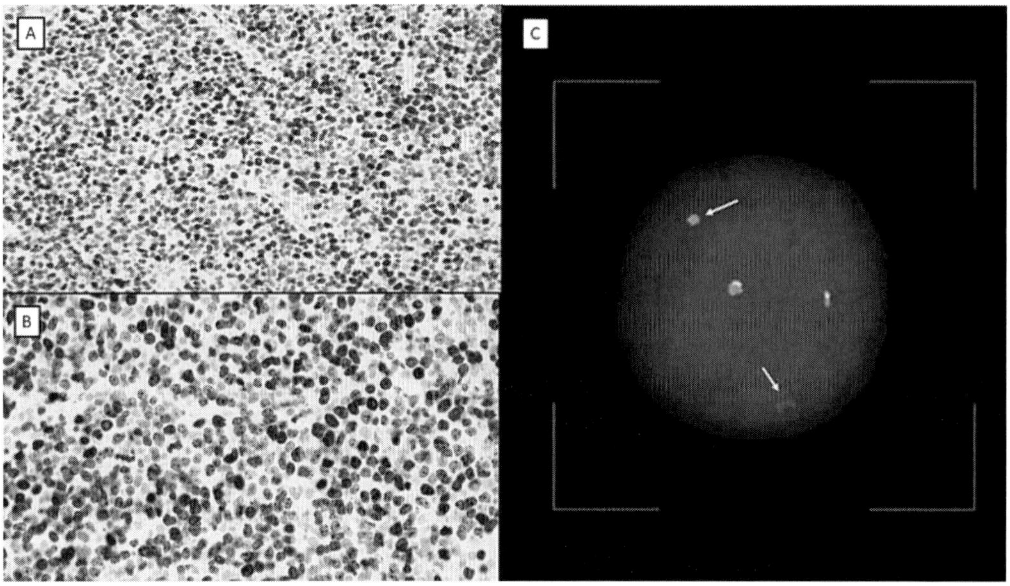

Figure 2. (A). Burkitt lymphoma with almost 100% Ki-67 positive cells. (B). Double hit lymphoma with >95% Ki-67 positive cells. (C). FISH analysis using the c-MYC break-apart probe. A c-MYC rearrangement is present as indicated by splitting apart of the normal red-green fusion signal into one red (centromeric end of MYC) and green (telomeric end of MYC) signal (arrows identify break-apart of MYC).

Prognosis and Treatment

DLBCL is curable with chemotherapy in the majority of cases [24] with the exception of DHL. DHL is known to be a highly aggressive lymphoma with inferior overall survival independent of the International Prognostic Index (IPI) score. In a retrospective analysis of 245 patients with DLBCL [3], MYC rearrangement was present in 35 patients and MYC/BCL2 were rearranged in 26 patients. MYC/BCL6 were rearranged in 10 patients and 7 patients had rearrangements in all three genes. Patients with any MYC rearrangement had significantly worse overall survival (OS), with survival of 35% vs 61% at 2 years (HR 2.03) [3]. The worse outcome was independent of the clinical risk factors, which makes the IPI score of limited value in DHL. Given this, attempts have been made to identify a more accurate prognostic scale in DHL.

In a retrospective study at MD Anderson Cancer Center (MDACC), Oki et al. developed a double-hit IPI (DHIPI) which used performance status >2 and bone marrow involvement as independent risk factors for adverse outcomes [11]. In another large multicenter retrospective study, a multivariate analysis was performed to assess what factors affected overall survival. In this study, factors associated with an increased risk of death were leukocytosis, LDH > 3X upper limit of normal, advanced Ann Arbor stage, and CNS involvement. Based on this information, a prognostic scoring system was formulated (DHL Prognostic Index-DPI). Patients were risk stratified into low risk (0 points), intermediate risk (1 point), and high risk (>2 points). This scoring system resulted in OS curves of the population with a 2 year OS rate of 91%, 59%, and 41% in low risk, intermediate risk, and high risk groups, respectively [4]. In addition to DHL, single hit lymphomas with only MYC rearrangement and triple hit lymphomas with three rearrangements are also described in the literature. Single hit lymphoma, while less common than DHL, also has similar adverse prognosis as the DHL group [10]. It remains unclear if patients with THL have different outcomes than those with DHL [25]. More recently, it has been noted that patients with DLBCL with increased expression of both MYC and BCL2 protein by IHC have inferior OS compared to patients without double expression [13]. DLBCLs with overexpression of MYC and BCL2 proteins seem to share a similar biology with DHLs. A retrospective study showed significantly inferior OS and progression free survival (PFS) for those double expression lymphomas treated with R-CHOP compared to those patients expressing one or neither (3 year OS 43% vs 86%, respectively HR 4.48, $P < 0.001$). The 3 year PFS was 39% in double expression group vs 75% in those without (HR 3.06, $P < 0.001$). Additionally, overexpression of either BCL2 or MYC alone is not significantly associated with outcome [8].

Given the adverse prognosis of DHL, it is important to find appropriate treatment strategy to improve outcomes in this population. There is sufficient data to show that patients with DHL respond poorly to standard therapies for DLBCL. Retrospective studies have shown that patients with DHL treated with R-CHOP chemotherapy have a median overall survival of 12 months or less [14]. In a retrospective study by MDACC, there was only a 40% complete response rate in the group of DHL patients who received R-CHOP. Of those who received R-CHOP, the 2 year event free survival (EFS) was 20% and the 5 year OS was 22% [11]. This is in stark contrast to all patients with DLBCL, who have been reported to have a 2 year PFS of 69% with standard therapy of R-CHOP [26]. Similarly, a retrospective study identified 330 patients with DLBCL that were treated with R-CHOP chemotherapy; the study analyzed tissue samples that were frozen prior to treatment and identified 35 patients with DHL. The probability of survival at 2 years was 35% compared to 61% for all other patients with DLBCL [3]. As a result, it is imperative that more aggressive chemotherapy regimens than standard R-CHOP be employed for DHL. Given its high tendency to involve the CNS, an intensified approach such as rituxan with hyperfractionated cyclophosphamide, vincristine, adriamycin, dexamethasone alternating with cycles of high dose methotrexate (HyperCVAD Part A and B), cyclophosphamide, oncovincristine, adriamycin, methotrexate, cytarabine, ifosfamide, etoposide (CODOX-M/IVAC), or DA-R-EPOCH may be appropriate. There are no prospective studies for analysis; however, the retrospective study by MDACC of patients with DHL treated with R-HyperCVAD regimen showed a complete response (CR) rate of 68% compared to 40% CR in those treated with R-CHOP, although OS and EFS were similar to those treated with R-CHOP [11]. The CR rate in patients treated with R-EPOCH in the same study was similar to R-HyperCVAD with high dose methotrexate at 68%, however the

EFS and OS were improved compared to both R-HyperCVAD and R-CHOP (P = 0.004 and P = 0.057, respectively) [11]. Still, other retrospective studies have not been able to demonstrate an effect on OS despite significantly improved CR rates in intensified chemotherapy regimens compared to R-CHOP. In a large multicenter retrospective study, patients with DHL treated with intensified chemotherapy regimens had improved EFS, with a median of 21.6 months compared to 7.8 months in those treated with R-CHOP. However, this study failed to show an overall survival benefit in the intensified chemotherapy arm. All of the intensive chemotherapy regimens that patients received in the study showed improved PFS (HyperCVAD, CODOX-M/IVAC, and DA-EPOCH), but none of these intensive chemotherapy regimens showed superiority over the others. A multivariate analysis identified a survival benefit of intensive chemotherapy regimens compared to R-CHOP with a hazard ratio of 0.53 [4]. In a meta-analysis of 401 patients, PFS was improved in DA-EPOCH compared to other intensive chemotherapy regimens, although no intensive chemotherapy regimen showed improved OS in this particular study [27].

Treatment options are limited given the median age at diagnosis as some are not able to tolerate more aggressive chemotherapy regimens. Unfortunately, patients face a very grim prognosis if they develop recurrent or refractory disease with an OS of 8 months in one retrospective study, although patients who received some sort of salvage regimen had an improved OS to 17 months [4].

CNS Prophylaxis

As noted above, DHL has a propensity for CNS involvement. In two retrospective studies, the CNS involvement at presentation was 4-7% [4, 11]. In the MDACC retrospective analysis, the 3 year cumulative risk of CNS involvement was 13%; the patients who received intrathecal methotrexate had a lower rate of CNS progression at 3 years compared to patients who did not receive intrathecal chemotherapy (5% vs 15%) [11]. Patients presenting with CNS involvement had an inferior OS compared to those without CNS involvement, with a median OS of 6 months vs 36 months [4]. Those patients without CNS involvement at presentation who received CNS prophylaxis, with either intrathecal methotrexate or systemic methotrexate, had a significantly improved OS of 45 months compared to 14 months in those who did not receive CNS prophylaxis [4]. While the importance of CNS prophylaxis in the treatment of DHL is clear, there is insufficient data to support one prophylactic regimen over another.

Role of Autologous Stem Cell Transplant

The role of autologous stem cell transplant (ASCT) is not well established in the literature in the treatment of DHL. In Petrich's large retrospective analysis of patients with DHL, median OS was not significantly different in patients achieving a CR to frontline therapy who went on to have an autologous stem cell transplant compared to those without ASCT [4]. In the MDACC retrospective study, 20% of patients underwent frontline transplantation. However, frontline transplant was unable to demonstrate an improved EFS or

OS, with 2-year EFS of 68% in patients who received transplant vs 53% in patients who did not receive transplant (P = 0.133), and OS was the same across both groups at 70% (P = 0.563) [11]. When the analysis was limited to patients with advanced disease, upfront autologous stem cell transplant was associated with marginally longer EFS (HR 0.42, P = 0.065) [11].

FUTURE DIRECTIONS

Patients with DHL do not perform well with conventional chemotherapy alone. MYC driven lymphomas also have a proclivity towards CNS spread. About 4-7% of patients have CNS involvement at baseline in one report [11]. As previously discussed, MDACC studies have shown 13% risk of CNS involvement at 3 year follow up [11]. CNS directed treatments need to be incorporated into treatment regimens. Hyperfractionated cyclophosphamide with doxorubicin, vincristine, dexamethasone, methotrexate, cytarabine and rituximab is a viable option as this regimen also incorporates intrathecal chemotherapy. Another option is the similar McGrath regimen. Both of these regimens incorporate high dose methotrexate and intrathecal treatments in their treatment scheme. There is no prospective randomized data; however, Oki et al. have shown that patients treated with HyperCVAD had a 68% CR as opposed to 40% CR seen in the R-CHOP arms [11]. Another study by Savage et al. which looked at 135 patients with newly diagnosed DLBCL patients found that MYC/BCL2 coexpression was an independent predictor of CNS involvement [10]. The 2 year CNS progression risk was found to be 17% in MYC/BCL coexpression cases and this was significantly higher than in cases without MYC/BCL2 coexpression. The role of transplant is unclear, though the role of chemotherapy which is more aggressive than R-CHOP is becoming well defined. There are currently various novel approaches that are being studied to target this resistant disease in ways other than cytotoxic chemotherapy.

Ibrutinib

BTK inhibitors, such as ibrutinib, have shown promise in the treatment of patients with refractory lymphomas, including several types of non-Hodgkin's lymphoma and Hodgkin's lymphoma. It is currently being evaluated in a clinical trial at M.D. Anderson in the post-transplant maintenance setting in patients with DHL. Ibrutinib may have a role in the refractory/relapsed setting in patients with DHL. It has been shown to induce responses in 41% of patients with relapsed ABC DLBCL, though how many of those were DHL is not known.

KPT-330

KPT-330, also known as Selinexor, is the first class selective inhibitor which binds to the nuclear export protein XPO1, leading to activation of tumor suppressor proteins and forcing nuclear retention [28]. Phase I study, presented at ASCO 2014 by Gutierrez et al., looked at

32 patients and showed that post treatment tumor biopsies confirmed reduction in MYC expression, improved tumor suppressor protein nuclear localization and increased apoptosis. Objective responses were noted in all subtypes of refractory NHL including patients with transformed FL, Richter's transformation and Mantle cell lymphoma. This drug needs to be further studied in Phase 2 and 3 clinical trials for relapsed refractory lymphoma and DHL.

BET Bromodomain Inhibitors

This class of drugs has shown preclinical activity and is in early clinical development stages. BET bromodomain inhibitors appear to interfere with cell cycle inhibitor, have pro-apoptotic activity, and interfere with MYC-inducing cell differentiation.

ABT-199

This is a small molecule of oral BCL2 inhibitor and a first in its class. ABT-199 is being studied in the phase I clinical trials, in combination with chemotherapy, for relapsed refractory non-Hodgkin's lymphoma.

Conclusion

It is well-established that patients with DHL have inferior PFS and OS compared to patients with conventional DLBCL. Despite its well-known prognosis, limited information is available regarding treatment of this lymphoma. Studies are limited due to lack of prospective trials, and the small sample sizes. It is important for patients to be referred for clinical trials whenever possible. Novel approaches, as discussed in the preceding section, may improve survival in this unique population of patients.

References

[1] Morton, L. M., Wang, S. S., Devesa, S. S., Hartge, P., Weisenburger, D. D., Linet, M. S. 2006. "Lymphoma incidence patterns by WHO subtype in the United States, 1992-2001." *Blood* 107:265-276.

[2] Dave, S. S., Fu, K., Wright, G. W., Lam, L. T., Kluin, P., Boerma, E. J., Greiner, T. C., et al. 2006. "Molecular diagnosis of Burkitt's lymphoma." *N Engl J Med* 354:2431-2442.

[3] Barrans, S., Crouch, S., Smith, A., Turner, K., Owen, R., Patmore, R., Roman, E., Jack, A. 2010. "Rearrangement of MYC is associated with poor prognosis in patients with diffuse large B-cell lymphoma treated in the era of rituximab." *J Clin Oncol* 28:3360-3365.

[4] Petrich, A. M., Nabhan, C., Smith, S. M. 2014. "MYC-associated and double-hit lymphomas: a review of pathobiology, prognosis, and therapeutic approaches." *Cancer* 120:3884-3895.

[5] Niitsu, N., Okamoto, M., Miura, I., Hirano, M. 2009. "Clinical features and prognosis of de novo diffuse large B-cell lymphoma with t(14;18) and 8q24/c-MYC translocations." *Leukemia* 23:777-783.

[6] Snuderl, M., Kolman, O. K., Chen, Y. B., Hsu, J. J., Ackerman, A. M., Dal Cin, P., Ferry, J. A., et al. 2010. "B-cell lymphomas with concurrent IGH-BCL2 and MYC rearrangements are aggressive neoplasms with clinical and pathologic features distinct from Burkitt lymphoma and diffuse large B-cell lymphoma." *Am J Surg Pathol* 34:327-340.

[7] Hu, S., Xu-Monette, Z. Y., Tzankov, A., Green, T., Wu, L., Balasubramanyam, A., Liu, W. M., et al. 2013. "MYC/BCL2 protein coexpression contributes to the inferior survival of activated B-cell subtype of diffuse large B-cell lymphoma and demonstrates high-risk gene expression signatures: a report from The International DLBCL Rituximab-CHOP Consortium Program." *Blood* 121:4021-4031; quiz 4250.

[8] Green, T. M., Young, K. H., Visco, C., Xu-Monette, Z. Y., Orazi, A., Go, R. S., Nielsen, O., et al. 2012. "Immunohistochemical double-hit score is a strong predictor of outcome in patients with diffuse large B-cell lymphoma treated with rituximab plus cyclophosphamide, doxorubicin, vincristine, and prednisone." *J Clin Oncol* 30:3460-3467.

[9] Pedersen, M. O., Gang, A. O., Poulsen, T. S., Knudsen, H., Lauritzen, A. F., Nielsen, S. L., Klausen, T. W., Norgaard, P. 2014. "MYC translocation partner gene determines survival of patients with large B-cell lymphoma with MYC- or double-hit MYC/BCL2 translocations." *Eur J Haematol* 92:42-48.

[10] Savage, K. J., Johnson, N. A., Ben-Neriah, S., Connors, J. M., Sehn, L. H., Farinha, P., Horsman, D. E., Gascoyne, R. D. 2009. "MYC gene rearrangements are associated with a poor prognosis in diffuse large B-cell lymphoma patients treated with R-CHOP chemotherapy." *Blood* 114:3533-3537.

[11] Oki, Y., Noorani, M., Lin, P., Davis, R. E., Neelapu, S. S., Ma, L., Ahmed, M., et al. 2014. "Double hit lymphoma: the MD Anderson Cancer Center clinical experience." *Br J Haematol* 166:891-901.

[12] Li, S., Lin, P., Young, K. H., Kanagal-Shamanna, R., Yin, C. C., Medeiros, L. J. 2013. "MYC/BCL2 double-hit high-grade B-cell lymphoma." *Adv Anat Pathol* 20:315-326.

[13] Horn, H., Ziepert, M., Becher, C., Barth, T. F., Bernd, H. W., Feller, A. C., Klapper, W., et al. 2013. "MYC status in concert with BCL2 and BCL6 expression predicts outcome in diffuse large B-cell lymphoma." *Blood* 121:2253-2263.

[14] Johnson, N. A., Slack, G. W., Savage, K. J., Connors, J. M., Ben-Neriah, S., Rogic, S., Scott, D. W., et al. 2012. "Concurrent expression of MYC and BCL2 in diffuse large B-cell lymphoma treated with rituximab plus cyclophosphamide, doxorubicin, vincristine, and prednisone." *J Clin Oncol* 30:3452-3459.

[15] Tomita, N., Tokunaka, M., Nakamura, N., Takeuchi, K., Koike, J., Motomura, S., Miyamoto, K., et al. 2009. "Clinicopathological features of lymphoma/leukemia patients carrying both BCL2 and MYC translocations." *Haematologica* 94:935-943.

[16] Ott, G., Rosenwald, A., Campo, E. 2013. "Understanding MYC-driven aggressive B-cell lymphomas: pathogenesis and classification." *Blood* 122:3884-3891.

[17] Cheah, C. Y., Oki, Y., Westin, J. R., Turturro, F. 2015. "A clinician's guide to double hit lymphomas." *Br J Haematol* 168:784-795.

[18] Sewastianik, T., Prochorec-Sobieszek, M., Chapuy, B., Juszczynski, P. 2014. "MYC deregulation in lymphoid tumors: molecular mechanisms, clinical consequences and therapeutic implications." *Biochim Biophys Acta* 1846:457-467.

[19] Lin, P., Medeiros, L. J. 2013. "The impact of MYC rearrangements and "double hit" abnormalities in diffuse large B-cell lymphoma." *Curr Hematol Malig Rep* 8:243-252.

[20] Song, M. K., Chung, J. S., Shin, D. H., Seol, Y. M., Shin, H. J., Choi, Y. J., Cho, G. J. 2009. "Prognostic significance of the Bcl-2 negative germinal centre in patients with diffuse large B cell lymphoma treated with R-CHOP." *Leuk Lymphoma* 50:54-61.

[21] Alizadeh, A. A., Eisen, M. B., Davis, R. E., Ma, C., Lossos, I. S., Rosenwald, A., Boldrick, J. C., et al. 2000. "Distinct types of diffuse large B-cell lymphoma identified by gene expression profiling." *Nature* 403:503-511.

[22] Swerdlow, Steven H. 2014. "Diagnosis of 'Double Hit' Diffuse Large B-Cell Lymphoma and B-Cell Lymphoma, Unclassifiable, with Features Intermediate between DLBCL and Burkitt Lymphoma: When and How, FISH versus IHC." *Hematology/the Education Program of the American Society of Hematology. American Society of Hematology. Education Program* 1:90.

[23] Pillai, R. K., Sathanoori, M., Van Oss, S. B., Swerdlow, S. H. 2013. "Double-hit B-cell lymphomas with BCL6 and MYC translocations are aggressive, frequently extranodal lymphomas distinct from BCL2 double-hit B-cell lymphomas." *Am J Surg Pathol* 37:323-332.

[24] Friedberg, J. W., Fisher, R. I. 2008. "Diffuse large B-cell lymphoma." *Hematol Oncol Clin North Am* 22:941-952, ix.

[25] Aukema, S. M., Siebert, R., Schuuring, E., van Imhoff, G. W., Kluin-Nelemans, H. C., Boerma, E. J., Kluin, P. M. 2011. "Double-hit B-cell lymphomas." *Blood* 117:2319-2331.

[26] Sehn, L. H., Donaldson, J., Chhanabhai, M., Fitzgerald, C., Gill, K., Klasa, R., MacPherson, N., et al. 2005. "Introduction of combined CHOP plus rituximab therapy dramatically improved outcome of diffuse large B-cell lymphoma in British Columbia." *J Clin Oncol* 23:5027-5033.

[27] Howlett, C., Snedecor, S. J., Landsburg, D. J., Svoboda, J., Chong, E. A., Schuster, S. J., Nasta, S. D., et al. 2015. "Front-line, dose-escalated immunochemotherapy is associated with a significant progression-free survival advantage in patients with double-hit lymphomas: a systematic review and meta-analysis." *Br J Haematol* 170:504-514.

[28] Gutierrez, Martin., Andre Goy, John C., Byrd, Joseph M. , Flynn, Morten Sorensen. , Brown, Peter, Gabrail, Nashat Y. 2014. "A Phase 1 Dose-Escalation Study of the Oral Selective Inhibitor of Nuclear Export (SINE) KPT-330 (selinexor) in Patients (pts) with Heavily Pretreated Non-Hodgkin Lymphoma (NHL)." *In ASCO Annual Meeting. J Clin Oncol* 32:5s.

EDITOR'S CONTACT INFORMATION

Dr. Haipeng Shao, MD, PhD
Assistant Member
Department of Hematopathology and Laboratory Medicine
Moffitt Cancer Center
12902 Magnolia Drive, Tampa, FL 33612
Email: Haipeng.Shao@moffitt.org

INDEX

A

B

D

E

F

G

H

I

J

K

L

M

N

O

P

T